ACP AMERICAN COLLEGE OF PHYSICIANS®
INTERNAL MEDICINE | *Doctors for Adults*

MKSAP® 16

Medical Knowledge Self-Assessment Program®

Infectious Disease

Welcome to the Infectious Disease Section of MKSAP 16!

Here, you will find updated information on central nervous system infection, skin and soft tissue infection, community-acquired pneumonia, tick-borne disease, urinary tract infection, *Mycobacterium tuberculosis* and nontuberculous mycobacterial infection, sexually transmitted infection, health care–associated infection, HIV infection, and many other clinical challenges. All of these topics are uniquely focused on the needs of generalists and subspecialists *outside* of infectious disease.

The publication of the 16th edition of Medical Knowledge Self-Assessment Program heralds a significant event, culminating 2 years of effort by dozens of leading subspecialists across the United States. Our authoring committees have strived to help internists succeed in Maintenance of Certification, right up to preparing for the MOC examination, and to get residents ready for the certifying examination. MKSAP 16 also helps you update your medical knowledge and elevates standards of self-learning by allowing you to assess your knowledge with 1,200 all-new multiple-choice questions, including 108 in Infectious Disease.

MKSAP began more than 40 years ago. The American Board of Internal Medicine's examination blueprint and gaps between actual and preferred practices inform creation of the content. The questions, refined through rigorous face-to-face meetings, are among the best in medicine. A psychometric analysis of the items sharpens our educational focus on weaknesses in practice. To meet diverse learning styles, we offer MKSAP 16 online and in downloadable apps for PCs, tablets, laptops, and smartphones. We are also introducing the following:

High-Value Care Recommendations: The Infectious Disease section starts with several recommendations based on the important concept of health care value (balancing clinical benefit with costs and harms) to address the needs of trainees, practicing physicians, and patients. These recommendations are part of a major initiative that has been undertaken by the American College of Physicians, in collaboration with other organizations.

Content for Hospitalists: This material, highlighted in blue and labeled with the familiar hospital icon (◧), directly addresses the learning needs of the increasing number of physicians who work in the hospital setting. MKSAP 16 Digital will allow you to customize quizzes based on hospitalist-only questions to help you prepare for the Hospital Medicine Maintenance of Certification Examination.

We hope you enjoy and benefit from MKSAP 16. Please feel free to send us any comments to mksap_editors@acponline.org or visit us at the MKSAP Resource Site (mksap.acponline.org) to find out how we can help you study, earn CME, accumulate MOC points, and stay up to date. I know I speak on behalf of ACP staff members and our authoring committees when I say we are honored to have attracted your interest and participation.

Sincerely,

Patrick Alguire, MD, FACP
Editor-in-Chief
Senior Vice President
Medical Education Division
American College of Physicians

Infectious Disease

Committee

Allan R. Tunkel, MD, PhD, MACP, Editor[2]
Professor of Medicine
Drexel University College of Medicine
Chair, Department of Medicine
Monmouth Medical Center
Long Branch, New Jersey

Thomas Fekete, MD, FACP, Associate Editor[1]
Professor of Medicine
Chief, Infectious Diseases
Section of Infectious Diseases
Temple University Medical School
Philadelphia, Pennsylvania

Karen C. Bloch, MD, MPH [1]
Assistant Professor
Department of Infectious Disease and Preventive Medicine
Division of Infectious Diseases
Vanderbilt University Medical Center
Nashville, Tennessee

Patricia D. Brown, MD, FACP[1]
Associate Professor of Medicine
Division of Infectious Diseases
Wayne State University School of Medicine
Chief of Medicine
Detroit Receiving Hospital
Detroit, Michigan

Larry M. Bush, MD, FACP[2]
Affiliated Professor of Biomedical Sciences
Charles E. Schmidt College of Medicine
Florida Atlantic University
Boca Raton, Florida
Affiliated Associate Professor of Medicine
University of Miami-Miller School of Medicine
JFK Medical Center
Palm Beach County, Florida

Michael Frank, MD, FACP[1]
Professor of Medicine
Residency Program Director
Vice Chair for Education
Department of Medicine
Medical College of Wisconsin
Milwaukee, Wisconsin

Keith S. Kaye, MD, MPH, FACP[2]
Professor of Medicine
Wayne State University
Corporate Medical Director, Infection Prevention, Epidemiology and Antimicrobial
   Stewardship, Detroit Medical Center
Detroit, Michigan

Fred A. Lopez, MD, FACP[2]
Richard Vial Professor and Vice Chair
Department of Medicine
Louisiana State University Health Sciences Center
New Orleans, Louisiana

Annette C. Reboli, MD, FACP[2]
Founding Vice Dean
Professor of Medicine
Cooper Medical School of Rowan University
Cooper University Hospital
Camden, New Jersey

Editor-in-Chief

Patrick C. Alguire, MD, FACP[1]
Senior Vice President, Medical Education
American College of Physicians
Philadelphia, Pennsylvania

Deputy Editor-in-Chief

Philip A. Masters, MD, FACP[1]
Senior Medical Associate for Content Development
American College of Physicians
Philadelphia, Pennsylvania

Senior Medical Associate for Content Development

Cynthia D. Smith, MD, FACP[2]
American College of Physicians
Philadelphia, Pennsylvania

Infectious Disease Clinical Editor

Mary Jane Barchman, MD, FACP[2]

Infectious Disease Reviewers

Robert D. Arbeit, MD[2]
Richard A. Fatica, MD[1]
Gloria T. Fioravanti, DO, FACP[1]

John D. Goldman, MD, FACP[1]
Duane R. Hospenthal, MD, PhD, FACP[1]
Richard H. Moseley, MD, FACP[1]
Mark E. Pasanen, MD, FACP[1]

Infectious Disease Reviewer Representing the American Society for Clinical Pharmacology & Therapeutics

Kevin Leary, MD, FACP[1]

Infectious Disease ACP Editorial Staff

Margaret Wells[1], Managing Editor
Sean McKinney[1], Director, Self-Assessment Programs
John Haefele[1], Assistant Editor

ACP Principal Staff

Patrick C. Alguire, MD, FACP[1]
Senior Vice President, Medical Education

D. Theresa Kanya, MBA[1]
Vice President, Medical Education

Sean McKinney[1]
Director, Self-Assessment Programs

Margaret Wells[1]
Managing Editor

Valerie Dangovetsky[1]
Program Administrator

Becky Krumm[1]
Senior Staff Editor

Ellen McDonald, PhD[1]
Senior Staff Editor

Katie Idell[1]
Senior Staff Editor

Randy Hendrickson[1]
Production Administrator/Editor

Megan Zborowski[1]
Staff Editor

Linnea Donnarumma[1]
Assistant Editor

John Haefele[1]
Assistant Editor

Developed by the American College of Physicians

---

1. Has no relationships with any entity producing, marketing, re-selling, or distributing health care goods or services consumed by, or used on, patients.

2. Has disclosed relationships with entities producing, marketing, re-selling, or distributing health care goods or services consumed by, or used on, patients. See below.

Conflicts of Interest

The following committee members, reviewers, and ACP staff members have disclosed relationships with commercial companies:

Robert D. Arbeit, MD
Employment
Idera Pharmaceuticals
Stock Options/Holdings
Idera Pharmaceuticals

Mary Jane Barchman, MD, FACP
Speakers Bureau
Novartis

Larry Bush, MD, FACP
Speakers Bureau
Cubist, Sanofi-Pasteur

Keith S. Kaye, MD, MPH, FACP
Speakers Bureau
Cubist, Merck, Pfizer, OrthoMcNeil
Consultantship
Merck, Pfizer, OrthoMcNeil, Forest Pharmaceuticals, Theradoc
Research Grants/Contracts
Merck, Pfizer, Cubist, Sage Products, Inc.

Fred A. Lopez, MD, FACP
Royalties
UpToDate

Annette C. Reboli, MD, FACP
Research Grants/Contracts
Merck, Pfizer, T2 BioSystems, Astellas
Royalties
UpToDate
Other
Pfizer, Merck

Cynthia D. Smith, MD, FACP
Stock Options/Holdings
Merck and Company

Allan R. Tunkel, MD, PhD, MACP
Employment
Food and Drug Administration
Research Grants/Contracts
UpToDate
Other
NIH, Infectious Diseases Society of America

Acknowledgments

The American College of Physicians (ACP) gratefully acknowledges the special contributions to the development and production of the 16th edition of the Medical Knowledge Self-Assessment Program® (MKSAP® 16) made by the following people:

Graphic Services: Michael Ripca (Technical Administrator/Graphic Designer) and Willie-Fetchko Graphic Design (Graphic Designer).

Production/Systems: Dan Hoffmann (Director, Web Services & Systems Development), Neil Kohl (Senior Architect), and Scott Hurd (Senior Systems Analyst/Developer).

MKSAP 16 Digital: Under the direction of Steven Spadt, Vice President, ACP Digital Products & Services, the digital version of MKSAP 16 was developed within the ACP's Digital Product Development Department, led by Brian Sweigard (Director). Other members of the team included Sean O'Donnell (Senior Architect), Dan Barron (Senior Systems Analyst/Developer), Chris Forrest (Senior Software Developer/Design Lead), Jon Laing (Senior Web Application Developer), Brad Lord (Senior Web Developer), John McKnight (Senior Web Developer), and Nate Pershall (Senior Web Developer).

The College also wishes to acknowledge that many other persons, too numerous to mention, have contributed to the production of this program. Without their dedicated efforts, this program would not have been possible.

Introducing the MKSAP Resource Site (mksap.acponline.org)

The MKSAP Resource Site (mksap.acponline.org) is a continually updated site that provides links to MKSAP 16 online answer sheets for print subscribers; access to MKSAP 16 Digital, Board Basics® 3, and MKSAP 16 Updates; the latest details on Continuing Medical Education (CME) and Maintenance of Certification (MOC) in the United States, Canada, and Australia; errata; and other new information.

ABIM Maintenance of Certification

Check the MKSAP Resource Site (mksap.acponline.org) for the latest information on how MKSAP tests can be used to apply to the American Board of Internal Medicine for Maintenance of Certification (MOC) points.

RCPSC Maintenance of Certification

In Canada, MKSAP 16 is an Accredited Self-Assessment Program (Section 3) as defined by the Maintenance of Certification Program of The Royal College of Physicians and Surgeons of Canada (RCPSC) and approved by the Canadian Society of Internal Medicine on December 9, 2011. Approval of Part A sections of MKSAP 16 extends from July 31, 2012, until July 31, 2015. Approval of Part B sections of MKSAP 16 extends from December 31, 2012, to December 31, 2015. Fellows of the Royal College may earn three credits per hour for participating in MKSAP 16 under Section 3. MKSAP 16 will enable Fellows to earn up to 75% of their required 400 credits during the 5-year MOC cycle. A Fellow can achieve this 75% level by earning 100 of the maximum of 174 *AMA PRA Category 1 Credits*™ available in MKSAP 16. MKSAP 16 also meets multiple CanMEDS Roles for RCPSC MOC, including that of Medical Expert, Communicator, Collaborator, Manager, Health Advocate, Scholar, and Professional. For information on how to apply MKSAP 16 CME credits to RCPSC MOC, visit the MKSAP Resource Site at mksap.acponline.org.

The Royal Australasian College of Physicians CPD Program

In Australia, MKSAP 16 is a Category 3 program that may be used by Fellows of The Royal Australasian College of Physicians (RACP) to meet mandatory CPD points. Two CPD credits are awarded for each of the 174 *AMA PRA Category 1 Credits*™ available in MKSAP 16. More information about using MKSAP 16 for this purpose is available at the MKSAP Resource Site at mksap.acponline .org and at www.racp.edu.au. CPD credits earned through MKSAP 16 should be reported at the MyCPD site at www.racp.edu.au/mycpd.

Continuing Medical Education

The American College of Physicians is accredited by the Accreditation Council for Continuing Medical Education (ACCME) to provide continuing medical education for physicians.

The American College of Physicians designates this enduring material, MKSAP 16, for a maximum of 174 *AMA PRA Category 1 Credits*™. Physicians should claim only the credit commensurate with the extent of their participation in the activity.

Up to 16 *AMA PRA Category 1 Credits*™ are available from December 31, 2012, to December 31, 2015, for the MKSAP 16 Infectious Disease section.

Learning Objectives

The learning objectives of MKSAP 16 are to:
- Close gaps between actual care in your practice and preferred standards of care, based on best evidence
- Diagnose disease states that are less common and sometimes overlooked and confusing
- Improve management of comorbid conditions that can complicate patient care
- Determine when to refer patients for surgery or care by subspecialists

- Pass the ABIM Certification Examination
- Pass the ABIM Maintenance of Certification Examination

Target Audience

- General internists and primary care physicians
- Subspecialists who need to remain up-to-date in internal medicine
- Residents preparing for the certifying examination in internal medicine
- Physicians preparing for maintenance of certification in internal medicine (recertification)

Earn "Same-Day" CME Credits Online

For the first time, print subscribers can enter their answers online to earn CME credits in 24 hours or less. You can submit your answers using online answer sheets that are provided at mksap.acponline.org, where a record of your MKSAP 16 credits will be available. To earn CME credits, you need to answer all of the questions in a test and earn a score of at least 50% correct (number of correct answers divided by the total number of questions). Take any of the following approaches:

1. Use the printed answer sheet at the back of this book to record your answers. Go to mksap.acponline.org, access the appropriate online answer sheet, transcribe your answers, and submit your test for same-day CME credits. There is no additional fee for this service.

2. Go to mksap.acponline.org, access the appropriate online answer sheet, directly enter your answers, and submit your test for same-day CME credits. There is no additional fee for this service.

3. Pay a $10 processing fee per answer sheet and submit the printed answer sheet at the back of this book by mail or fax, as instructed on the answer sheet. Make sure you calculate your score and fax the answer sheet to 215-351-2799 or mail the answer sheet to Member and Customer Service, American College of Physicians, 190 N. Independence Mall West, Philadelphia, PA 19106-1572, using the courtesy envelope provided in your MKSAP 16 slipcase. You will need your 10-digit order number and 8-digit ACP ID number, which are printed on your packing slip. Please allow 4 to 6 weeks for your score report to be emailed back to you. Be sure to include your email address for a response.

If you do not have a 10-digit order number and 8-digit ACP ID number or if you need help creating a username and password to access the MKSAP 16 online answer sheets, go to mksap.acponline.org or email custserv@acponline.org.

Permission/Consent for Use of Figures Shown in MKSAP 16 Infectious Disease Multiple-Choice Questions

Figure shown in Self-Assessment Test Item 25 reproduced with permission from the Massachusetts Medical Society. From Baker DJ, Reboli AC. [Images in Clinical Medicine]. N Engl J Med. 1997;998. Copyright © 1997 Massachusetts Medical Society.

Disclosure Policy

It is the policy of the American College of Physicians (ACP) to ensure balance, independence, objectivity, and scientific rigor in all of its educational activities. To this end, and consistent with the policies of the ACP and the Accreditation Council for Continuing Medical Education (ACCME), contributors to all ACP continuing medical education activities are required to disclose all relevant financial relationships with any entity producing, marketing, re-selling, or distributing health care goods or services consumed by, or used on, patients. Contributors are required to use generic names in the discussion of therapeutic options and are required to identify any unapproved, off-label, or investigative use of commercial products or devices. Where a trade name is used, all available trade names for the same product type are also included. If trade-name products manufactured by companies with whom contributors have relationships are discussed, contributors are asked to provide evidence-based citations in support of the discussion. The information is reviewed by the committee responsible for producing this text. If necessary, adjustments to topics or contributors' roles in content development are made to balance the discussion. Further, all readers of this text are asked to evaluate the content for evidence of commercial bias and send any relevant comments to mksap_editors@acponline.org so that future decisions about content and contributors can be made in light of this information.

Resolution of Conflicts

To resolve all conflicts of interest and influences of vested interests, the ACP precluded members of the content-creation committee from deciding on any content issues that involved generic or trade-name products associated with proprietary entities with which these committee members had relationships. In addition, content was based on best evidence and updated clinical care guidelines, when such evidence and guidelines were available. Contributors' disclosure information can be found with the list of contributors' names and those of ACP principal staff listed in the beginning of this book.

Hospital-Based Medicine

For the convenience of subscribers who provide care in hospital settings, content that is specific to the hospital setting has been highlighted in blue. Hospital icons (▣) highlight where the hospital-only content begins, continues over more than one page, and ends.

Educational Disclaimer

The editors and publisher of MKSAP 16 recognize that the development of new material offers many opportunities for error. Despite our best efforts, some errors may persist in print. Drug dosage schedules are, we believe, accurate and in accordance with current standards. Readers are advised, however, to ensure that the recommended dosages in MKSAP 16 concur with the information provided in the product information material. This is especially important in cases of new, infrequently used, or highly toxic drugs. Application of the information in MKSAP 16 remains the professional responsibility of the practitioner.

The primary purpose of MKSAP 16 is educational. Information presented, as well as publications, technologies, products, and/or services discussed, is intended to inform subscribers about the knowledge, techniques, and experiences of the contributors. A diversity of professional opinion exists, and the views of the contributors are their own and not those of the ACP. Inclusion of any material in the program does not constitute endorsement or recommendation by the ACP. The ACP does not warrant the safety, reliability, accuracy, completeness, or usefulness of and disclaims any and all liability for damages and claims that may result from the use of information, publications, technologies, products, and/or services discussed in this program.

Publisher's Information

Unauthorized Use of This Book Is Against the Law

MKSAP 16 ISBN: 978-1-938245-00-8
(Infectious Disease) ISBN: 978-1-938245-09-1

Printed in the United States of America.

For order information in the U.S. or Canada call 800-523-1546, extension 2600. All other countries call 215-351-2600. Fax inquiries to 215-351-2799 or email to custserv@acponline.org.

Errata and Norm Tables

Errata for MKSAP 16 will be available through the MKSAP Resource Site at mksap.acponline.org as new information becomes known to the editors.

MKSAP 16 Performance Interpretation Guidelines with Norm Tables, available July 31, 2013, will reflect the knowledge of physicians who have completed the self-assessment tests before the program was published. These physicians took the tests without being able to refer to the syllabus, answers, and critiques. For your convenience, the tables are available in a printable PDF file through the MKSAP Resource Site at mksap.acponline.org.

Table of Contents

Infectious Disease High-Value Care Recommendations

The American College of Physicians, in collaboration with multiple other organizations, is embarking on a national initiative to promote awareness about the importance of stewardship of health care resources. The goals are to improve health care outcomes by providing care of proven benefit and reducing costs by avoiding unnecessary and even harmful interventions. The initiative comprises several programs that integrate the important concept of health care value (balancing clinical benefit with costs and harms) for a given intervention into various educational materials to address the needs of trainees, practicing physicians, and patients.

To integrate discussion of high-value, cost-conscious care into MKSAP 16, we have created recommendations based on the medical knowledge content that we feel meet the below definition of high-value care and bring us closer to our goal of improving patient outcomes while conserving finite resources.

High-Value Care Recommendation: A recommendation to choose diagnostic and management strategies for patients in specific clinical situations that balances clinical benefit with cost and harms with the goal of improving patient outcomes.

Below are the High-Value Care Recommendations for the Infectious Disease section of MKSAP 16.

- Do not use latex agglutination tests to identify the cause of bacterial meningitis because results of these tests rarely change treatment.
- Pre-lumbar puncture CT scans are only recommended in patients with a suspected mass lesion; who are immunocompromised; who have a history of central nervous system disease; or who present with new-onset seizures, decreased level of consciousness, focal neurologic deficits, or papilledema.
- The diagnosis of skin infections is typically based on clinical findings, not blood, skin, or biopsy cultures.
- Incision and drainage is the primary therapy for a cutaneous abscess, and possibly, antibiotic treatment, depending on extent and severity of infection.
- Ulcers that are clinically uninfected (that is, without purulence or inflammation) should not be treated with antibiotics.
- Blood cultures, sputum Gram stain and culture, and pneumococcal and *Legionella* urine antigen testing are optional in outpatients with community-acquired pneumonia (see Item 79).

- Once patients with pneumonia are ready to switch to oral therapy, most can be safely discharged without observation (see Item 46).
- Follow-up chest imaging is not indicated in most patients with pneumonia who improve with treatment but should be considered in those who are older than 40 years of age and smokers.
- Serologic testing is not recommended for patients with early Lyme disease because a measurable antibody response may not have had time to develop (see Item 23).
- Serologic testing for Lyme disease should be restricted to patients with clinically suggestive signs or symptoms who either reside in or have traveled to an endemic area.
- Urine culture is usually not needed for patients with an uncomplicated urinary tract infection because results rarely change management.
- Urologic investigation, including CT and/or ultrasonography, should be restricted to those with pyelonephritis who have persistent flank pain or fever after 72 hours of antimicrobial therapy.
- Screening for and treatment of asymptomatic bacteriuria is indicated only in pregnant women and patients undergoing invasive urologic procedures (see Item 85).
- Do not obtain MRIs to follow treatment response of patients with osteomyelitis because results are not very specific and can lead to additional unwarranted therapy.
- Do obtain blood cultures in patients with suspected vertebral osteomyelitis because such culture results are positive in more than 50% of patients and can minimize the extent of the evaluation.
- Do not obtain stool cultures in otherwise healthy patients with diarrhea unless they have had symptoms for longer than 3 days, associated fever, or bloody or mucoid stools because results rarely change management (see Item 48).
- Do not obtain stool cultures in hospitalized patients with diarrhea after they have been in the hospital longer than 3 days.
- Do not send formed stool for *Clostridium difficile* toxin testing because positive results are more likely to reflect colonization than active infection.
- Do not send stool for ova and parasites testing in patients with diarrhea lasting fewer than 7 days.
- HIV viral load testing should only be used to diagnose patients with suspected acute-phase HIV and to monitor the efficacy of antiretroviral treatment.

- When influenza virus infection has been documented in the community, a diagnosis can be established clinically and rapid influenza diagnostic tests are unnecessary.
- Prophylactic or therapeutic antiviral therapy should be avoided in persons at low risk for or with equivocal clinical findings of influenza virus infection (see Item 43).
- Use newer antimicrobial agents only when clearly indicated and when appropriate treatment options are unavailable because they are expensive and need to be reserved for the most serious infections.

Infectious Disease

Central Nervous System Infections

Meningitis

Viral Meningitis

Epidemiology and Cause

The aseptic meningitis syndrome is defined as the presence of clinical and laboratory findings consistent with meningitis in a patient who has normal cerebrospinal fluid (CSF) stains and culture on initial evaluation. Viruses are the major cause, and enteroviruses are diagnosed in 85% to 95% of cases. Approximately 30,000 to 75,000 cases are reported annually in the United States, although the actual number is likely underrepresented. Enteroviral meningitis usually occurs in the summer and fall and is spread by the fecal-oral route. Although enteroviral meningitis occurs most often in infants and children, it is also the most common cause of aseptic meningitis in adults.

Meningitis develops in 10% to 30% of patients infected with mumps virus, although mumps is rare in a highly immunized population. Herpes simplex viruses (HSV) account for 0.5% to 3% of cases of aseptic meningitis and are most often associated with primary genital infection due to herpes simplex virus type 2 (HSV-2). HSV-2 is also the most common cause of the syndrome of benign recurrent lymphocytic meningitis (previously termed Mollaret meningitis). Although encephalitis is the most common neurologic manifestation of West Nile virus infection (seen in fewer than 1% of patients), aseptic meningitis may also occur.

Diagnosis

Adult patients with enteroviral meningitis usually present with the sudden onset of fever, headache, nuchal rigidity, and photophobia. The duration of illness is usually less than 1 week, and many patients report improvement after diagnostic lumbar puncture. Patients with mumps meningitis usually report fever, vomiting, and headache. Salivary gland enlargement occurs in only 50% of these patients. Patients with the syndrome of benign recurrent lymphocytic meningitis characteristically develop approximately 10 episodes of meningitis lasting 2 to 5 days followed by spontaneous recovery.

CSF findings in patients with viral meningitis are shown in **Table 1**. Viral cultures of CSF are insensitive for diagnosis and are not routinely recommended. Nucleic acid amplification tests, such as polymerase chain reaction (PCR), are both sensitive (86% to 100%) and specific (92% to 100%) for diagnosing enteroviral meningitis. PCR has also been useful for diagnosing HSV-induced meningitis and for associating HSV-2

TABLE 1. Typical CSF Findings in Patients with Viral and Bacterial Meningitis

CSF Parameter	Viral Meningitis[a]	Bacterial Meningitis
Opening pressure	≤250 mm H_2O	200-500 mm H_2O[b]
Leukocyte count	50-1000/µL (50-1000 × 10^6/L)	1000-5000/µL (1000-5000 × 10^6/L)[c]
Leukocyte differential	Lymphocytes[d]	Neutrophils
Glucose	>45 mg/dL (2.5 mmol/L)	<40 mg/dL (2.2 mmol/L)[e]
Protein	<200 mg/dL (2000 mg/L)	100-500 mg/dL (1000-5000 mg/L)
Gram stain	Negative	Positive in 60%-90%[f,g]
Culture	Negative	Positive in 70%-85%[g]

CSF = cerebrospinal fluid; µL= microliter.

[a]Primarily nonpolio enteroviruses (echoviruses and coxsackieviruses).

[b]Values exceeding 600 mm H_2O suggest the presence of cerebral edema, intracranial suppurative foci, or communicating hydrocephalus.

[c]Range may be <100/µL (100 × 10^6/L) to >10,000/µL (10,000 × 10^6/L).

[d]May have neutrophil predominance early in infection, but lymphocyte predominance occurs after the first 6 to 48 hours.

[e]The CSF:plasma glucose ratio is ≤0.40 in most patients.

[f]The likelihood of a positive Gram stain correlates with number of bacteria in the CSF.

[g]The yield of positive results is significantly reduced by prior administration of antimicrobial therapy.

CONT.

with the presence of benign recurrent lymphocytic meningitis. West Nile virus meningitis is best diagnosed by detection of IgM antibodies in CSF.

Treatment

Treatment of patients with enteroviral meningitis is supportive. Whether antiviral therapy alters the course of mild HSV-2 meningitis is unclear. Antiviral suppressive therapy may be considered in patients with benign recurrent lymphocytic meningitis, although there are no clinical trials to date that support the safety and efficacy of this approach. ◻

KEY POINTS

- Aseptic meningitis syndrome is defined as the presence of clinical and laboratory findings consistent with meningitis in a patient who has normal cerebrospinal fluid stains and culture on initial evaluation.
- Polymerase chain reaction is both sensitive and specific for diagnosing enteroviral meningitis and is also useful for diagnosing aseptic meningitis due to herpes simplex virus.
- Treatment of enteroviral meningitis is supportive.

Bacterial Meningitis

Cause

Streptococcus pneumoniae is the most common cause of bacterial meningitis in the United States. Approximately 70% of patients with *S. pneumoniae* meningitis have otitis media, sinusitis, pneumonia, basilar skull fracture with CSF leak, or are immunocompromised (splenectomy or asplenia, hypogammaglobulinemia, multiple myeloma, alcoholism, chronic liver or kidney disease, malignancy, or HIV infection).

Neisseria meningitidis meningitis most often occurs in children and young adults and in patients with properdin and terminal complement (C5, C6, C7, C8, and perhaps C9) deficiencies. *Listeria monocytogenes* meningitis develops most frequently in neonates, older adults (>50 years of age), and in those who are immunocompromised (diabetes mellitus, liver or kidney disease, collagen vascular disorders, disorders of iron overload, HIV infection, transplant recipients, and patients taking anti–tumor necrosis factor α agents such as infliximab and etanercept), although cases have been reported in patients with no underlying disorders. Outbreaks have been associated with ingestion of contaminated coleslaw, soft cheeses, raw vegetables, alfalfa tablets, cantaloupes, and frankfurters and other processed meats. The incidence of invasive listeriosis has been decreasing, most likely as a result of decreased contamination by *L. monocytogenes* in ready-to-eat foods.

Meningitis due to group B streptococci (*Streptococcus agalactiae*) most commonly occurs in neonates. Because of this risk, the Centers for Disease Control and Prevention (CDC) and the American College of Obstetricians and Gynecologists have established guidelines for the prevention of early-onset disease. These guidelines recommend universal screening of all pregnant women for rectovaginal colonization at 35 to 37 weeks' gestation and the administration of antimicrobial prophylaxis to carriers.

Meningitis caused by gram-negative bacilli (*Escherichia coli, Klebsiella* species, *Serratia marcescens, Pseudomonas aeruginosa*) may occur following head trauma, after neurosurgical procedures, and after placement of ventricular drains. Older adults, immunocompromised patients, and patients with gram-negative bacteremia or disseminated strongyloidiasis are also at risk for gram-negative meningitis. *Haemophilus influenzae*–induced bacterial meningitis in children or adults suggests the presence of sinusitis, otitis media, epiglottitis, pneumonia, diabetes mellitus, alcoholism, splenectomy or asplenia, head trauma with CSF leak, and immunodeficiencies such as hypogammaglobulinemia.

Recurrent bacterial meningitis accounts for about 1% to 6% of cases of community-acquired meningitis. The most common predisposing conditions in adults are remote head trauma and/or CSF leakage. Immunodeficient disorders such as complement deficiencies, asplenia, and HIV infection may also predispose to recurrent bacterial meningitis.

Health care–associated (nosocomial) bacterial meningitis usually occurs in the setting of head trauma, recent neurosurgery, or placement of external or internal ventricular drains and is usually caused by a different spectrum of pathogens than those causing community-acquired bacterial meningitis. Likely pathogens include staphylococci (*Staphylococcus aureus* and coagulase-negative staphylococci), gram-negative bacilli (*P. aeruginosa*), and *Propionibacterium acnes* (especially in patients with internal ventricular drains).

Epidemiology

The epidemiology of bacterial meningitis in the United States has changed significantly since the introduction of conjugate vaccines (**Table 2**). Since licensure of the 7-valent

TABLE 2. Causes of Bacterial Meningitis in the United States

	Percentage of Total Cases		
Pathogen	1986[a]	1995[b]	2003-2007
Haemophilus influenzae	45	7	7
Neisseria meningitidis	14	25	14
Streptococcus pneumoniae	18	47	58
Streptococcus agalactiae	6	12	18
Listeria monocytogenes	3	8	3

[a]Other bacteria represent 14% of total cases.

[b]Because of rounding, the percentage does not total 100%.

pneumococcal conjugate vaccine for children (covering serotypes 4, 6B, 9V, 14, 18C, 19F, and 23F) in 2000, one study reported that the incidence of pneumococcal meningitis decreased from 1.13 cases per 100,000 population between 1998 and 1999 to 0.79 case per 100,000 population between 2004 and 2005. However, the incidence of meningitis caused by serotypes 19A, 22F, and 35B (not covered by the vaccine) increased during this time. In a recent surveillance study conducted by the CDC in eight states representing 17 million persons of all ages, the incidence of bacterial meningitis declined from 2.0 to 1.38 cases per 100,000 population between 1998 and 1999 and 2006 and 2007; the median age of patients with meningitis increased from 30.3 years to 41.9 years. A 13-valent pneumococcal conjugate vaccine has recently been licensed in the United States, which offers additional protection against serotype 19A, but not serotypes 22F and 35B.

A quadrivalent meningococcal conjugate vaccine that provides coverage against four of the five major meningococcal serogroups (A, C, Y, and W135) was licensed for use in the United States in 2005. Routine single-dose vaccination is recommended for all children and adolescents ages 11 to 18 years, and revaccination is recommended for persons at prolonged increased risk of developing meningococcal disease. This vaccine does not provide coverage against serogroup B meningococci, which are responsible for almost one third of cases of invasive meningococcal infection in the United States. Vaccination against *H. influenzae* type b infection has almost eradicated what was once the most common form of bacterial meningitis. Remaining cases of *H. influenzae* meningitis are usually caused by other serotypes or nontypeable strains.

Diagnosis

Patients with bacterial meningitis usually present with some combination of fever, headache, stiff neck, and signs of cerebral dysfunction (confusion, delirium, or a decreased level of consciousness). Clinical features in patients with health care–associated bacterial meningitis most often include fever and a decreased level of consciousness, although these findings may be difficult to recognize in patients who are sedated, have recently undergone a neurosurgical procedure, or have an underlying disease that may mask the signs and symptoms.

Bacterial meningitis is diagnosed by CSF examination (see Table 1). Use of latex agglutination tests, which detect antigens of common meningeal pathogens, is no longer recommended because of the frequency of false-positive and false-negative results and because antigen testing does not modify the decision as to whether to administer antimicrobial therapy. A rapid immunochromatographic test that detects the C polysaccharide cell wall antigen of all strains of *S. pneumoniae* has an overall sensitivity of 95% to 100% and specificity of 100% for the rapid diagnosis of pneumococcal meningitis, although more studies are needed to demonstrate its usefulness. PCR has a sensitivity of 92% to 100% and specificity of 100% for diagnosing pneumococcal meningitis. Use of PCR for this indication has not been extensively evaluated, and false-positive results have been reported. However, modifications to the technique may make PCR useful in diagnosing patients with bacterial meningitis, especially when CSF Gram stain and culture are negative.

Management

A management algorithm for patients with suspected bacterial meningitis is shown in **Figure 1**.

When acute bacterial meningitis is suspected, blood cultures and lumbar puncture must be performed immediately because lumbar puncture is needed to determine whether CSF findings are consistent with the clinical manifestations and suspected diagnosis. Emergent lumbar puncture should not be performed, however, in patients whose clinical presentation is consistent with a central nervous system (CNS) mass lesion. A CT scan of the head should be done before lumbar puncture in these patients, as well as in patients who are immunocompromised, have a history of CNS disease, present with new-onset seizures, or have a decreased level of consciousness, focal neurologic deficits, or papilledema. Some experts also suggest delaying lumbar puncture in patients with clinical signs of impending brain herniation because of the risk of precipitating herniation even when CT findings are normal. Clinical signs of impending herniation include deteriorating level of consciousness (especially a Glasgow Coma Scale score of ≤11), brainstem signs (including papillary changes, posturing, or irregular respirations), and a seizure.

Empiric antimicrobial therapy is started immediately for all patients after CSF is obtained by lumbar puncture, and adjunctive dexamethasone is also begun for most adult patients. Recommendations for selecting empiric antimicrobial agents are based on the patient's age and underlying condition (**Table 3, see page 5**). For patients in whom the lumbar puncture is delayed, blood culture specimens are obtained and appropriate adjunctive and empiric antimicrobial therapy is started before the lumbar puncture is performed. For all patients, targeted antimicrobial therapy can be initiated after the presumptive pathogen is identified on CSF Gram stain following lumbar puncture (**Table 4, see page 5**). Once the pathogen is positively identified and in vitro susceptibility is known, the antimicrobial regimen can be modified to provide optimal therapy (**Table 5, see page 6**).

Most adult patients with bacterial meningitis should be started on adjunctive dexamethasone when empiric antimicrobial therapy is begun. Adjunctive corticosteroids have been shown to decrease mortality and negative short-term neurologic sequelae in patients in developed countries, although their efficacy in resource-poor countries with significant prevalence of HIV infection and other comorbid diseases has not been established. Use of adjunctive dexamethasone may also be a concern in patients for whom

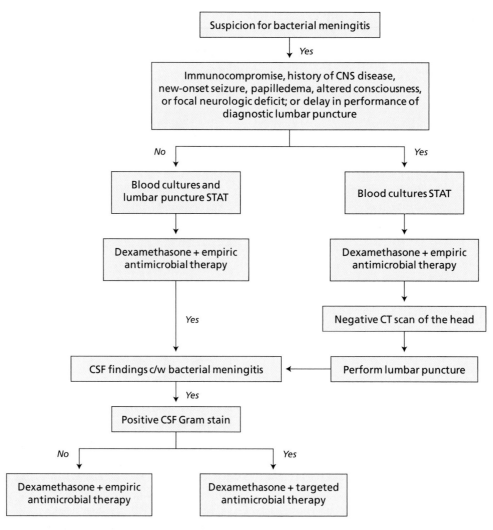

FIGURE 1. Management algorithm for adults with suspected bacterial meningitis.

CNS = central nervous system; c/w = consistent with; CSF = cerebrospinal fluid.

Reprinted with permission from Tunkel AR, Hartman BJ, Kaplan SL, et al. Practice guidelines for the management of bacterial meningitis. Clin Inf Dis. 2004; 39:1267–84. Copyright 2004 Oxford University Press.

vancomycin is the most appropriate antimicrobial agent, because vancomycin's ability to penetrate the CSF may be reduced when dexamethasone is also administered. However, adjustment of the vancomycin dose to achieve serum trough concentrations of 15 to 20 micrograms/mL may help to overcome this problem. For patients receiving adjunctive dexamethasone and standard antimicrobial therapy with vancomycin and a third-generation cephalosporin (either cefotaxime or ceftriaxone) for treatment of pneumococcal meningitis who do not improve as expected or whose isolate has a cefotaxime or ceftriaxone minimal inhibitory concentration greater than 2.0 micrograms/mL, a repeat lumbar puncture is recommended 36 to 48 hours after initiation of therapy to document CSF sterility.

Outpatient intravenous antimicrobial therapy may be appropriate for selected patients with acute bacterial meningitis because outpatient therapy is associated with decreased costs of hospitalization, decreased risk of hospital-acquired infections, and better quality of life. The following criteria can be used for selecting patients for outpatient intravenous therapy: (1) completion of inpatient therapy for more than 6 days; (2) absence of fever for at least 24 to 48 hours; (3) no significant neurologic dysfunction, focal findings, or seizure activity; (4) clinical stability or improving infection; (5) ability to take fluids by mouth; (6) access to home health nursing for administration of antimicrobial therapy; (7) reliable intravenous line and infusion device (if needed); (8) daily availability of a physician; (9) established plan for physician visits, nurse visits, laboratory monitoring, and emergencies; (10) patient and/or family compliance; and (11) a safe environment with access to a telephone, utilities, food, and a refrigerator.

KEY POINTS

- Approximately 70% of patients with *Streptococcus pneumoniae* meningitis are immunocompromised or have an underlying disorder such as otitis media, sinusitis, or pneumonia.

- Patients with bacterial meningitis may have some combination of fever, headache, stiff neck, and signs of cerebral dysfunction.

- When acute bacterial meningitis is suspected, immediate blood cultures and lumbar puncture must be performed unless lumbar puncture is contraindicated.

- Empiric antimicrobial therapy is started immediately for all patients with suspected bacterial meningitis after lumbar puncture is performed followed by targeted antimicrobial therapy after presumptive identification of the pathogen on cerebrospinal fluid Gram stain.

- Adjunctive dexamethasone should be started immediately for most adult patients with suspected bacterial meningitis who are living in developed countries.

TABLE 4. Recommended Targeted Antimicrobial Therapy for Bacterial Meningitis[a]

Pathogen	Antimicrobial Therapy
Streptococcus pneumoniae[b]	Vancomycin plus a third-generation cephalosporin[c,d]
Neisseria meningitidis	Third-generation cephalosporin[c]
Listeria monocytogenes	Ampicillin or penicillin G[e]
Haemophilus influenzae type b[f]	Third-generation cephalosporin[c]

[a]Based on identification of presumptive pathogen by cerebrospinal fluid Gram stain.

[b]Pending in vitro susceptibility testing, assume that the pneumococcal isolate is highly resistant to penicillin and use combination therapy.

[c]Cefotaxime or ceftriaxone.

[d]Addition of rifampin should be considered.

[e]Addition of an aminoglycoside should be considered.

[f]Pending in vitro susceptibility testing, assume that the pathogen produces β-lactamase.

TABLE 3. Recommended Empiric Antimicrobial Therapy for Suspected Bacterial Meningitis[a]

Community-acquired Meningitis		
Predisposing Factor	**Common Bacterial Pathogens**	**Antimicrobial Therapy**
Age <1 month	*Streptococcus agalactiae, Escherichia coli, Listeria monocytogenes, Klebsiella* species	Ampicillin plus cefotaxime or ampicillin plus an aminoglycoside
Age 1-23 months	*Streptococcus pneumoniae, Haemophilus influenzae, S. agalactiae, Neisseria meningitidis, E. coli*	Vancomycin plus a third-generation cephalosporin[b,c,d]
Age 2-50 years	*S. pneumoniae, N. meningitidis*	Vancomycin plus a third-generation cephalosporin[b,c,d]
Age >50 years	*S. pneumoniae, N. meningitidis, L. monocytogenes,* aerobic gram-negative bacilli	Vancomycin plus ampicillin plus a third-generation cephalosporin[b,c]
Immunocompromised state	*S. pneumoniae, N. meningitidis, L. monocytogenes,* aerobic gram-negative bacilli (including *Pseudomonas aeruginosa*)	Vancomycin plus ampicillin plus either cefepime or meropenem
Health care–associated Meningitis		
Predisposing Factor	**Common Bacterial Pathogens**	**Antimicrobial Therapy**
Basilar skull fracture	*S. pneumoniae, H. influenzae,* group A β-hemolytic streptococci	Vancomycin plus a third-generation cephalosporin[b]
Postneurosurgery or head trauma	*Staphylococcus aureus,* coagulase-negative staphylococci (especially *Staphylococcus epidermidis*), aerobic gram-negative bacilli (including *P. aeruginosa*)	Vancomycin plus either ceftazidime or cefepime or meropenem
Ventricular catheters (external or internal)	*S. aureus,* coagulase-negative staphylococci (especially *S. epidermidis*), aerobic gram-negative bacilli (including *P. aeruginosa*), diphtheroids (including *Propionibacterium acnes*)	Vancomycin plus either ceftazidime or cefepime or meropenem

[a]Based on the patient's age and underlying condition.

[b]Cefotaxime or ceftriaxone.

[c]Some experts would add rifampin if adjunctive dexamethasone is given.

[d]Add ampicillin if the patient has risk factors for or infection with *L. monocytogenes* is suspected.

TABLE 5. Recommended Specific Antimicrobial Therapy for Bacterial Meningitis Based on Pathogen and in vitro Susceptibility Testing

Pathogen/Susceptibilities	Standard Therapy	Alternative Therapies
Streptococcus pneumoniae		
Penicillin MIC ≤0.06 µg/mL	Penicillin G or ampicillin	Third-generation cephalosporin[a]; chloramphenicol
Penicillin MIC ≥0.12 µg/mL		
Cefotaxime or ceftriaxone MIC <1.0 µg/mL	Third-generation cephalosporin[a]	Meropenem; cefepime
Cefotaxime or ceftriaxone MIC ≥1.0 µg/mL	Vancomycin plus a third-generation cephalosporin[a,b]	Moxifloxacin[b,c]
Neisseria meningitidis		
Penicillin MIC <0.1 µg/mL	Penicillin G or ampicillin	Third-generation cephalosporin[a]; chloramphenicol
Penicillin MIC 0.1-1.0 µg/mL	Third-generation cephalosporin[a]	Chloramphenicol; a fluoroquinolone; meropenem
Listeria monocytogenes	Ampicillin or penicillin G[d]	Trimethoprim-sulfamethoxazole
Streptococcus agalactiae	Ampicillin or penicillin G[d]	Third-generation cephalosporin[a]; vancomycin
Haemophilus influenzae		
β-lactamase-negative	Ampicillin	Third-generation cephalosporin[a]; cefepime; aztreonam; chloramphenicol; a fluoroquinolone
β-lactamase-positive	Third-generation cephalosporin[a]	Chloramphenicol; cefepime; aztreonam; a fluoroquinolone
Escherichia coli and other Enterobacteriaceae[e]	Third-generation cephalosporin[a]	Aztreonam; meropenem; a fluoroquinolone; trimethoprim-sulfamethoxazole
Pseudomonas aeruginosa[e]	Ceftazidime[d] or cefepime[d]	Aztreonam[d]; meropenem[d]; ciprofloxacin[d]
Staphylococcus aureus		
Methicillin-sensitive	Nafcillin or oxacillin	Vancomycin; meropenem; linezolid; daptomycin
Methicillin-resistant	Vancomycin[f]	Trimethoprim-sulfamethoxazole; linezolid; daptomycin
Staphylococcus epidermidis	Vancomyin[f]	Linezolid

MIC = minimal inhibitory concentration; µg = micrograms.

[a]Cefotaxime or ceftriaxone.

[b]Addition of rifampin should be considered if the pathogen is sensitive and if the ceftriaxone MIC is >2 micrograms/mL.

[c]Has not been studied in patients with pneumococcal meningitis, but efficacy has been demonstrated in experimental animal models; if used, administering in combination with either a third-generation cephalosporin (cefotaxime or ceftriaxone) or vancomycin should be considered.

[d]Addition of an aminoglycoside should be considered.

[e]Choice of specific antimicrobial therapy should be guided by in vitro susceptibility test results.

[f]Addition of rifampin should be considered.

Focal Central Nervous System Infections

Brain abscess, cranial subdural empyema, and spinal epidural abscess are discussed below.

Brain Abscess

The most common pathogenetic mechanism of brain abscess formation is direct extension from a contiguous focus of infection, most often the middle ear, mastoid cells, or paranasal sinuses (**Table 6**). A second mechanism is

TABLE 6. Predisposing Conditions, Etiologic Agents, and Empiric Antimicrobial Therapy in Patients with Bacterial Brain Abscess

Predisposing Condition	Usual Bacterial Isolates	Empiric Antimicrobial Therapy
Otitis media or mastoiditis	Streptococci (aerobic or anaerobic); *Bacteroides* species; *Prevotella* species; Enterobacteriaceae	Metronidazole plus a third-generation cephalosporin[a]
Sinusitis	Streptococci; *Bacteroides* species; Enterobacteriaceae; *Staphylococcus aureus*; *Haemophilus* species	Metronidazole plus a third-generation cephalosporin[a,b]
Dental sepsis	Mixed *Fusobacterium, Prevotella,* and *Bacteroides* species; streptococci	Penicillin plus metronidazole
Penetrating trauma or after neurosurgery	*S. aureus*, streptococci, Enterobacteriaceae, *Clostridium* species	Vancomycin plus a third-generation cephalosporin[a,c]
Lung abscess, empyema, bronchiectasis	*Fusobacterium, Actinomyces, Bacteroides,* and *Prevotella* species; streptococci; *Nocardia* species	Penicillin plus metronidazole plus a sulfonamide[d]
Endocarditis	*S. aureus*, streptococci	Vancomycin plus gentamicin

[a]Cefotaxime or ceftriaxone; the fourth-generation cephalosporin cefepime may also be used.

[b]Add vancomycin if infection caused by methicillin-resistant *Staphylococcus aureus* is suspected.

[c]Use ceftazidime or cefepime if infection caused by *Pseudomonas aeruginosa* is suspected.

[d]Use trimethoprim-sulfamethoxazole if infection caused by *Nocardia* species is suspected.

hematogenous dissemination from a distant focus of infection; primary sources are chronic pyogenic lung diseases, wound and skin infections, osteomyelitis, pelvic infections, cholecystitis, intraabdominal infections, and infective endocarditis. Patients with congenital heart disease and hereditary hemorrhagic telangiectasia are also at increased risk. Trauma is a third pathogenetic mechanism, occurring secondary to an open cranial fracture with dural breach, as a result of neurosurgery, or after a foreign body injury. The cause of brain abscess is unknown in 10% to 35% of patients.

Most symptoms and signs are related to the size and location of the space-occupying lesion within the brain. Headache is the most common symptom; sudden worsening of the headache may signify rupture of the abscess into the ventricular space and is associated with a high mortality rate. Less than 50% of patients with brain abscess present with the triad of headache, fever, and focal neurologic deficit.

MRI is the diagnostic procedure of choice. Diffusion-weighted MRI can be used to help discriminate between abscess lesions and neoplasms. CT is reserved for patients unable to undergo MRI.

The optimal management of brain abscess requires a multidisciplinary approach. All lesions larger than 2.5 cm should be excised or stereotactically aspirated, and specimens should undergo microbiologic and histopathologic analysis. For abscesses in the early cerebritis stage (that is, the earliest stage of purulent brain infection when there is little or no enhancement on neuroimaging) or when all the abscesses are smaller than 2.5 cm, the largest lesion should be aspirated for diagnosis and microbiologic identification. Following specimen retrieval, it is appropriate to initiate empiric antimicrobial therapy based on the patient's predisposing conditions

and the presumed pathogenesis of brain abscess formation (see Table 6). In patients with significant cerebral edema and mass effect, initiation of corticosteroids is warranted.

Antimicrobial therapy usually lasts 6 to 8 weeks, and parenteral agents are preferred to ensure achievement of adequate tissue levels. Depending on the patient's response clinically and as demonstrated on imaging, this regimen may be followed by prolonged oral antimicrobial therapy if an appropriate agent is available. Shorter courses of therapy (3 to 4 weeks) may be adequate for patients who have undergone complete surgical excision of the brain abscess. Repeat neuroimaging biweekly up to 3 months after completion of therapy is recommended to monitor for re-expansion of the abscess or failure to respond.

KEY POINTS

- To establish the diagnosis and cause of brain abscess, a lesion should be stereotactically aspirated or surgically excised, and specimens should undergo culture and histopathologic analysis.

- In patients with brain abscess, intravenous antimicrobial therapy is usually continued for 6 to 8 weeks, followed by prolonged oral therapy if an appropriate agent is available.

Cranial Subdural Empyema

Paranasal sinusitis is the most common condition (40% to 80% of cases) predisposing to the development of cranial subdural empyema. Bacterial species that are most often isolated include aerobic streptococci, staphylococci, aerobic gram-negative bacilli, and anaerobic streptococci and other anaerobes; polymicrobial infections are common.

CONT.

Cranial subdural empyema can be rapidly progressive in its clinical presentation, with symptoms and signs related to increased intracranial pressure, meningeal irritation, or focal cortical inflammation. Headache is a prominent symptom and becomes generalized as the infection progresses. The diagnostic neuroimaging procedure of choice is MRI, which is preferred to CT because it provides better clarity of morphologic detail; may detect empyemas not seen on CT, such as those located at the base of the brain, along the falx cerebri, or in the posterior fossa; and can differentiate extraaxial empyemas from most sterile effusions and subdural hematomas.

Cranial subdural empyema is a medical and surgical emergency. Given the potential for polymicrobial infection, empiric antimicrobial therapy with vancomycin, metronidazole, and a third- or fourth-generation cephalosporin is warranted. The goals of surgical therapy are to achieve adequate decompression of the brain and evacuate the empyema. The optimal surgical approach is not clearly defined, although craniotomy is most often recommended because it allows wide exposure and better drainage of the empyema, which may be more loculated, tenacious, and extensive than that demonstrated by neuroimaging studies. Retrospective analyses have shown a lower mortality rate in patients with cranial subdural empyema who were treated with craniotomy compared with those who had drainage through craniectomy or burr holes. However, a limited drainage procedure (burr holes) may be preferable in patients with septic shock, those with localized parafalcine collections, and in children with subdural empyema secondary to meningitis. **H**

KEY POINTS

- The clinical presentation of cranial subdural empyema can be rapidly progressive, with symptoms and signs related to increased intracranial pressure, meningeal irritation, or focal cortical inflammation.
- Craniotomy is most often recommended in patients with cranial subdural empyema because it allows wide exposure and better drainage of the empyema compared to more limited procedures.

H Spinal Epidural Abscess

Spinal epidural abscess most often occurs secondary to hematogenous dissemination to the epidural space from foci elsewhere in the body. Therefore, the most common infecting microorganism is *Staphylococcus aureus* (50% to 90% of cases). Gram-negative bacilli and anaerobes may be seen if the infection has a urinary or gastrointestinal source. The clinical presentation progresses through four stages: backache and focal vertebral pain; nerve root pain, manifested by radiculopathy or paresthesias; spinal cord dysfunction; and paraplegia. MRI with gadolinium enhancement is the diagnostic procedure of choice; it can enable visualization of the spinal cord and the epidural space in sagittal and transverse sections and can also identify accompanying osteomyelitis, intramedullary spinal cord lesions, and diskitis.

The principles of therapy for spinal epidural abscess are surgical decompression, drainage of the abscess, and antimicrobial therapy. Empiric antimicrobial therapy should always include an antistaphylococcal agent (usually vancomycin pending organism identification and in vitro susceptibility testing) plus coverage for gram-negative bacilli with agents such as an antipseudomonal cephalosporin or carbapenem, especially for patients with a history of injection drug use or a spinal procedure. Spinal epidural abscess is a surgical emergency requiring surgical drainage with decompression to minimize the likelihood of permanent neurologic sequelae. Antimicrobial therapy alone can be considered in patients who have localized pain and radicular symptoms without long-tract signs; these patients require frequent neurologic examinations and serial MRI studies to demonstrate resolution of the abscess. Emergent surgery is required in patients with increasing neurologic deficit, persistent severe pain, or increasing fever or peripheral leukocyte count. Surgery is not likely to be effective in patients who have experienced complete paralysis for longer than 24 to 36 hours, although some authorities have performed surgery when complete paralysis has lasted less than 72 hours. **H**

KEY POINTS

- The clinical presentation of spinal epidural abscess begins with backache and focal vertebral pain and progresses to nerve root pain, spinal cord dysfunction, and paraplegia.
- The principles of spinal epidural abscess management are surgical decompression, drainage of the abscess, and antimicrobial therapy.
- Antimicrobial therapy alone can be considered in patients with spinal epidural abscess who have localized pain and radicular symptoms without long-tract signs; frequent follow-up neurologic examinations and serial MRI studies to demonstrate abscess resolution are necessary.

Encephalitis

Encephalitis refers to infection of the brain parenchyma with associated neurologic dysfunction. The meninges are also frequently involved, and the terms "encephalitis" and "meningoencephalitis" are used interchangeably. Although more than 100 microorganisms are associated with encephalitis, the most commonly diagnosed causes in the United States are herpes simplex virus and West Nile virus. In more than 50% of patients, however, a cause is not identified despite intensive diagnostic evaluation (**Table 7**).

Clinically, encephalitis is defined by an altered mental status lasting for at least 24 hours. Decreased consciousness may range from mild confusion to coma, and seizures occur in up to 40% of patients. Other common manifestations include hallucinations, ataxia, and cranial neuropathies. Focal neurologic

TABLE 7. Selected Viral Causes of Encephalitis Among Adults in the United States

Cause	Epidemiology	Clinical Features	Diagnosis	Treatment
Eastern equine encephalitis virus	Mosquito-borne infection	Case fatality rate, 50%-70%	Serology	Supportive
Herpes simplex virus-1	Reactivation of latent virus in about two thirds of cases	Temporal lobe seizures, fever	CSF PCR	Acyclovir
Human herpes virus-6	Immunocompromise, particularly bone marrow transplantation	Seizures	CSF PCR	Ganciclovir or foscarnet
JC virus (PML)	AIDS, immunomodulating therapy (natalizumab, rituximab)	Focal neurologic findings, subacute onset	CSF PCR	Decrease immunosuppression, start ART (in patients with AIDS)
Rabies virus	Transmitted by bite of infected animal	Agitation, paresthesias at site of inoculation, hydrophobia, autonomic instability	Serology (serum or CSF), RT-PCR of saliva, immuno-fluorescence staining of nuchal biopsy specimen	Supportive
St. Louis encephalitis virus	Mosquito-borne infection, endemic to United States west of the Mississippi River	Seizures, altered mentation, urinary tract symptoms, SIADH	Serology	Supportive
West Nile virus	Mosquito-borne infection, widely distributed worldwide	Acute flaccid paralysis, parkinsonian symptoms, myoclonus	Serology	Supportive

CSF PCR = cerebrospinal fluid polymerase chain reaction; PML = progressive multifocal leukoencephalopathy; ART = antiretroviral therapy; RT-PCR = reverse transcriptase polymerase chain reaction; SIADH = syndrome of inappropriate antidiuretic hormone secretion.

findings may be present when a localized anatomic region of the brain is involved.

Neuroimaging is required to define the location and extent of central nervous system involvement. MRI is more sensitive than CT scanning for this purpose. Lumbar puncture should be performed in all patients without contraindications. The cerebrospinal fluid (CSF) typically exhibits a lymphocytic pleocytosis, although the CSF may be acellular. All patients should be tested for herpes simplex virus. Other serologic studies and molecular testing are based on the season of the year, geographic location, history of exposures, predisposing conditions, and clinical findings (for example, rash). ◱

Herpes Simplex Encephalitis

Herpes simplex encephalitis is the most common cause of endemic encephalitis in the United States, with a predilection for the very young and the elderly. Herpes simplex virus type 1 (HSV-1) accounts for greater than 90% of cases in adults; herpes simplex virus type 2 (HSV-2) causes the remaining cases. More than two thirds of infections are due to reactivation of latent HSV-1 virus rather than to primary infection. Even with antiviral therapy, the mortality rate for herpes simplex encephalitis ranges from 15% to 30%, and neuropsychiatric sequelae are common.

Most patients present within a week of onset of symptoms, most commonly alterations in mental status and fever.

Orolabial herpetic lesions are present in less than 10% of patients. Because the virus most often infects the temporal lobes, partial complex seizures may occur. Without treatment, infection progresses to bilateral temporal lobe hemorrhagic necrosis, resulting in severe neurologic impairment or death.

Results of routine laboratory studies are nonspecific. CSF pleocytosis is generally present, with a lymphocytic predominance. However, the CSF leukocyte count is normal (0-5/microliter [0-5 × 10⁶/L]) in approximately 5% of patients. Neuroimaging findings that localize inflammation to one or both temporal lobes are strongly suggestive of this diagnosis (**Figure 2**). MRI is superior to CT scanning for identifying early infection when radiographic abnormalities may be subtle. An electroencephalogram may show characteristic periodic lateralizing epileptiform discharges localizing to the temporal lobes.

Microbiologic diagnosis requires detection of HSV in the CSF or brain tissue. HSV polymerase chain reaction (PCR) of CSF has a sensitivity of greater than 95% and specificity approaching 100% for diagnosis. False-negative HSV PCR results may occur early in the course of infection. In most patients, HSV PCR results remain positive for more than 7 days after antiviral therapy is begun. Because CSF viral culture is insensitive and HSV serologic studies are nonspecific, these tests are not indicated for diagnosis.

Intravenous acyclovir is the treatment of choice for herpes simplex encephalitis. Because delay in initiating treatment

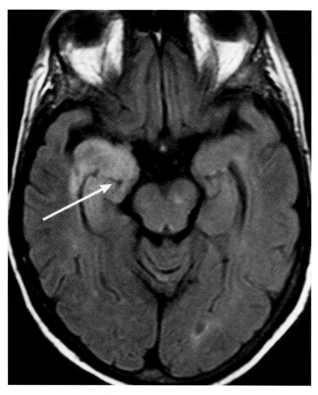

FIGURE 2. Brain MRI exhibiting right temporal lobe enhancement (arrow) in a patient with herpes simplex encephalitis.

is associated with adverse neurologic outcomes or death, beginning empiric acyclovir before HSV PCR results are available is recommended. A positive HSV PCR result is diagnostic, and intravenous acyclovir is continued for 14 to 21 days. Oral antivirals such as valacyclovir have poor CSF penetration and result in subtherapeutic levels, mandating continuation of intravenous therapy for the entire treatment course. In patients with a low clinical suspicion for herpes simplex encephalitis, acyclovir may be discontinued when HSV PCR results are negative. Patients with an initially negative HSV PCR in whom there is a strong clinical suspicion for herpes simplex encephalitis should undergo repeat HSV PCR on a second CSF sample 3 to 7 days after the initial lumbar puncture or be treated with a full course of acyclovir. **H**

KEY POINTS

- Herpes simplex virus polymerase chain reaction of cerebrospinal fluid is diagnostic of herpes simplex encephalitis and should be performed in all patients with suspected infection.
- Intravenous acyclovir is the treatment of choice for patients with herpes simplex encephalitis.

West Nile Virus Encephalitis

West Nile virus encephalitis, first detected in the United States in 1999, has become an important cause of epidemic encephalitis nationally, although the regional incidence varies considerably from year to year. The virus is spread by the bite of an infected *Culex* mosquito, with the peak incidence in the late summer and early fall.

West Nile virus encephalitis is asymptomatic in 80% of patients. Symptomatic infections include West Nile fever, occurring in 20% of patients, and West Nile neuroinvasive disease (WNND), occurring in less than 1% of patients, with adults over 50 years of age being disproportionately affected. Patients with West Nile fever develop a self-limited febrile illness associated with fatigue, rash, headache, anorexia, back pain, and myalgia. Clinical manifestations of WNND include meningitis, encephalitis, and myelitis, either alone or as overlapping findings. An objective finding of focal weakness is an important clue to diagnosing WNND. In the most severe cases, this manifests as acute flaccid paralysis and may lead to diaphragmatic involvement with respiratory failure similar to poliomyelitis. Other neurologic findings suggestive of WNND include extrapyramidal signs, which may mimic the tremors and bradykinesia of Parkinson disease. Rash may be present but is more common with West Nile fever than with WNND. Standard laboratory studies in WNND typically reveal a lymphocyte-predominant CSF pleocytosis, although in contrast to most viral encephalitides, neutrophils constitute a substantial proportion of the differential count. MRI of the brain is often normal or shows nonspecific abnormalities. Bilateral enhancement of the thalamus and basal ganglia on T2-weighted MRI images has been reported in a subset of patients with WNND.

Detection of West Nile virus IgM antibody in the CSF of symptomatic patients is diagnostic of WNND. The antibody is reliably detected within 9 days of onset of fever and often persists for more than 1 year. Serologic cross-reactivity with other flaviviruses (for example, St. Louis encephalitis virus, Japanese encephalitis virus, dengue virus, yellow fever virus) may cause false-positive West Nile virus IgM antibody results following recent infection with or immunization against one of these viruses. Nucleic acid amplification techniques are insensitive in diagnosing WNND because of the very brief period of viremia occurring in WNND.

Treatment of West Nile virus infection is supportive, although ongoing studies are evaluating the role of immunotherapy. There are no commercially available human vaccines against this virus. Prevention involves minimizing the risk of transmission from infected mosquitoes. **H**

KEY POINTS

- Clinical manifestations of West Nile neuroinvasive disease include meningitis, encephalitis, and myelitis, either alone or in combination; an objective finding of focal weakness is characteristic.
- The diagnosis of West Nile neuroinvasive disease is established by detection of West Nile virus IgM antibody in the CSF of symptomatic patients.
- Treatment of West Nile virus infection is supportive.

Prion Diseases of the Central Nervous System

Introduction

Prions are novel pathogens composed of transmissible proteins that lack associated genetic material and cause five recognized clinical syndromes in humans (**Table 8**). Creutzfeldt-Jakob disease and variant Creutzfeldt-Jakob disease occur most often. Common features of all prion diseases include progressive neurologic impairment, the absence of inflammatory cerebrospinal fluid (CSF) findings, and the presence of spongiform changes on neuropathologic examination. There are currently no treatments available for these conditions, which are invariably fatal.

Creutzfeldt-Jakob Disease

Creutzfeldt-Jakob disease (CJD) is classified as sporadic (sCJD), familial (fCJD), iatrogenic (iCJD), and variant (vCJD). The most common form is sCJD (85% of cases), followed by fCJD (10% to 15% of cases); iCJD and vCJD each account for approximately 1% of cases.

sCJD typically affects older adults with onset between 50 and 70 years of age. Patients may present with psychiatric manifestations, cognitive decline, or motor dysfunction. Extrapyramidal signs are present in approximately 65% of patients. Myoclonus and rapidly progressive dementia are hallmarks of this disease (**Table 9**). The median survival after symptom onset is 5 months.

The diagnosis of sCJD is challenging because routine laboratory testing is unrevealing. The CSF is typically acellular, although the total protein level may be elevated. Detection of elevated levels of 14-3-3 protein, a specific neuronal protein, in the cerebrospinal fluid may be an indirect marker of sCJD, but

this test has low sensitivity and specificity and is only available through the National Prion Disease Pathology Surveillance Center (www.cjdsurveillance.com). The electroencephalogram may show a characteristic periodic sharp wave pattern in the later stages of disease. MRI is a useful diagnostic tool, with findings of areas of focal cortical hyperintensity on diffusion-weighted imaging or fluid-attenuated inversion recovery (FLAIR) sequences predictive of infection. Neural tissue evaluation demonstrating spongiform changes and histopathologic staining for prion protein (PrPsc) confirm the diagnosis, but results are rarely available pre-mortem.

In general, invasive neurosurgical procedures for patients with suspected prion disease are discouraged because of the potential for contamination of surgical instruments and exposure of health care workers to infectious tissues. If necessary, disposable instruments or those able to be specially sterilized

---

TABLE 9. World Health Organization Criteria for Probable Sporadic Creutzfeldt-Jakob Disease (All Four Criteria Must Be Met)

1. Progressive dementia

2. Clinical signs (requires at least two of the following with duration <2 years):
   a. Myoclonus
   b. Pyramidal or extrapyramidal dysfunction
   c. Visual or cerebellar disturbance
   d. Akinetic mutism

3. Laboratory or EEG findings (at least one of the following):
   a. Characteristic EEG findings (1- to 2-Hz periodic sharp waves)
   b. Cerebrospinal fluid positive for 14-3-3 protein

4. No alternative diagnosis identified by routine investigation

EEG = electroencephalogram.

TABLE 8. Classification of Prion Diseases

Disease	Epidemiology	Pathophysiology	Clinical Findings	Time to Death
Kuru	Papua New Guinea (Fore tribe)	Exposure to human brain tissue by cannibalism	Tremors, ataxia, movement disorders, dementia	<2 years
Gerstmann-Sträussler-Scheinker syndrome	Inherited, autosomal dominant	PRNP gene mutation	Progressive cerebellar degeneration with dementia	<5 years
Fatal familial insomnia	Inherited	PRNP gene mutation	Insomnia, myoclonus, autonomic dysfunction, endocrinopathy (dementia rare)	<1 year
Sporadic Creutzfeldt-Jakob disease	Mean age of onset, 65 years	Spontaneous mutation of host protein to form prion protein PrPsc	Rapidly progressive dementia, myoclonus, extrapyramidal signs	<6 months
Variant Creutzfeldt-Jakob disease	Most cases identified in the United Kingdom and Europe. Mean age of onset, 29 years	Dietary consumption of meat contaminated with brain tissue from animals with bovine spongiform encephalopathy	Paresthesias, psychiatric symptoms, delayed onset of dementia	~1 year

should be used; involvement by infection prevention practitioners is essential. Similarly, harvesting tissues from patients with suspected spongiform encephalopathy should be avoided.

Variant Creutzfeldt-Jakob Disease

In the late 1990s, a cluster of cases suggestive of sCJD was reported from the United Kingdom. In contrast to patients with sCJD, patients with this disorder were younger, had primarily psychiatric presentations, and had less rapid disease progression. These findings ultimately led to recognition of this outbreak as a unique prion disease, termed vCJD.

Neuropathologic findings unique to vCJD include heavy concentrations of amyloid plaque in the cerebrum and cerebellum that stain for a type of prion protein (PrPsc type 4 pattern) that is not found in other human prion diseases but is described in animals and animal products infected with bovine spongiform encephalopathy. Coupled with epidemiologic data, the consumption of animal protein, particularly beef, during a large-scale epidemic of bovine spongiform encephalopathy supports animal-to-human transmission.

The diagnosis is made by radiographic and neuropathologic examination. Characteristic findings on MRI (pulvinar sign) and identification of the PrPsc protein in tonsillar tissue facilitate pre-mortem diagnosis. Changes in animal feeding and butchering practices have led to sharp decreases in the incidence of vCJD.

KEY POINTS

- Common features of all prion diseases include progressive neurologic impairment, the absence of inflammatory cerebrospinal fluid findings, and the presence of spongiform changes on neuropathologic examination.

- Neural tissue evaluation demonstrating spongiform changes and histopathologic staining for prion protein (PrPsc) confirm the diagnosis of sporadic Creutzfeldt-Jakob disease, but results are rarely available pre-mortem, and invasive neurosurgical procedures pose a risk of secondary transmission.

- Patients with variant Creutzfeldt-Jakob disease have prion protein (PrPsc) that can be identified in tonsillar tissue, allowing pre-mortem confirmatory pathologic diagnosis.

Skin and Soft Tissue Infections

Introduction

The most common microorganisms causing skin infection are streptococci, particularly group A β-hemolytic streptococci (GABHS), and *Staphylococcus aureus*. The presence of lymphangitis and a "peau d'orange" appearance of the skin are more consistent with streptococcal infection, whereas an abscess or drainage from an existing wound or site of previous penetrating trauma suggests *S. aureus* as the likely pathogen.

Erysipelas is a superficial infection involving the upper dermis and is primarily due to infection with GABHS. Tender, warm, intensely erythematous plaques with well-demarcated, indurated borders and associated edema are characteristic findings. Fever is often present. Although erysipelas usually involves the lower extremities, the upper extremities and face also may be affected.

Cellulitis involves the deep dermis and subcutaneous fat tissue. In contrast to erysipelas, cellulitis is characterized by spreading erythema that is not well demarcated (**Figure 3**). As in erysipelas, edema, redness, warmth, fever, and leukocytosis often occur. If furuncles, carbuncles, or abscesses are present, cellulitis is usually due to *S. aureus*. **Table 10** provides additional cellulitis risk factors with microbiologic associations that should be considered in the appropriate clinical situation.

The diagnosis of skin infections is often based on clinical findings because a microbial diagnosis is established in only a few patients. Blood culture results are positive in only about 5% of patients and appear most helpful in those who appear toxic or are immunocompromised. Because of low yield and questionable accuracy, cultures obtained by punch biopsy or needle aspiration of a lesion are not routinely performed. Most cases of diffuse, nontraumatic cellulitis with nondiagnostic culture results are due to β-hemolytic streptococci and typically respond to β-lactam antibiotics. Purulent cellulitis is more suggestive of staphylococcal disease and should be treated empirically with effective therapy against methicillin-resistant *S. aureus* (MRSA) infection. Recommended empiric antimicrobial agents for outpatients with a community-associated (CA)-MRSA skin or soft tissue infection include trimethoprim-sulfamethoxazole, a tetracycline (for example, doxycycline), clindamycin, and linezolid. **H**

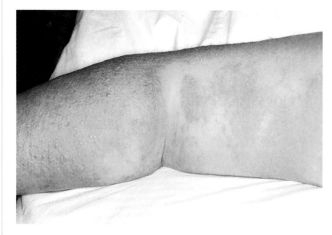

FIGURE 3. Spreading, undemarcated erythema of cellulitis; purulent drainage or exudate may also be present.

TABLE 10. Cellulitis Pathogens Associated with Specific Behaviors/Risk Factors

Pathogen	Risk Factor	Comment
Aeromonas hydrophila	Contact with or participation in recreational sports in freshwater lakes, streams, rivers (including brackish water); contact with leeches	Cellulitis nonspecific in clinical appearance; minor trauma to skin usually leads to inoculation of organism
Vibrio vulnificus, other *Vibrio* species	Contact with salt water or brackish water; contact with drippings from raw seafood	May cause cellulitis through direct inoculation into skin or may be ingested, leading to bacteremia with secondary skin infection. Hallmark is hemorrhagic bullae in area of cellulitis lesion(s)
Erysipelothrix rhusiopathiae	Contact with saltwater marine life (can also infect freshwater fish)	Cellulitis usually involves the hand or arm, and occurs in those handling fish, shellfish, or occasionally, poultry or meat contaminated with bacterium. Causes erysipeloid disease
Pasteurella multocida	Contact primarily with cats	Cellulitis occurs as a result of cat scratch or bite
Capnocytophaga canimorsus	Contact primarily with dogs	Cellulitis and sepsis particularly in patients with hyposplenism
Bacillus anthracis	Target of bioterrorism	Edematous pruritic lesion with central eschar; spore-forming organism
Francisella tularensis	Contact with or bite from infected animal (particularly cats); arthropod bites (particularly ticks)	Ulceroglandular syndrome characterized by ulcerative lesion with central eschar and localized tender lymphadenopathy; constitutional symptoms often present
Mycobacterium marinum	Contact with fresh water or salt water, including fish tanks and swimming pools	Lesion often trauma-associated and often involving upper extremity; papular lesions become ulcerative at site of inoculation; ascending lymphatic spread can be seen ("sporotrichoid" appearance); systemic toxicity usually absent

KEY POINTS

- The presence of lymphangitis and a "peau d'orange" appearance of the skin are more consistent with streptococcal infection, whereas an abscess or drainage from an existing wound or site of previous penetrating trauma is more suggestive of staphylococcal infection.

- The diagnosis of skin infections is often clinical because a microbial diagnosis is established in only a few patients.

Community-Associated Methicillin-Resistant *Staphylococcus aureus*

CA-MRSA is a significant public health problem. Most CA-MRSA isolates contain genes encoding for multiple toxins, including cytotoxins that result in leukocyte destruction and tissue necrosis. CA-MRSA most often causes purulent skin and soft tissue infections (SSTI) and, less commonly, pneumonia. Healthy young persons tend to be infected, and outbreaks occur in athletes, prison inmates, men who have sex with men, children in day care centers, injection drug users, homeless persons, and military personnel, particularly when close contact or crowded conditions exist. CA-MRSA is now the most common identifiable cause of SSTI in patients seen in the emergency department. These genetically distinct CA-MRSA strains are also replacing MRSA strains as causes of infection in hospitals and other health care settings. The emergence of CA-MRSA has affected empiric treatment of SSTI because these new strains have distinct antibiotic susceptibility patterns.

Clinical practice guidelines by the Infectious Diseases Society of America have been published for the management of SSTI in the era of CA-MRSA. Incision and drainage is the primary therapy for a cutaneous abscess. Antibiotic treatment is also recommended when (1) patients are very young or elderly; (2) multiple sites of infection, systemic illness, comorbidities, or immunosuppression is present; (3) infection quickly progresses and is associated with concomitant cellulitis; (4) there is poor response to incision and drainage; or (5) abscesses are in locations where they are difficult to drain, such as the face, genitalia, or hand. Empiric therapy for CA-MRSA is indicated for patients with purulent cellulitis.

Oral antibiotic agents for outpatient treatment of CA-MRSA include clindamycin, trimethoprim-sulfamethoxazole, tetracyclines, and linezolid. However, clindamycin resistance among patients with CA-MRSA should be monitored locally, and some experts recommend avoiding empiric therapy with clindamycin when local resistance rates exceed 10% to 15%. In addition, results of susceptibility testing for clindamycin may be misleading, with treatment failures reported in patients in whom the isolate was shown to be susceptible to clindamycin but resistant to erythromycin. Fluoroquinolones are not recommended because of the concern for development of MRSA resistance during treatment as well as the increased prevalence of resistance already observed in many areas. Only linezolid and clindamycin also provide reliable coverage for β-hemolytic streptococci. When patients require hospitalization for a complicated SSTI, such as deep infection, infected burns and ulcers, and surgical wound infections, surgical debridement and broad-spectrum antibiotics, including those with coverage for MRSA, should be considered. Appropriate antibiotics for empiric MRSA coverage in this setting include vancomycin, daptomycin, telavancin, ceftaroline, and linezolid. **H**

KEY POINTS

- Community-associated methicillin-resistant *Staphylococcus aureus* most often causes purulent skin and soft tissue infection and, less commonly, pneumonia.
- The emergence of community-associated methicillin-resistant *Staphylococcus aureus* has affected empiric treatment of skin and soft tissue infections because these new strains have distinct antibiotic susceptibility patterns.
- Incision and drainage is the primary therapy for a cutaneous abscess in patients with community-associated methicillin-resistant *Staphylococcus aureus* infection, and possibly, depending on the extent and severity of infection, antibiotic treatment.

Necrotizing Fasciitis

Necrotizing fasciitis is an SSTI that extends beyond the epidermis, dermis, and subcutaneous fat tissues to involve the fascia and, potentially, the underlying muscle. This life-threatening infection is often classified according to its associated microbiologic findings. Type I necrotizing fasciitis is a polymicrobial infection usually encompassing a combination of streptococci, staphylococci, aerobic gram-negative bacilli, and anaerobes such as *Clostridium*, *Bacteroides*, and *Peptostreptococcus* species. One example of type I necrotizing fasciitis is perineal fasciitis, also known as Fournier gangrene. Type II necrotizing fasciitis is a monomicrobial infection typically caused by *Streptococcus pyogenes* ("flesh-eating bacteria"). Other bacteria that can cause a similar infection are *Vibrio vulnificus*, *S. aureus*, and *Streptococcus agalactiae*. *V. vulnificus* is a curved gram-negative rod found in warm coastal waters such as the Gulf of Mexico. Patients who are immunocompromised, especially those with iron overload syndromes such as cirrhosis, are at increased risk for developing necrotizing fasciitis secondary to *V. vulnificus* after ingestion of raw or undercooked shellfish or after traumatized skin is exposed to contaminated sea water (**Figure 4**). Clostridial myonecrosis, or gas gangrene, is a similarly presenting necrotizing infection that is differentiated by muscle involvement. This infection is usually associated with trauma, recent surgery, or injection drug use and is caused primarily by *Clostridium perfringens*, although other *Clostridium* species have been reported.

Necrotizing fasciitis is often associated with a preexisting skin infection or trauma, including chronic vascular or pressure ulcers (for example, diabetic foot ulcers) and surgical wounds. However, an obvious portal of entry may not be evident. Necrotizing fasciitis usually involves the lower extremities, followed by the upper extremities, but any site can be affected (**Figure 5**).

Cutaneous manifestations may initially include erythematous lesions associated with significant pain and edema. The severity of pain is often disproportionate to the visible skin findings. The lesions may rapidly increase in size and develop a violaceous, bullous, and gangrenous appearance. Palpation of affected areas may demonstrate "woody" induration and crepitus as a result of soft tissue–associated gas. Patients may be toxic, with fever, hypotension, mental status changes, tachycardia, leukocytosis, and laboratory evidence of multi-organ dysfunction. Streptococcal-associated necrotizing fasciitis is associated with toxic shock syndrome in up to 50% of patients. Anesthesia may develop in the affected area as a result of localized nerve necrosis.

Clinical suspicion of necrotizing fasciitis is important in directing early evaluation, including surgical consultation. Evidence of systemic inflammation, including elevations of the total leukocyte count, erythrocyte sedimentation rate, and serum C-reactive protein level, is often present, and the serum creatine kinase level may also be increased. MRI of the

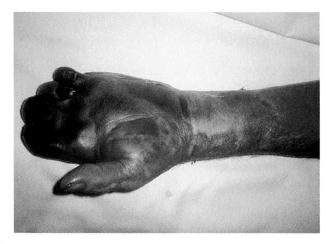

FIGURE 4. Necrotizing fasciitis secondary to *Vibrio vulnificus*, manifested as hemorrhagic bullous lesions.

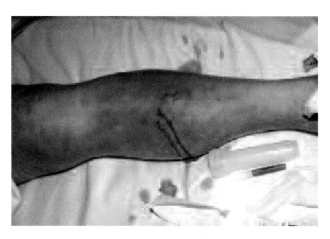

FIGURE 5. Necrotizing fasciitis of the left calf of an elderly patient with peripheral arterial disease.

affected area can localize and determine the extent of fascial plane involvement. Blood cultures and staining of wound-associated tissue may be helpful.

Because mortality rates range from 30% to 70% and are increased when surgery is delayed, timely surgical exploration is essential to determine the extent of necrosis and debride all necrotic tissue; sometimes, surgery is pursued when the diagnosis is uncertain. Cultures of infected tissue should be obtained during surgical intervention. Repeat surgical evaluation is pursued in most patients 24 to 36 hours later and continued daily as indicated.

In addition to supportive care and surgery, empiric broad-spectrum antibiotics are appropriate for patients with suspected necrotizing fasciitis. Initial therapy should include coverage for *S. aureus* (including MRSA), streptococci, gram-negative bacilli, and anaerobes. Regimens consisting of an anti-MRSA agent such as vancomycin or daptomycin or linezolid plus (1) piperacillin-tazobactam, (2) cefepime and metronidazole, or (3) a carbapenem (for example, meropenem or imipenem) are reasonable. Clindamycin should be part of the initial regimen when infection due to GABHS or clostridia is suspected. When type II necrotizing fasciitis secondary to GABHS or clostridial myonecrosis is present, combined therapy with both penicillin and clindamycin is indicated. Clindamycin may be beneficial in early treatment because of its ability to suppress toxin production, although 5% or more of streptococci and staphylococci may be resistant to this drug. Antibiotics can be discontinued once surgical debridement is no longer needed and clinical improvement is evident.

Studies regarding use of intravenous immune globulin (IVIG) to treat streptococcal necrotizing fasciitis are conflicting. To date, there are no definitive recommendations for use of IVIG in patients with necrotizing fasciitis, although some experts recommend its use in patients with associated toxic shock or a high risk of death. **H**

KEY POINTS

- Cutaneous manifestations of necrotizing fasciitis often initially include erythematous lesions associated with significant pain and edema.
- Timely surgical exploration is essential in patients with necrotizing fasciitis to determine the extent of necrosis and debride all necrotic tissue.
- Empiric broad-spectrum antibiotics are appropriate for patients with suspected necrotizing fasciitis.

Toxic Shock Syndrome

Toxic shock syndrome (TSS) is an uncommon, and potentially fatal, infection caused by toxin-producing staphylococci and streptococci. Menstruation-associated staphylococcal TSS was described in the 1980s in women who used tampons. Nonmenstruation-associated staphylococcal TSS occurs in patients with surgical and obstetrical wound infections, sinus infection with nasal packings, osteomyelitis, skin ulcers, burns, and pneumonia and in injection drug users. Clinical features may include chills, malaise, fever, hypotension, erythematous rash, and multi-organ involvement (**Table 11**). Patients may have no localizing signs of infection when systemic toxicity develops.

TABLE 11. Diagnostic Criteria for Staphylococcal Toxic Shock Syndrome

The presence of:

Fever >38.9 °C (102.0 °F)

Systolic blood pressure less than 90 mm Hg

Diffuse macular rash with subsequent desquamation, especially on palms and soles

Involvement of three of the following organ systems:

Gastrointestinal (nausea, vomiting, diarrhea)

Muscular (severe myalgia or fivefold or greater increase in serum creatine kinase level)

Mucous membrane (hyperemia of the vagina, conjunctivae, or pharynx)

Kidney (blood urea nitrogen or serum creatinine level at least twice the upper limit of normal)

Liver (bilirubin, aspartate aminotransferase or alanine aminotransferase concentration twice the upper limit of normal)

Blood (platelet count <100,000/µL [100 × 10⁹/L])

Central nervous system (disorientation without focal neurologic signs)

Negative serologies for Rocky Mountain spotted fever, leptospirosis, and measles; negative cerebrospinal fluid cultures for organisms other than *Staphylococcus aureus*

µL = microliter.

Adapted with permission from Moreillon P, Aue Y-A, Glauser MP. *Staphylococcus aureus*. In: Mandell GL, Dolin R, Bennett JE, eds. Principles and Practice of Infectious Disease. 6th ed. Philadelphia, PA: Churchill Livingstone; 2005:2331. Copyright 2005, Elsevier.

Streptococcal TSS can occur secondary to infection with any β-hemolytic streptococcus, although *S. pyogenes* is most common. Most cases occur in the setting of SSTIs, although streptococci may also gain entry through mucous membranes such as in pharyngitis. Surgical procedures, blunt trauma with hematoma and ecchymoses, influenza and varicella infections, and NSAID use have also been associated with this syndrome. A portal of entry may not be evident in about 50% of patients. The diagnostic criteria for streptococcal TSS are found in **Table 12**. Bacteremia is more common and mortality rates are higher in patients with streptococcal TSS than in those with staphylococcal TSS.

Patients with TSS require early supportive therapy and treatment of any underlying infection. Site management may include debridement and removal of foreign bodies. Empiric broad-spectrum antibiotics similar to those given for necrotizing fasciitis should be administered until the pathogen or pathogens are identified. Once culture results are known, antibiotic coverage can be targeted. Because of its ability to inhibit toxin production and modulate production of tumor necrosis factor, clindamycin is also included when either staphylococcal or streptococcal involvement is suspected. IVIG is sometimes recommended for treatment of streptococcal TSS based on observational data that showed better survival in patients treated with IVIG. Hyperbaric oxygen may also be helpful as adjunctive therapy, but more studies are needed before its standard use is recommended.

Secondary transmission of GABHS-induced TSS to close contacts of patients has been reported. Contact isolation precautions should be initiated for patients with suspected or known invasive GABHS-induced disease, including TSS and necrotizing fasciitis, until 24 hours of antibiotic therapy has been completed. Although not routinely recommended, postexposure penicillin-based prophylaxis may be considered for household contacts of patients with invasive GABHS

infection, including those who are older than 65 years of age or have conditions associated with an increased risk of developing invasive infection (for example, diabetes mellitus, cardiac disease, varicella infection, cancer, HIV infection, corticosteroid use, or injection drug use). **H**

KEY POINT

- Patients with toxic shock syndrome require early supportive care, treatment of any underlying infection, possible debridement and removal of foreign bodies, and administration of empiric broad-spectrum antibiotics until microbial identification is made.

Animal Bites

Animal bites are responsible for 1% of all visits to the emergency department in the United States. Approximately 5% to 20% of these bites are infected. Complications include formation of abscesses, soft tissue infection, tenosynovitis, septic arthritis, osteomyelitis, and bacteremia. The animal involved and the location of the bite are important. Dog bites are less likely to become infected than cat bites. Infections after a bite are due to oral flora of the animal and microorganisms present on the skin of the patient. Infections after dog and cat bites are usually due to a mix of aerobic and anaerobic microorganisms. Staphylococci and streptococci are reported in approximately 40% of bite wounds, and anaerobes commonly found in the oral flora of both cats and dogs, including *Bacteroides*, *Porphyromonas*, and *Prevotella* species, are reported in these infections. *Pasteurella* species, particularly *P. multocida*, are gram-negative coccobacilli that are frequently isolated from wounds after cat and dog bites, scratches, or licks. *Capnocytophaga canimorsus* is a gram-negative rod that can cause overwhelming sepsis, most often in patients with asplenia, following a dog or cat bite or scratch.

A thorough history of both the patient and the animal is needed in the evaluation of patients with animal bites. The type of animal involved, the circumstances under which the attack occurred, the timing of the bite, and the health status of the animal are important. The patient's immune status, including tetanus and rabies immunization history, use of immunosuppressive medications, and presence of any immunocompromising disorders, should be determined. Physical examination should identify the location and extent of injury; evidence of necrosis or crush injury; presence of edema, erythema, or purulent discharge; nerve involvement; and range of motion and function. Adequate wound irrigation and debridement are required, and the need for additional tetanus and rabies prophylaxis is determined. Radiographic evaluation is obtained when bone involvement is possible, crepitus is present, or foreign bodies are suspected.

TABLE 12. Diagnostic Criteria for Streptococcal Toxic Shock Syndrome
Definite Case:
Isolation of GABHS from a sterile site
Probable Case:
Isolation of GABHS from a nonsterile site
Hypotension
The presence of two of the following findings:
Kidney (acute kidney insufficiency or failure)
Liver (elevated aminotransferase concentrations)
Skin (erythematous macular rash, soft tissue necrosis)
Blood (coagulopathy, including thrombocytopenia and disseminated intravascular coagulation)
Pulmonary (acute respiratory distress syndrome)
GABHS = group A β-hemolytic streptococci.

Antibiotic prophylaxis should be considered for any immunocompromised patient and for patients who have wounds on the hands or near a joint or bone, moderate or severe wounds at any site, significant crush injuries, or wounds with associated edema. A 3- to 5-day course of amoxicillin-clavulanate is recommended. Patients with a β-lactam allergy may be given a fluoroquinolone or doxycycline or trimethoprim-sulfamethoxazole plus an anti-anaerobic agent such as clindamycin.

Antibiotics are given when wounds are infected. Patients not requiring hospitalization can be treated with the same oral agents used for prophylaxis. Hospitalization is needed for patients with severe or deep infections; nerve, tendon, or crush injuries; or infected hand bites. Intravenous antibiotic regimens may include β-lactam/β-lactamase combinations, cefoxitin, or carbapenems. Patients who are allergic to penicillin can be treated with a fluoroquinolone plus clindamycin. The addition of agents such as vancomycin can be considered in patients with suspected infection caused by MRSA. Therapy is usually required for less than 2 weeks, although longer courses of 3 to 4 weeks for joint infection and at least 4 to 6 weeks for bone infection are appropriate.

Cat-scratch disease is an infection that most often occurs in immunocompetent children and young adults following inoculation of the fastidious gram-negative bacterium *Bartonella henselae* after a cat scratch or bite. A pustule or papule or erythema develops at the site of inoculation several days to 2 weeks after the scratch or bite. Significant tender regional lymphadenopathy, occasionally suppurative, develops 2 to 3 weeks after inoculation in areas that drain the infected site. The lymphadenopathy generally resolves within months, and extranodal disease is rare. The diagnosis is often made clinically, although a laboratory diagnosis is possible through culture, serology, histopathology, or nucleic acid–based testing. Although cat-scratch disease is generally a self-limited infection when antibiotics are not given, some experts recommend a short course of antibiotic therapy, usually with azithromycin.

KEY POINTS

- Dog bites are less likely to become infected than cat bites.
- Following a dog or cat bite, adequate wound irrigation and debridement are required, and the need for tetanus and rabies prophylaxis is determined.
- Antibiotic prophylaxis following a dog or cat bite should be considered for any immunocompromised patient and for patients who have wounds on the hands or near a joint or bone, moderate or severe wounds at any site, significant crush injuries, or wounds with associated edema.
- Antibiotics should be given to all patients with an infected dog or cat bite.

Human Bites

Human bite wounds are categorized as self-inflicted, occlusional, or clenched-fist injuries. Self-inflicted wounds such as paronychia are incidental and result from thumb sucking or nail biting. Occlusional bite wounds result from intentional bites, usually in the setting of a confrontation, and often involve the fingers (in particular the index or middle finger), hand, and other upper extremity locations. Clenched-fist injuries result from a punch to the mouth of another person and commonly cause a traumatic laceration of the third, fourth, or fifth metacarpal head.

Infection caused by human oral flora is typically polymicrobial, including α-hemolytic streptococci, staphylococci, *Haemophilus* species, and *Eikenella corrodens,* as well as anaerobes, many of which produce β-lactamases.

Initial evaluation and management are similar to that for animal bites and should also include evaluation for potentially transmissible pathogens, including those causing HIV infection, herpes simplex virus infection, syphilis, and hepatitis B and C virus infection. Patients who have human bite wounds without evidence of infection should receive prophylactic amoxicillin-clavulanate for 3 to 5 days. Patients with clenched-fist injuries require particular attention because such injuries are prone to deeper infection involving the tendons, joints, and bone. In these patients, radiographic evaluation, consultation with a hand surgeon to determine the need for exploration of the wound, and possibly, hospitalization, are indicated. Broad-spectrum antibiotics with anaerobic coverage such as β-lactam/β-lactamase inhibitors, cefoxitin, or carbapenems can be administered empirically. Vancomycin can be considered for patients with risk factors for MRSA infection.

KEY POINTS

- Patients who have human bite wounds without evidence of infection should receive prophylactic amoxicillin-clavulanate for 3 to 5 days.
- Patients with clenched-fist injuries usually require radiographic evaluation, consultation with a hand surgeon, and possibly, hospitalization.

Diabetic Foot Infections

Foot infections are common in patients with diabetes mellitus because of the neuropathy, vascular insufficiency, and immunodeficiency associated with this disease. Most infections begin after trauma and are categorized as mild, moderate, or severe.

Mild infections are most often caused by staphylococci and streptococci.

Findings include purulence or inflammation (pain, tenderness, warmth, erythema, and induration) and cellulitis that extends no deeper than the superficial soft tissue and spreads 2 cm or less around the ulcer. Systemic findings are absent.

Patients with moderate infections have cellulitis that extends beyond 2 cm around the ulcer, gangrene, lymphangitic spread, deep tissue abscess, or deep tissue spread, including extension to the muscle, joint, tendon, or bone. Systemic findings are absent. Severe infections are limb-threatening and are associated with metabolic instability or systemic toxicity, such as fever, tachycardia, hypotension, kidney insufficiency, mental status changes, and leukocytosis. These more extensive infections are usually polymicrobial, including staphylococci, streptococci, enteric gram-negative bacilli, *Pseudomonas aeruginosa*, and anaerobes.

Ulcers that are clinically uninfected (that is, without purulence or inflammation) should not be treated with antibiotics. In the absence of recent antibiotic use, most patients with mild and many with moderate diabetic foot infections can receive empiric treatment with a short course of oral antibiotics directed against aerobic gram-positive staphylococci and streptococci, similar to skin infections in nondiabetic individuals. Severe limb-threatening infections require surgical evaluation and initial broad-spectrum antibiotic coverage commensurate with the severity of the systemic findings. Definitive antibiotic treatment should be adjusted based on results of cultures obtained from deeper tissue during surgical debridement or by aspiration. Superficial swab cultures are misleading and should be avoided.

Two common problems are usually encountered in patients with significant diabetic foot infections: (1) arterial insufficiency from macrovascular complications of diabetes, and (2) osteomyelitis. An assessment for possible arterial insufficiency (see MKSAP 16 Cardiovascular Medicine) should be undertaken. Evaluation for potential bone infection is more challenging, because bone changes related to neuropathy and Charcot changes (bony abnormalities due to repeated trauma) can mimic osteomyelitis. The role of MRI to identify occult osteomyelitis has not been fully resolved, but the presence of bone infection usually becomes apparent over time, as wound healing is poor or drainage recurs after ulcer closure. Wound care consisting of wound cleansing, debridement, and off-loading of local foot pressure is essential for optimal healing of all diabetic foot wounds and is often best managed with close involvement of podiatrists and wound care specialists. **H**

KEY POINTS

- Diabetic foot ulcers that are clinically uninfected should not be treated with antibiotics.

- Mild and many moderate diabetic foot infections can be treated with a short course of oral antibiotics directed against aerobic gram-positive staphylococci and streptococci.

- Severe diabetic foot infections are limb-threatening and require surgical evaluation and initial broad-spectrum antibiotic coverage commensurate with the severity of the systemic findings.

Community-Acquired Pneumonia

Epidemiology

Community-acquired pneumonia (CAP) is defined as an acute pneumonia occurring in persons who have not been hospitalized recently and are not living in facilities such as nursing homes. Underlying disease such as chronic bronchitis and COPD, cardiovascular disease, and diabetes mellitus increases the risk of CAP. Smokers are at increased risk for invasive pneumococcal infections even if they do not have structural lung disease. Other risk factors include alcoholism and the presence of neurologic diseases that increase the risk of aspiration. With few exceptions (for example, *Legionella* pneumonia due to inhalation of contaminated aerosolized water), CAP is caused by microaspiration of organisms that may colonize the oropharynx, which often occurs during sleep. In contrast, aspiration pneumonia refers to pneumonia that occurs following a large-volume aspiration of gastric contents, which results in a chemical pneumonitis followed by a bacterial infection.

CAP occurs most commonly in elderly patients; 60% of all hospitalizations for pneumonia occur in patients over 65 years of age. Additional risk factors in this age group include cardiopulmonary disease, poor functional status, low weight, and recent weight loss. Pneumonia is the eighth leading cause of death in the United States and the most common cause of death from an infectious disease. The mortality rate for outpatients with CAP is less than 5%; the mortality rate for inpatients is 10% but can be as high as 30% for patients who are admitted to the intensive care unit (ICU).

The cost of caring for patients with CAP is estimated to exceed 17 billion dollars annually. Various aspects of caring for hospitalized patients are considered quality indicators, and hospital performance influences reimbursement to health care institutions by Medicare and other third-party payers. Guidelines are available to direct antibiotic selection in patients with CAP and are discussed later. Numerous studies have shown that use of guideline-concordant antibiotics is associated with decreased mortality rates in hospitalized patients. A marked reduction in 30-day mortality rates in elderly patients with CAP from 1987 to 2005 has recently been reported. Greater use of pneumococcal and influenza vaccination and use of guideline-concordant antibiotics are hypothesized as possible explanations for this reduction, although it has never been shown that pneumococcal vaccination reduces mortality from pneumonia in this population.

KEY POINT

- Community-acquired pneumonia occurs most often in elderly patients; 60% of all hospitalizations for pneumonia are in patients over 65 years of age.

Microbiology

Streptococcus pneumoniae is the most commonly documented pathogen in patients with CAP and the most frequent cause of bacteremic pneumonia acquired in the community. *Haemophilus influenzae* and *Moraxella catarrhalis* are also common pathogens. Other gram-negative organisms are responsible for a small proportion of cases of CAP. Enteric gram-negative bacilli can cause CAP in patients with chronic medical comorbidities, chronic liver disease, and alcoholism. *Klebsiella pneumoniae* is reported in patients with alcoholism. *Pseudomonas aeruginosa* is a potential cause of CAP in patients with chronic underlying structural lung disease (such as bronchiectasis or cystic fibrosis), frequent exacerbations of severe COPD, and a history of long-term corticosteroid therapy, but many such patients have risk factors for health care–associated pneumonia. *Staphylococcus aureus*, including community-associated methicillin-resistant *S. aureus* infection (CA-MRSA), is a less common potential cause of CAP. *S. aureus* should be considered when CAP occurs following influenza, in patients with cavitary pneumonia in whom there are no risk factors for aspiration, in injection drug users, and in patients with a recent history of a CA-MRSA skin and soft tissue infection.

Regardless of antimicrobial susceptibility, CAP due to *S. aureus* is associated with a higher mortality rate and more prolonged length of stay compared with CAP from other causes. *Mycoplasma pneumoniae* and *Chlamydophila pneumoniae* infection are more likely to occur in outpatients with CAP. *Legionella* infection must be considered, especially in cases of severe CAP and in patients with a recent history of travel. *Legionella* infections are more common in the summer and sometimes occur in epidemics when a common-source reservoir aerosolizes bacteria that are inhaled by susceptible patients. Respiratory viruses, including influenza, parainfluenza, respiratory syncytial virus, and adenovirus, may cause CAP. Outbreaks of severe CAP due to adenovirus type 14 have recently been described. Epidemiologic history that should prompt consideration of less common pathogens is outlined in **Table 13**. 🄷

KEY POINTS

- *Streptococcus pneumoniae* is the most frequently documented pathogen in patients with community-acquired pneumonia; *Haemophilus influenzae* and *Moraxella catarrhalis* are also common.
- Community-acquired pneumonia due to *Staphylococcus aureus* is associated with higher mortality rates and more prolonged hospitalizations compared with community-acquired pneumonia due to other pathogens.

Diagnosis

The acute onset of cough (especially with purulent sputum production), fever, chills, pleuritic chest pain, and dyspnea is characteristic of pneumonia. The presentation may be much more nonspecific in elderly patients, who may present with confusion or an exacerbation of an underlying chronic cardiopulmonary disease. Tachypnea is the most sensitive finding suggesting pneumonia in this age group.

When obtaining a history in patients with suspected CAP, risk factors for health care–associated pneumonia, such as antibiotic therapy or hospitalization in the preceding 90 days, must be excluded. Any epidemiologic exposures that might suggest the possibility of unusual pathogens must also be determined.

Clinical findings alone are not sufficient to confirm a diagnosis of pneumonia; a chest radiograph should be obtained in all patients. In patients who have a clinical presentation compatible with pneumonia and focal auscultatory findings on chest examination, an initial normal chest radiograph, although uncommon, should not exclude the diagnosis of CAP. A repeat chest radiograph in 24 to 48 hours may show airspace disease.

The role of routine diagnostic testing to determine the 🄷 microbial cause of CAP is controversial. The Infectious Diseases Society of America/American Thoracic Society (IDSA/ATS) Consensus Guidelines suggest that microbiologic diagnostic testing is optional in outpatients. In patients who are hospitalized but not in the ICU, diagnostic testing is recommended for those in whom outpatient antibiotic therapy was ineffective and for those with cavitary infiltrates, alcoholism, chronic liver disease, functional or anatomic asplenia, severe obstructive or structural lung disease, or leukopenia. The *Legionella* urine antigen test should also be performed in patients with a recent travel history. Diagnostic testing is considered optional in other hospitalized patients.

There is strong consensus that patients with CAP who require ICU admission should have blood cultures, sputum Gram stain and culture (or culture of an endotracheal aspirate in intubated patients), and pneumococcal and *Legionella* urine antigen testing. The sensitivity of the pneumococcal urine antigen test is 70%, with a specificity as high as 96%, and the test has a rapid turnaround time. Although the *Legionella* urine antigen test detects only *L. pneumophila* serogroup 1, this strain is responsible for 85% or more of cases of legionellosis. Reported sensitivity of this test varies from 70% to 90%, with a specificity of 99%.

Blood culture results are positive in 5% to 14% of hospitalized patients with CAP. Obtaining blood culture samples before antibiotic therapy is begun is one of the Medicare quality of care indicators for CAP. Data indicate that obtaining blood cultures is associated with lower mortality rates in patients older than 65 years of age. Patients with a large pleural effusion on presentation (typically defined as an effusion occupying half or more of the hemithorax on an upright chest radiograph or a fluid level of more than 1 cm on lateral decubitus films) should undergo thoracentesis; in addition, these patients should have blood and sputum cultures and pneumococcal and *Legionella* urine antigen tests. Studies to date have not demonstrated a significant

TABLE 13. Possible Microbial Causes of Community-Acquired Pneumonia

Clinical Presentation	Commonly Encountered Pathogens
Aspiration	Gram-negative enteric pathogens, oral anaerobes
Cough >2 weeks with whoop or posttussive vomiting	*Bordetella pertussis*
Lung cavity infiltrates	Community-associated methicillin-resistant *Staphylococcus aureus*, oral anaerobes, endemic fungal pathogens, *Mycobacterium tuberculosis*, atypical mycobacteria

Epidemiology or Risk Factor	Commonly Encountered Pathogens
Alcoholism	*Streptococcus pneumoniae*, oral anaerobes, *Klebsiella pneumoniae*, *Acinetobacter* species, *M. tuberculosis*
COPD and/or smoking	*Haemophilus influenzae, Pseudomonas aeruginosa, Legionella* species, *S. pneumoniae, Moraxella catarrhalis, Chlamydophila pneumoniae*
Exposure to bat or bird droppings	*Histoplasma capsulatum*
Exposure to birds	*Chlamydophila psittaci*
Exposure to rabbits	*Francisella tularensis*
Exposure to farm animals or parturient cats	*Coxiella burnetii*
Exposure to rodent excreta	Hantavirus
HIV infection (early)	*S. pneumoniae, H. influenzae, M. tuberculosis*
HIV infection (late)	Those with early HIV infection plus *Pneumocystis jirovecii, Cryptococcus, Histoplasma, Aspergillus*, atypical mycobacteria (especially *Mycobacterium kansasii*), *P. aeruginosa*
Hotel or cruise ship stay in previous 2 weeks	*Legionella* species
Travel or residence in southwestern United States	*Coccidioides* species, hantavirus
Travel or residence in Southeast and East Asia	*Burkholderia pseudomallei*
Influenza activity in community	Influenza, *S. pneumoniae, Staphylococcus aureus, H. influenzae*
Injection drug use	*S. aureus*, anaerobes, *M. tuberculosis, S. pneumoniae*
Endobronchial obstruction	Anaerobes, *S. pneumoniae, H. influenzae, S. aureus*
Bronchiectasis or cystic fibrosis	*Burkholderia cepacia, P. aeruginosa, S. aureus*
Bioterrorism	*Bacillus anthracis, Yersinia pestis, Francisella tularensis*

Adapted with permission from Mandell LA, Wunderink RG, Anzueto A, et al; Infectious Diseases Society of America; American Thoracic Society. Infectious Diseases Society of America/American Thoracic Society consensus guidelines on the management of community-acquired pneumonia in adults. Clin Infect Dis. 2007;44 Suppl 2:S27-72. [PMID: 17278083] Copyright 2007, Oxford University Press.

CONT. difference between empiric therapy and pathogen-directed therapy, except among patients in the ICU. Pathogen-directed therapy, however, does allow for focusing and reducing antibiotic coverage, which may be associated with fewer adverse effects. Confirming an etiologic diagnosis may be especially helpful when patients fail to respond to antibiotic therapy.

The role of inflammatory biomarkers such as procalcitonin in the diagnosis and management of pneumonia remains investigational. **H**

KEY POINTS

- The acute onset of cough (especially with purulent sputum production), fever, chills, pleuritic chest pain, and dyspnea is characteristic of community-acquired pneumonia.
- The presence of tachypnea is the most sensitive finding suggesting pneumonia in elderly patients.

- Blood cultures, sputum Gram stain and culture, and pneumococcal and *Legionella* urine antigen testing are indicated for patients with community-acquired pneumonia who require admission to an intensive care unit.

Management
Site of Care

Deciding whether to hospitalize a patient for treatment of CAP has a major impact on the cost of care, because the greatest expenditure for treating CAP occurs among hospitalized patients. Studies have shown that most patients with CAP prefer outpatient treatment, if possible.

Several scoring systems are available to help determine mortality risk to guide decisions regarding the need for hospitalization. The CURB-65 score uses five indicators of severity of illness (confusion, blood urea nitrogen level >20 mg/dL (7.14 mmol/L), respiration rate ≥30/min, systolic blood pressure <90 mm Hg or diastolic blood pressure <60 mm Hg, and age ≥65 years). One point is scored for each positive indicator. Patients with a score of 0 or 1 have a low mortality risk and can be considered for outpatient treatment. Those with a score of 2 or more should be hospitalized. Patients with a score of 3 or more should be considered for admission to the ICU. The Pneumonia Severity Index (PSI) assigns patients to one of five mortality risk groups. Patients in PSI risk groups I and II are generally treated as outpatients. Those in risk group III may require brief hospitalization for observation, whereas those in risk groups IV and V generally require hospital admission. The calculation of the PSI score includes 20 different variables and therefore requires access to a decision support tool (http://pda.ahrq.gov/clinic/psi/psicalc.asp).

Studies have shown that both scoring systems perform well in terms of predicting mortality. For predicting the risk of mortality, recent investigation suggests that the negative predictive value of these scoring systems is greater than the positive predictive value. Both the PSI and the CURB-65 scores have been shown to predict the time to clinical stability in hospitalized patients with CAP.

Prediction rules are only one part of clinical decision-making concerning when and whether to hospitalize patients with pneumonia. Some patients with a low mortality risk may still require admission because of inadequate social support, exacerbation of underlying chronic pulmonary or cardiovascular disease, inability to tolerate oral therapy, or other indicators of severity of illness not accounted for in the scoring systems. Pulse oximetry should be performed to document the adequacy of oxygenation in individuals who will be managed as outpatients.

CAP is considered severe when a patient requires initial admission to the ICU or early transfer to the ICU. Ways of identifying patients with severe CAP at the time of presentation are being studied because delayed ICU admission is an independent predictor of in-hospital mortality in such patients, and greater than 50% of ICU deaths due to CAP occurs in patients who were initially admitted to the medical ward. The IDSA/ATS guidelines propose major and minor criteria for admission to the ICU. The major criteria include the need for mechanical ventilation and vasopressor support. The minor criteria incorporate the original ATS minor criteria for severe CAP and the CURB-65 criteria (**Table 14**). It is currently proposed that patients with three or more minor criteria should be admitted to the ICU. These criteria have not undergone extensive prospective validation, although recent investigation has shown that the negative predictive value of the severe CAP minor criteria is greater than 90%.

TABLE 14. IDSA/ATS Minor Criteria for Severe Community-Acquired Pneumonia

Clinical Criteria
Confusion (new-onset disorientation to person, place, or time)
Hypothermia (core temperature <36.0 °C [96.8 °F])
Respiration rate ≥30/min[a]
Hypotension necessitating aggressive fluid resuscitation
Multilobar pulmonary infiltrates

Laboratory Criteria
Arterial Po_2/Fio_2 ratio ≤250[a]
Leukopenia (<4000 cells/μL [4.0 × 10⁹/L])
Thrombocytopenia (<100,000 /μL [10 × 10⁹/L])
Blood urea nitrogen >20 mg/dL (7.1 mmol/L)

μL = microliter; IDSA/ATS = Infectious Diseases Society of America/American Thoracic Society.

[a]A patient who requires noninvasive positive-pressure ventilation should be considered to meet this criterion.

Reprinted with permission from Mandell LA, Wunderink RG, Anzueto A, et al; Infectious Diseases Society of America; American Thoracic Society. Infectious Diseases Society of America/American Thoracic Society consensus guidelines on the management of community-acquired pneumonia in adults. Clin Infect Dis. 2007;44 Suppl 2:S27-72. [PMID: 17278083] Copyright 2007, Oxford University Press.

Antibiotic Therapy

Most patients with CAP are treated empirically. Even if a microbial diagnosis is eventually confirmed, initial antibiotic therapy needs to be chosen based on limited information. The selection of antibiotic therapy depends on the site of care (outpatient, medical ward, or ICU) and the presence of risk factors for certain pathogens.

In outpatients, risk factors for drug-resistant *S. pneumoniae* influence the selection of empiric therapy. These risk factors include age older than 65 years, recent (within the past 3 months) β-lactam therapy, medical comorbidities, immunocompromising conditions and immunosuppressive therapy, alcoholism, and exposure to a child in day care. Recommendations for outpatient antibiotic therapy for CAP are provided in **Table 15**. A treatment duration of 5 to 7 days is appropriate for most outpatients.

TABLE 15. Antibiotic Therapy for Community-Acquired Pneumonia in Outpatients

Risk Factors	Treatment
Previously healthy and no risk factor(s) for drug-resistant *Streptococcus pneumoniae*	Macrolide (azithromycin, clarithromycin, or erythromycin) or doxycycline
Risk factor(s) for drug-resistant *S. pneumoniae* or underlying comorbidities	Respiratory fluoroquinolone (moxifloxacin, gemifloxacin, or levofloxacin) **or** β-lactam[a] plus a macrolide or doxycycline

[a]Amoxicillin, 1 g every 8 hours, or amoxicillin-clavulanate, 2 g every 12 hours (preferred), or cefpodoxime or cefuroxime, 500 mg twice daily (alternative).

Recommendations for empiric antibiotic therapy for inpatients (medical ward and ICU) are provided in **Table 16**. The selection of empiric antibiotics for patients with severe CAP is influenced by the presence of risk factors for *P. aeruginosa* and CA-MRSA infection. Antibiotic coverage for possible *P. aeruginosa infection* is appropriate for patients with severe CAP who have a sputum Gram stain that shows gram-negative rods. Empiric antibiotics should include coverage for CA-MRSA in patients with a compatible sputum Gram stain.

For patients with a confirmed microbial cause of CAP, therapy is directed at the isolated pathogen (**Table 17**). Several retrospective studies have suggested that combined β-lactam and macrolide therapy is potentially beneficial in patients with bacteremic pneumococcal pneumonia. Suggested explanations for this benefit include the possibility of coinfection with an atypical pathogen and the anti-inflammatory effect of macrolides, independent of their antimicrobial activity. No prospective clinical trials of combination therapy have been undertaken to date.

The timing of initial empiric antibiotic therapy for hospitalized patients is one of the quality of care indicators by Medicare and other third-party payers. Starting antibiotics within 6 hours of presentation is indicated, based on studies that showed decreased mortality rates among Medicare patients who received antibiotic therapy within 8 hours of presentation and a second analysis that showed decreased mortality rates if antibiotic therapy was begun within 4 hours of presentation. Some experts, however, are concerned that too much emphasis on meeting time criteria for antibiotic administration may increase unnecessary antibiotic use. The IDSA/ATS guidelines simply recommend giving the first dose of antibiotics while the patient is still in the emergency department.

In hospitalized patients, intravenous antibiotic therapy can be changed to oral therapy when criteria for clinical stability are met (temperature ≤37.8 °C [100.0 °F], pulse rate ≤100/min, respiration rate ≤24/min, systolic blood pressure ≥90 mm Hg, arterial oxygen saturation ≥90% or PO_2 ≥ 60 mm Hg [7.9 kPa] on ambient air, ability to tolerate oral intake, and normal mental status). Once patients are ready to switch to oral therapy, they can be safely discharged without observation on oral therapy unless an underlying comorbidity is present requiring continued hospitalization. A 7-day course of therapy (including therapy received during hospitalization) is sufficient for most patients, provided the initial antibiotic was active against the isolated pathogen. More prolonged therapy is required for patients who take longer to become clinically stable, those with cavitary pneumonia, and those with pneumonia due to *S. aureus* or *P. aeruginosa*. Patients with pneumococcal bacteremia do not require a more prolonged course of intravenous antibiotic therapy, although they may take longer to become clinically stable. When indicated, patients should receive pneumococcal and influenza vaccination during their hospitalization for CAP, as vaccination is part of the pneumonia quality of care indicators.

Complications

Failure to improve after initial empiric therapy may be because of misdiagnosis of CAP (for example, cryptogenic organizing pneumonia, vasculitis, pulmonary embolism) or to a resistant pathogen. Patients with persistent fever and those who initially improve and then relapse require evaluation for a

---

TABLE 16. Empiric Antibiotic Therapy for Community-Acquired Pneumonia in Inpatients

Inpatient Setting	Treatment
Medical ward	β-lactam[a] plus a macrolide or doxycycline; **or** respiratory fluoroquinolone (moxifloxacin, gemifloxacin or levofloxacin)
Intensive care unit	β-lactam[b] plus either azithromycin or a fluoroquinolone[c]; if penicillin-allergic, a respiratory fluoroquinolone[d] plus aztreonam
If risk factor(s) for *Pseudomonas aeruginosa* or gram-negative rods on sputum Gram stain	Antipseudomonal β-lactam with pneumococcal coverage (cefepime, imipenem, meropenem, or piperacillin-tazobactam) plus ciprofloxacin or levofloxacin (750 mg); **or** antipseudomonal β-lactam with pneumococcal coverage plus an aminoglycoside plus azithromycin; **or** antipseudomonal[e] β-lactam with pneumococcal coverage plus an aminoglycoside plus a respiratory fluoroquinolone
If risk factor(s) for CA-MRSA or compatible sputum Gram stain	Add vancomycin or linezolid to β-lactam[b] plus either azithromycin or a fluoroquinolone[c]

CA-MRSA = community-associated methicillin-resistant *Staphylococcus aureus*.

[a]Cefotaxime, ceftriaxone, or ampicillin; ertapenem is an alternative in patients with an increased risk of enteric gram-negative pathogens (not *P. aeruginosa*).

[b]Cefotaxime, ceftriaxone, or ampicillin-sulbactam.

[c]Moxifloxacin, gemifloxacin, ciprofloxacin, or levofloxacin.

[d]Moxifloxacin, gemifloxacin, or levofloxacin.

[e]Aztreonam can be used in a patient with a severe β-lactam allergy.

TABLE 17. Pathogen-Specific Therapy for Community-Acquired Pneumonia

Pathogen	Preferred Therapy	Alternative Therapy
Streptococcus pneumoniae		
Penicillin MIC <2 μg/mL	Penicillin G, amoxicillin	Macrolide, oral[a] or parenteral[b] cephalosporin, doxycycline, respiratory fluoroquinolone[c]
Penicillin MIC ≥2 μg/mL	Cefotaxime, ceftriaxone, respiratory fluoroquinolone[c]	Vancomycin, linezolid, and 3 g/d amoxicillin if penicillin MIC ≤4 μg/mL
Haemophilus influenzae		
β-Lactamase negative	Amoxicillin	Fluoroquinolone, doxycycline, azithromycin, clarithromycin[d]
β-Lactamase positive	Second- or third-generation cephalosporin, amoxicillin-clavulanate	Fluoroquinolone, doxycycline, azithromycin, clarithromycin
Mycoplasma pneumoniae, Chlamydophila pneumoniae	Macrolide, tetracycline	Fluoroquinolone
Legionella species	Fluoroquinolone, azithromycin	Doxycycline
Enterobacteriaceae	Use the most appropriate narrow-spectrum agent appropriate for treatment of pneumonia based on susceptibility test results in vitro	
Pseudomonas aeruginosa	Antipseudomonal β-lactam plus aminoglycoside or ciprofloxacin or levofloxacin (based on susceptibility test results in vitro)	Aminoglycoside plus ciprofloxacin or levofloxacin (based on susceptibility test results in vitro)
Staphylococcus aureus		
Methicillin susceptible	Nafcillin	Cefazolin, clindamycin[e]
Methicillin resistant	Vancomycin[f] or linezolid	Trimethoprim-sulfamethoxazole

MIC = minimal inhibitory concentration; μg = micrograms.

[a]Cefpodoxime, cefprozil, cefuroxime, cefdinir, cefditoren.

[b]Cefuroxime, cefotaxime, ceftriaxone.

[c]Levofloxacin, gemifloxacin, moxifloxacin.

[d]Azithromycin is more active in vitro than clarithromycin against *H. influenzae*.

[e]If susceptibility is documented, including disk diffusion test (D-test) if erythromycin resistant.

[f]Consider alternative if vancomycin MIC is ≥2 micrograms/mL.

Adapted with permission from Mandell LA, Wunderink RG, Anzueto A, et al. Infectious Diseases Society of America/American Thoracic Society consensus guidelines on the management of community-acquired pneumonia in adults. Clin Infect Dis. 2007;44(Suppl 2):S27-72. Copyright 2007, Oxford University Press.

possible parapneumonic effusion or empyema. Up to one third of patients hospitalized for the treatment of CAP develop a parapneumonic effusion. Thoracentesis to exclude a complicated parapneumonic effusion or empyema is necessary only if patients fail to respond clinically. Drug fever or a nosocomial infection should be considered in patients who have a persistent fever.

Follow-up

Follow-up chest imaging is not indicated in most patients who improve with treatment. However, a follow-up chest radiograph should be considered to document clearance of pulmonary infiltrates and determine the presence of a possible pulmonary malignancy 6 to 8 weeks after completing treatment for patients who are older than 40 years of age and for smokers. In a recent study, 9.2% of patients hospitalized for pneumonia were diagnosed with a pulmonary malignancy following hospitalization. The median time to diagnosis was 297 days; only 27% were diagnosed within 90 days of admission. Smokers should receive counseling regarding smoking cessation. Such counseling is one of the quality of care indicators for pneumonia. The success of any smoking intervention is modest, but the association of smoking with pneumonia and with progressive lung disease makes this a logical time for counseling.

Outpatients and hospitalized patients who were treated for CAP should generally have a follow-up office visit 10 to

CONT.

14 days after completing therapy. Hospitalized patients who required more than 3 days to become clinically stable are at increased risk for rehospitalization and death and require early follow-up after initial discharge. Studies have shown that the median time for resolution of respiratory symptoms in patients with CAP is 14 days. However, one third of patients continue to have at least one pneumonia-related symptom at 28 days. Patients who recover from an episode of CAP are at significantly increased risk of dying, although the leading causes of death are comorbidities such as COPD and cardiovascular disease. H

KEY POINTS

- Most patients with community-acquired pneumonia are treated empirically; the selection of antibiotic therapy depends on the site of care and the presence of risk factors for certain pathogens.

- In outpatients with community-acquired pneumonia, risk factors for drug-resistant *Streptococcus pneumoniae* influence the selection of empiric antibiotic therapy.

- When indicated, hospitalized patients with community-acquired pneumonia should receive pneumococcal and influenza vaccinations.

- In patients with community-acquired pneumonia, failure to improve after initial empiric therapy may be because of misdiagnosis of community-acquired pneumonia or a resistant pathogen.

Tick-Borne Diseases

Lyme Disease

Lyme disease is the most common arthropod-borne infection in the United States, with 22,561 confirmed cases reported in 2010. The incidence varies geographically, and hyperendemic areas in the northeast and north central United States reflect the geographic density of the vector deer tick, *Ixodes scapularis*, in these areas (**Figure 6**). The causative spirochete is *Borrelia burgdorferi sensu stricto*, which is transmitted to humans following vector tick attachment and feeding. Because the nymphal deer tick is so small, fewer than 50% of infected patients recall a tick attachment. Deer ticks may also serve as vectors for other tick-borne infections (**Table 18**), and coinfection may occur.

Lyme disease has three distinct stages: early localized, early disseminated, and late (**Table 19**). The clinical manifestations of Lyme disease depend on the stage of infection. Early localized Lyme disease typically occurs 1 to 2 weeks following infection. The initial clinical manifestation is erythema migrans (EM), an erythematous skin lesion at the site of tick attachment that is noted in 70% to 80% of patients with confirmed infection (**Figure 7**). Classically, the border of EM expands over several days, and the lesion often develops central clearing, leading to the description of a "target" or "bullseye" appearance. Atypical EM may present as a confluent erythematous macule that sometimes has a vesicular or necrotic

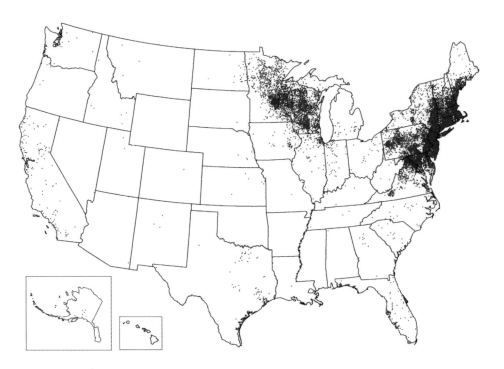

FIGURE 6. Geographic distribution of Lyme disease cases in the United States, 2010.

Courtesy of the Centers for Disease Control and Prevention. Accessed on June 14, 2012, at www.cdc.gov/ncidod/dvbid/lyme/ld_Incidence.htm.

TABLE 18. Selected Human Tick-Borne Diseases in the United States

Disease	Pathogen	Vector	Predominant United States Geographic Distribution
Lyme disease	*Borrelia burgdorferi*	Deer tick	Northeast and north central
Babesiosis	*Babesia microti*	Deer tick	Northeast and north central
Southern tick–associated rash illness	Unknown	Lone Star tick	Southeast, south central, and mid-Atlantic
Human monocytic ehrlichiosis	*Ehrlichia chaffeensis*	Lone Star tick	Southeast, south central, and mid-Atlantic
Human granulocytic anaplasmosis	*Anaplasma phagocytophilum*	Deer tick	Northeast and north central
Rocky Mountain spotted fever	*Rickettsia rickettsii*	Dog tick	Continental

eschar in the center. Secondary cellulitis that develops at the site of tick attachment may also mimic EM.

If early localized Lyme disease is not treated, progression to later stages may occur. Early disseminated Lyme disease is associated with spirochetemia that develops several weeks after the initial infection. Patients frequently present with a febrile illness associated with myalgia, headache, fatigue, and lymphadenopathy. Multiple EM lesions are common at this stage and are found at anatomic sites distinct from the initial tick attachment. Localized infection associated with early disseminated Lyme disease may involve the heart and central nervous system. Lyme myocarditis is reported in 5% of untreated patients and ranges from asymptomatic first-degree heart block to complete heart block. Conduction abnormalities due to Lyme disease are reversible and respond to antibiotics. Neurologic manifestations of early disseminated Lyme disease include cranial nerve palsy (unilateral or bilateral), aseptic meningitis, and radiculopathy.

TABLE 19. Clinical Presentation and Treatment of Lyme Disease

Clinical Manifestations	Diagnostic Testing	Antibiotic Formulation and Duration (see also Table 20)
Early Localized Stage (Incubation period: 3-30 days)		
EM at site of tick attachment	Visualization of EM	Oral , 14-21 days[a]
Early Disseminated Stage (Incubation period: 3-6 weeks)		
Multiple EM lesions distinct from site of tick attachment	ELISA with confirmatory Western blot	Oral, 14-21 days
Cranial nerve palsy (unilateral or bilateral)	ELISA with confirmatory Western blot	Oral, 14-21 days
Meningitis	ELISA with confirmatory Western blot	IV, 10-28 days
Myocarditis	ELISA with confirmatory Western blot	First-degree heart block, asymptomatic: oral, 14-21 days
		Second-degree AV or complete heart block: IV followed by oral (once patient is stabilized), 14-21 days
Late Stage (Incubation Period: Months to Years)		
Arthritis	ELISA with confirmatory Western blot, PCR of synovial fluid	Oral, 28 days
Recurrent arthritis after treatment	Western blot, PCR of synovial fluid	Oral or IV, 28 days
Encephalopathy or encephalomyelitis	ELISA with confirmatory Western blot, PCR of cerebrospinal fluid (low sensitivity)	IV, 14-28 days
Post-Lyme Disease Syndrome		
Nonspecific headache, arthralgia, fatigue	None	Supportive care; antibiotics not indicated

AV = atrioventricular; ELISA = enzyme-linked immunosorbent assay; EM = erythema migrans; IV = intravenous; PCR = polymerase chain reaction.

[a]Range of 10-21 days if doxycycline is used, 14-21 days for alternative agents.

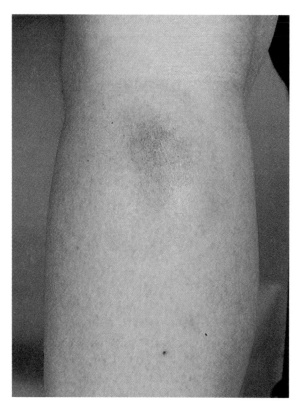

FIGURE 7. Erythema migrans lesion of early localized Lyme disease manifested as "target lesion" with central clearing.

Late-stage Lyme disease occurs in as many as 60% of untreated patients. Lyme arthritis is characterized by migratory monoarticular or oligoarticular inflammation, which often improves spontaneously and then recurs in the same joint or another joint months to years later. The knee is involved in 85% of patients. In the United States, late neurologic complications are rare, and affected patients usually present with an encephalopathy with deficits in cognition and short-term memory.

The diagnosis of early localized Lyme disease is clinical and is based on visualization of the EM skin lesion. Serologic testing is not recommended at this stage, because a measurable antibody response may not have had time to develop. However, laboratory confirmation of infection is required for all later stages of Lyme disease. Detection of antibodies against *B. burgdorferi* using a two-stage approach is recommended. The initial test is an enzyme-linked immunosorbent assay (ELISA), which is sensitive but not sufficiently specific for diagnosis. A positive or equivocal ELISA should therefore be followed by a confirmatory Western blot to detect antibodies directed against specific *B. burgdorferi* epitopes. Interpretation of the Western blot is standardized and is based on the absolute number of positive bands. Testing for IgM antibody to *B. burgdorferi* should be restricted to patients with less than 1 month of symptoms, because an isolated IgM antibody titer in the absence of detectable IgG

antibody after this period likely represents a false-positive test result. Neurologic involvement is supported by cerebrospinal fluid (CSF) pleocytosis and a positive ratio of CSF to serum antibodies or a positive CSF polymerase chain reaction (PCR), although CSF PCR must be considered experimental in the diagnosis of central nervous system Lyme disease.

Serologic testing for Lyme disease should be restricted primarily to patients with clinically suggestive signs or symptoms (other than erythema migrans) who reside in or have traveled to an endemic area. The finding of *B. burgdorferi* antibodies in patients who have nonspecific symptoms of fatigue or myalgia or who are unlikely to have been exposed to a vector tick likely represents a false-positive test result. Serologic testing following a tick bite in an asymptomatic patient is not indicated. Because *B. burgdorferi* antibodies remain positive indefinitely, serial testing is also not recommended.

Treatment recommendations vary and are based on the disease stage and organ involvement (**Table 20**); (see also Table 19). Empiric doxycycline is the recommended treatment of erythema migrans. Post–Lyme disease syndrome, sometimes erroneously called "chronic Lyme disease," presents a particular treatment challenge. This syndrome refers specifically to patients with confirmed Lyme disease, based on stringent clinical and laboratory criteria, who have persistent constitutional symptoms despite appropriate antibiotic treatment. Supportive therapy to ameliorate symptoms is appropriate for these patients, but prolonged durations or repeated courses of antibiotics (oral or intravenous) are ineffectual and strongly discouraged.

KEY POINTS

- The initial clinical manifestation of Lyme disease is erythema migrans, which is an erythematous skin lesion at the site of tick attachment.

- Although serologic studies are not recommended for diagnosing early localized Lyme disease, two-stage laboratory testing (enzyme-linked immunosorbent assay followed by confirmatory Western blot when the initial screening test is positive or equivocal) is required for the diagnosis of all later stages of infection.

- Serologic testing for Lyme disease should be restricted to patients with clinically suggestive signs or symptoms who either reside in or have traveled to an endemic area.

- The finding of *B. burgdorferi* antibodies in patients who have nonspecific symptoms of fatigue or myalgia or who are unlikely to have been exposed to a vector tick likely represents a false-positive test result for Lyme disease.

TABLE 20. Preferred Antibiotic Treatment of Lyme Disease

Antibiotic	Dosage
Oral regimens	
Doxycycline[a]	100 mg twice daily
Amoxicillin	500 mg three times daily
Cefuroxime	500 mg twice daily
Parenteral regimen	
Ceftriaxone	2 g daily

[a]Doxycycline is also active against *Anaplasma phagocytophilum* and is the preferred agent for patients ages 8 years and older who are not pregnant or breast-feeding.

Data from Wormser GP, Dattwyler RJ, Shapiro ED, et al. The clinical assessment, prevention, and treatment of Lyme disease, human granulocytic anaplasmosis, and babesiosis: clinical practice guidelines by the Infectious Diseases Society of America. Clin Infect Dis. 2006;43(9):1089-1134 [PMID: 17029130] Copyright 2006 Oxford University Press. Used with permission.

Babesiosis

Babesiosis is a tick-borne protozoal infection. The geographic distribution of babesiosis due to *Babesia microti*, the most common pathogen, corresponds to that of Lyme disease (see Figure 6) because both infections are transmitted by the same vector tick species. Other *Babesia* species cause clinically similar infections but are endemic to the northwestern and midwestern United States. Person-to-person transmission may occur after transfusion of infected blood products from an asymptomatic donor. Following infection, protozoa persist and replicate inside human erythrocytes. Most infections with *B. microti* are asymptomatic and, when infection is clinically apparent, symptoms range from a self-limited febrile illness to fulminant multiorgan system failure and death.

Patients with mild infection present with fever and findings related to hemolysis, including splenomegaly, hepatomegaly, and jaundice. Asplenic patients tend to have high levels of parasitemia and more severe disease. Other risk factors for more severe disease include older age, HIV infection, and other immunocompromised states. The clinical presentation in patients with severe babesiosis may include profound hemolytic anemia, acute kidney injury, disseminated intravascular coagulation, high-output heart failure, and circulatory collapse.

Laboratory findings reflect the presence of hemolysis and include a macrocytic anemia (due to increased numbers of reticulocytes), increased serum bilirubin level, decreased haptoglobin concentration, and increased serum lactate dehydrogenase level. Thrombocytopenia and elevated serum liver enzyme values are also common.

The preferred method for diagnosing babesiosis is PCR using whole blood specimens, which is more sensitive than direct microscopy. Visualization of intraerythrocytic ring forms on a thin-preparation blood smear is suggestive of babesiosis, but differentiation from falciparum malaria may be difficult if the patient has a compatible travel history for both infections. Serologic testing is not recommended because seroconversion may lag behind onset of clinical symptoms, or conversely, detectable antibodies may reflect a previous asymptomatic infection.

Treatment is indicated for all symptomatic patients with laboratory confirmation of infection as well as for asymptomatic patients with documented persistence of parasites for more than 3 months. Treatment regimens for patients with mild disease include the combination of atovaquone and azithromycin or quinine and clindamycin; the former regimen is better tolerated. Quinine combined with clindamycin is the treatment of choice for severe disease, and exchange transfusion is recommended for patients with greater than 10% parasitemia. Symptoms typically respond rapidly to therapy but may recur in immunocompromised patients.

KEY POINTS

- Babesiosis may be asymptomatic and when clinically apparent ranges from a self-limited febrile illness to fulminant multiorgan system failure and death.
- The preferred method for diagnosing babesiosis is polymerase chain reaction on whole blood specimens, which is more sensitive than direct microscopy.
- Treatment regimens for patients with mild babesiosis include the combination of atovaquone and azithromycin or quinine and clindamycin.

Southern Tick–Associated Rash Illness

Southern tick–associated rash illness (STARI) is clinically indistinguishable from the early localized form of Lyme disease. However, STARI occurs in a geographically distinct distribution in the southeast, mid-Atlantic, and south central United States. Results of testing in patients with STARI will be negative for *B. burgdorferi* infection. The causative agent has not been identified, but the vector appears to be the Lone Star tick, *Amblyomma americanum*.

The primary clinical manifestation of STARI is an EM skin lesion that is often associated with fever, headache, and myalgia. Much like the early localized form of Lyme disease, the diagnosis of STARI is clinical and is based on recognition of the classic EM lesion. Treatment with doxycycline is recommended, although disease progression to later stages has not been reported in untreated patients.

KEY POINTS

- The distinguishing clinical manifestation of Southern tick–associated rash illness is erythema migrans, which is often associated with fever, headache, and myalgia.
- Doxycycline is the recommended treatment for Southern tick–associated rash illness.

Ehrlichiosis and Anaplasmosis

Human monocytic ehrlichiosis (HME) and human granulocytic anaplasmosis (HGA) are clinically similar tick-borne rickettsial diseases that occur in geographically distinct areas of the United States. The different distribution is based on the endemicity of the vector ticks (see Table 18). Both diseases usually occur within 1 to 2 weeks after inoculation and are characterized by a nonfocal febrile illness with frequent headache, myalgia, and fatigue. Skin lesions are described in fewer than 30% of adults with HME and are very uncommon in patients with HGA. The most common skin lesion in patients with HME is a maculopapular rash, but a petechial eruption similar to that seen with Rocky Mountain spotted fever has been described (see Figure 8, discussed below). Meningoencephalitis is also more frequent in patients with HME, occurring in 20% of these patients.

Both HME and HGA are associated with leukopenia (particularly lymphopenia), thrombocytopenia, and elevated serum liver enzyme values. The abnormal liver enzyme findings may lead to the erroneous diagnosis of acute cholecystitis and possible unnecessary surgical intervention. In patients with clinical signs suggestive of meningoencephalitis, the CSF typically shows a lymphocytic pleocytosis with a mildly elevated protein concentration; rarely, CSF findings suggestive of bacterial meningitis have been reported.

The causative agents, *Ehrlichia chaffeensis* and *Anaplasma phagocytophilum*, are trophic for monocytes and neutrophils, respectively. In approximately 20% of patients, the diagnosis is suggested by the presence of intraleukocytic clusters of bacteria (morulae) on a buffy coat stain. Antibodies are seldom detected at the time of acute infection and appear 2 to 4 weeks following clinical illness. Because treatment delay has been associated with increased mortality rates for both HME and HGA, empiric antibiotics should be started when either infection is suspected clinically, followed by laboratory confirmation later if necessary.

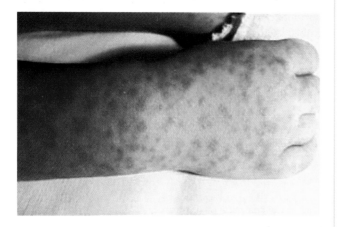

FIGURE 8. Petechial skin lesions associated with Rocky Mountain spotted fever.

Picture courtesy of Centers for Disease Control and Prevention. Accessed on June 14, 2012, at www.cdc.gov/rmsf/symptoms/index.html.

Doxycycline, 100 mg twice daily for 7 to 14 days, is used to treat HME and HGA. Symptoms respond to treatment within 24 to 72 hours, and an alternative diagnosis should be considered if defervescence does not occur during this time.

KEY POINTS

- Both human monocytic ehrlichiosis and human granulocytic anaplasmosis are characterized by a nonfocal febrile illness with frequent headache, myalgia, and fatigue.
- Results of serologic testing may be negative in patients with acute human monocytic ehrlichiosis and human granulocytic anaplasmosis infection but may be positive 2 to 4 weeks after development of clinical illness if the diagnosis requires confirmation.
- Treatment of human monocytic ehrlichiosis and human granulocytic anaplasmosis should be initiated when infection is suspected because treatment delays are associated with poorer outcomes.
- Doxycycline is the treatment of choice for both human monocytic ehrlichiosis and human granulocytic anaplasmosis.

Rocky Mountain Spotted Fever

Rocky Mountain spotted fever (RMSF) is a tick-borne rickettsial disease found throughout the contiguous United States. The incubation period following infection ranges from 2 to 14 days. Fever is almost always present and is variably accompanied by headache, myalgia, confusion, and gastrointestinal symptoms. The characteristic finding of RMSF is a petechial rash (**Figure 8**). The rash is ultimately identified in 90% of patients but is present at the onset of fever in only 15%. Initial skin findings are nonblanching macules on the wrists and ankles that progress over days to a petechial skin eruption involving the trunk, extremities, palms, and soles, but sparing the face. Skin lesions do not occur in 10% of patients, and the absence of lesions is a risk factor for an adverse outcome, presumably because of delay in recognizing the infection and initiating treatment.

Laboratory findings in patients with RMSF include thrombocytopenia and elevated serum liver enzyme values. In contrast to ehrlichiosis and anaplasmosis, leukocyte counts tend to be normal. Patients with RMSF meningoencephalitis typically have a lymphocytic pleocytosis.

Serologic testing is generally used for diagnosis. However, seroconversion often lags behind the onset of clinical symptoms. A fourfold rise in antibody titer or seroconversion noted on a convalescent serum sample obtained 2 to 4 weeks after the acute illness is considered diagnostic. Immunohistochemical studies of a skin biopsy specimen showing *Rickettsi rickettsii* may confirm the diagnosis at the time of presentation. Doxycycline should be started empirically whenever RMSF is suspected and should not be withheld or discontinued based on serologic test results.

Urinary Tract Infections

Epidemiology and Microbiology

Urinary tract infection (UTI) is defined as inflammation of the uroepithelium that involves the lower urinary tract (cystitis), upper urinary tract (pyelonephritis), or both. In the United States, UTIs account for approximately 100,000 hospital admissions each year at a cost of 1.6 billion dollars annually. UTIs are more common in women than in men, with most occurring between the ages of 16 and 35 years. One in three women will have a UTI by age 24 years, and recurrence rates are reported to be as high as 45%. Bacteremia develops in approximately 2% to 4% of patients with nosocomial UTIs, which is associated with a 13% mortality rate. In addition, increased antimicrobial resistance among causative pathogens is posing management challenges in outpatient and hospital settings.

Escherichia coli, the most common pathogen causing UTIs, is responsible for approximately 85% of cases. In addition, coagulase-negative staphylococci such as *Staphylococcus saprophyticus* may cause approximately 10% of UTIs. Gram-negative bacilli other than *E. coli* account for approximately 5% of UTIs. Gram-negative bacilli such as *Proteus, Pseudomonas, Klebsiella,* and *Enterobacter* species are frequent pathogens in recurrent UTIs and UTIs associated with structural urinary tract abnormalities. Multiple pathogens may be isolated when structural abnormalities are present.

Multidrug-resistant pathogens are more common in hospitalized patients, kidney transplant recipients, and patients with underlying urologic abnormalities, previous UTIs, recent antibiotic treatment, or immunocompromising conditions. Fungi, such as *Candida* species, are more frequent pathogens in patients with diabetes mellitus or chronic indwelling urinary catheters and those receiving antibiotics.

KEY POINTS

- Urinary tract infections are more common in women than in men; one in three women will have a urinary tract infection by age 24 years.
- *Escherichia coli* is the causative pathogen in 85% of urinary tract infections.

Diagnosis

UTIs are categorized as uncomplicated or complicated. An uncomplicated UTI is an infection occurring in a normal urinary tract and generally responds well to conventional antimicrobial treatment. Complicated UTIs are infections that occur in patients with structural or functional urinary tract abnormalities and are seen most often in infants, older patients, patients with indwelling urinary catheters, and those with renal calculi. Patients with spinal cord injuries, diabetes mellitus, multiple sclerosis, and AIDS are also more likely to develop complicated UTIs. In general, UTIs in pregnant women and men are considered to be complicated. Complicated UTIs may be associated with multidrug-resistant pathogens and require radiographic investigation more often than do uncomplicated UTIs.

Symptoms of UTI vary widely depending on patient age and severity of infection. Symptoms may include dysuria, frequency, nocturia, enuresis, urgency, hematuria, low back pain, suprapubic pain, flank pain, fever, chills, rigors, and in the elderly, new incontinence and altered mental status.

Definitive laboratory diagnosis requires microscopic urinalysis. The presence of 10 or more leukocytes/microliter of unspun urine from a midstream, clean-catch sample indicates significant pyuria and is indicative of a UTI. The presence of hematuria is helpful in the differential diagnosis because this finding is suggestive of a UTI but not of vaginitis or urethritis.

Urine dipsticks for detecting the presence of leukocyte esterase (suggesting pyuria) and nitrite (produced by bacteria in the urine) are clinically convenient and relatively reliable in confirming infection, particularly if both indicators are positive and the patient has signs or symptoms consistent with UTI. However, in clinical circumstances suggestive of UTI, negative or discordant findings cannot exclude infection, and microscopic analysis is warranted.

Urine culture is usually not needed for patients with an uncomplicated UTI because a treatment response to antimicrobial agents will have occurred before the results become available. A urine culture should be obtained in (1) patients with suspected pyelonephritis, a complicated UTI, or recurrent UTIs (not associated with sexual activity); (2) patients for whom routine treatment may not be available (for example, because of allergies); or (3) patients in whom the presence of a resistant organism is strongly suspected. Cultures are recommended for pregnant women with asymptomatic bacteriuria and for all patients before urologic manipulation. The presence of 10^5 or more colony-forming units (CFU) of bacteria/mL of urine from a midstream, clean-catch sample indicates significant bacteriuria and is diagnostic of UTI in most patients. However, in women with acute dysuria and pyuria, a urine culture yielding 10^2 or more CFU of bacteria/mL is diagnostic of UTI. Recovery of mixed bacteria from a single urine culture sample suggests contamination.

Urologic investigation, including CT and/or ultra-sonography, is not necessary for most patients with UTI but is indicated for those with pyelonephritis who have persistent flank pain or fever after 72 hours of antimicrobial therapy to exclude a perinephric or intrarenal abscess. Older men with recurrent UTIs should also undergo urologic investigation to rule out structural defects, including prostatitis.

KEY POINTS

- Uncomplicated urinary tract infections (UTIs) generally respond well to antimicrobial therapy, whereas complicated UTIs are often associated with multi-drug-resistant pathogens in patients with other comorbidities.

- The presence of 10 or more leukocytes/microliter of unspun urine from a midstream, clean-catch sample or a urine dipstick showing leukocyte esterase indicates significant pyuria and is indicative of a urinary tract infection.

- Urine culture is usually not needed for patients with an uncomplicated urinary tract infection because a treatment response to antimicrobial therapy will have occurred before the results become available.

Management

Cystitis in Women

Dysuria is the most frequent manifestation of cystitis in women and usually occurs together with one or more of the following: urgency, frequency, suprapubic pain, and hematuria. Fever is usually absent. The presence of pyuria is sufficient for diagnosing cystitis in young, sexually active, nonpregnant women. A urine culture should be performed if the diagnosis is unclear, the patient is pregnant, or the infection has recurred after treatment

Various antimicrobial agents are available for treating acute uncomplicated cystitis in women (**Table 21**). Fluoroquinolones and β-lactam agents are not recommended as first-line agents; the fluoroquinolones should be considered as alternative agents. Recommended antibiotics for treating cystitis in pregnant patients include amoxicillin and nitrofurantoin.

KEY POINTS

- Dysuria is the most common manifestation of acute cystitis in women, usually accompanied by urgency, frequency, suprapubic pain, or hematuria, but typically not fever.

- Trimethoprim-sulfamethoxazole, nitrofurantoin monohydrate macrocrystals, and fosfomycin are recommended for treating acute uncomplicated cystitis in women.

Recurrent Urinary Tract Infections in Women

Recurrent UTIs often occur in healthy, young, sexually active women who have a normal urinary tract. In some reports, more than 25% of women who experience their first UTI develop a recurrent infection within months. A recurrent UTI is classified as either a relapse or reinfection. A relapse is present if the current infection is caused by the same pathogen as the initial UTI and occurs within 2 weeks of completing the initial therapy. A reinfection is diagnosed if the current infection is caused by a different strain than that causing the initial UTI or if a urine culture sample was sterile between the two episodes of UTI. Most recurrences are reinfections. Risk factors that increase the likelihood for recurrent UTI include biologic (vaginal colonization with uropathogens), genetic (nonsecretor of ABH blood group antigens), and pelvic structure factors; frequency of sexual activity; spermicide use; a new sexual partner; a history of UTIs at or before age 15 years; and a family history of a mother with recurrent UTIs. Among postmenopausal women, risk factors include urinary incontinence, the presence of a cystocele or postvoid urine residual, and a history of UTIs before menopause.

Prevention strategies for recurrent UTIs include avoiding spermicides. Other factors that might decrease risk but have not been demonstrated to do so in controlled studies include postcoital voiding and liberal fluid intake. The role of cranberry juice in prevention remains unclear. Continuous or postcoital antimicrobial prophylaxis may be considered in patients with two or more symptomatic infections within 6 months or three or more episodes within 12 months. Management of these patients may also include early institution of self-treatment based on positive dipstick findings or clinical symptoms of UTI. Intravaginal estrogen cream is an option for postmenopausal women with recurrent UTIs.

TABLE 21. Recommended First-Line Antimicrobial Agents for Acute Uncomplicated Cystitis in Women		
Agent	**Dose and Duration**	**Comments**
Trimethoprim-sulfamethoxazole	160/800 mg (one double-strength tablet) orally twice daily for 3 days	Avoid if resistance rates to uropathogens are >20% or if used to treat a urinary tract infection in preceding 3 months
Nitrofurantoin monohydrate macrocrystals	100 mg orally twice daily for 5 days	Avoid if pyelonephritis is suspected
Fosfomycin	3 g orally (single dose)	Has lower efficacy compared with some other agents; avoid if pyelonephritis is suspected

A urologic workup is generally not required for recurrent UTIs unless a structural or physiologic abnormality is suspected. Recurrent UTIs due to *Proteus* species may be associated with nephrolithiasis and require additional diagnostic studies. Multiple relapses due to the same pathogenic strain are also an indication for urologic workup.

KEY POINT

- Antimicrobial prophylaxis may be considered if recurrent urinary tract infections develop in women who have two or more symptomatic infections within 6 months or three or more episodes within 12 months.

Acute Pyelonephritis

Pyelonephritis is an inflammation of the renal parenchyma typically resulting from an ascending bladder infection. Clinical manifestations may include flank pain radiating to the groin, fever, chills, nausea, vomiting, and concurrent or antecedent symptoms of a lower UTI.

Empiric antimicrobial therapy should be initiated after a urine culture is obtained. When a patient does not require hospitalization, ciprofloxacin, 500 mg orally twice daily for 7 days, with or without an initial loading dose of ciprofloxacin, 400 mg intravenously, is an appropriate choice in geographic areas where fluoroquinolone resistance rates are less than 10%. In areas where fluoroquinolone resistance rates are higher, an initial single parenteral dose of a long-acting cephalosporin (such as ceftriaxone, 1 g) or a consolidated 24-hour dose of an aminoglycoside is also recommended prior to oral fluoroquinolone therapy. Oral β-lactam agents are less effective than other available agents for the treatment of pyelonephritis.

Patients with pyelonephritis requiring hospitalization should be treated initially with intravenous antimicrobial agents, including a fluoroquinolone (with the exception of moxifloxacin); an aminoglycoside with or without ampicillin; an extended-spectrum cephalosporin or extended-spectrum penicillin with or without an aminoglycoside; or a carbapenem. Choices should be based on local resistance data. **H**

KEY POINTS

- Clinical manifestations of acute pyelonephritis include flank pain radiating to the groin, fever, chills, nausea, vomiting, and concurrent or antecedent symptoms of a lower urinary tract infection.
- In patients with acute pyelonephritis, empiric antimicrobial therapy should be administered after a urine culture is obtained.

Asymptomatic Bacteriuria

Asymptomatic bacteriuria is defined as the presence of specified numbers of bacteria in a urine specimen of an asymptomatic patient. Screening for and treatment of asymptomatic bacteriuria has been shown to be indicated only in pregnant women and men and women undergoing invasive urologic procedures. Screening for bacteriuria in other patient populations is not recommended and should not be a component of routine medical care.

KEY POINT

- Treatment of asymptomatic bacteriuria is recommended only for pregnant women and for men and women undergoing invasive urologic procedures.

Acute Prostatitis

Isolated bladder infection in men is rare. Often, bladder infection and symptoms of UTI are associated with acute bacterial prostatitis. Patients with acute prostatitis often develop a sudden febrile illness with chills, low back pain, or perineal pain accompanied by symptoms of a lower UTI. The diagnosis is based on clinical findings. Digital rectal examination often shows an edematous, tender prostate. Urinalysis often reveals pyuria and bacteriuria. A clean-catch urine culture is recommended to determine the causative pathogen. Enteric gram-negative pathogens are most common. Trimethoprim-sulfamethoxazole is the treatment of choice, and a fluoroquinolone (ciprofloxacin or levofloxacin) is an alternative option. The duration of therapy is typically 4 to 6 weeks. **H**

KEY POINTS

- Clinical manifestations of acute prostatitis include a sudden febrile illness with chills, low back pain, or perineal pain accompanied by symptoms of a lower urinary tract infection.
- Trimethoprim-sulfamethoxazole is the antimicrobial agent of choice for treating acute prostatitis.

Mycobacterium tuberculosis Infection

Introduction

About two billion people worldwide are believed to have latent tuberculosis infection (LTBI), and each year about nine million people develop active disease. Public health approaches to control tuberculosis include primary prevention (isolating and treating patients with active disease and administering bacillus Calmette-Guérin [BCG] vaccine to persons at risk) and secondary prevention (treating patients with LTBI). Despite these measures, about two million people worldwide die of active disease each year. About 25% of those who die are coinfected with HIV.

Epidemiology

The number of new cases of tuberculosis reported yearly in the United States declined by about 58% from 1993 through 2010, when 11,182 cases were reported, representing an all-time low since reporting began in the United States in 1953. However, the percentage of cases in foreign-born persons increased during this period and constituted 60% of all cases in the United States in 2010. The rate of infection in foreign-born persons is 11 times higher than that of persons born in the United States. Eighty percent of all cases of tuberculosis in foreign-born persons living in the United States develop in Hispanics and Asians, and Mexico, the Philippines, India, Vietnam, and China are the top five countries of origin. Racial and ethnic minority groups are also disproportionately affected. In 2010, blacks or African Americans represented 40% of all new reported cases of tuberculosis in U.S.-born persons. Hispanics represent the largest proportion of total cases reported (29%).

KEY POINTS

- In the United States, the number of new cases of tuberculosis reported yearly declined by about 58% from 1993 through 2010.

- The rate of tuberculosis infection in foreign-born persons living in the United States is 11 times higher than that of persons born in the United States.

Pathophysiology

Mycobacterium tuberculosis is an acid-fast bacillus that causes primary tuberculosis infection when airborne respiratory droplets are inhaled and delivered to the terminal airways. Macrophages ingest the mycobacteria, which continue to multiply intracellularly and can potentially spread to other organs through the lymphatics and bloodstream. Most persons remain asymptomatic because their immune system contains the mycobacteria, and the only clues to the presence of infection are new reactivity to the tuberculin skin test (or interferon-γ release assay) or radiographic evidence such as localized scarring of the pulmonary parenchyma and lymph nodes (the Ghon complex). These findings indicate the presence of LTBI, which is not contagious. Progression to active disease can occur after initial infection (primary progressive tuberculosis) or by reactivation of LTBI. Without treatment, about 10% of persons infected with *M. tuberculosis* develop active tuberculosis during their lifetime, and approximately 50% of these persons will develop active disease within the first 2 years after being infected. Impairment of host defenses, such as in patients receiving immunosuppressive agents (corticosteroids or tumor necrosis factor antagonists) or those with HIV infection, diabetes mellitus, chronic kidney disease, malnutrition, and malignancy, increases the risk for primary progressive tuberculosis and reactivation of LTBI.

KEY POINTS

- Progression to active tuberculosis can occur after initial infection (primary progressive tuberculosis) or by reactivation of latent tuberculosis infection.

- Without treatment, about 10% of persons infected with *Mycobacterium tuberculosis* will develop active tuberculosis during their lifetime.

Clinical Manifestations

As noted earlier, patients with LTBI are asymptomatic. Although patients with LTBI do not have systemic manifestations of active tuberculosis, they are at increased risk for future development of active disease. Active disease is characterized by pulmonary and constitutional signs and symptoms (fever, night sweats, cough, chest pain, weight loss, and anorexia) that can develop insidiously. The cough is often chronic and can be nonproductive or productive, bloody, and purulent.

Findings on physical examination are nonspecific and range from normal to subtle to overtly abnormal, depending on the extent of parenchymal and pleural involvement. Immunocompromised patients, including those with HIV infection, often do not have typical signs and symptoms of tuberculosis and are more likely to develop extrapulmonary or disseminated disease. Extrapulmonary disease commonly involves the lymph nodes, bones, joints, and pleura. However, any site, including genitourinary, peritoneal, meningeal, pericardial, and laryngeal tissue, may be involved, and infection at these sites may mimic various other diseases.

KEY POINTS

- Patients with latent tuberculosis infection are asymptomatic.

- Patients with active tuberculosis may have pulmonary and constitutional signs and symptoms that can develop insidiously.

- Immunocompromised patients, including those with HIV infection, often do not have typical signs and symptoms of tuberculosis and are more likely to develop extrapulmonary or disseminated disease.

Diagnostic Testing

Two tests (discussed below) are available to detect LTBI: the Mantoux tuberculin skin test (TST) and interferon-γ release assays (IGRAs). However, neither test is able to distinguish between latent and active infection. Therefore, any individual with a positive test for LTBI should be carefully evaluated for the possibility of active infection.

In patients presenting with clinical findings consistent with active infection, in addition to a thorough history and physical examination, a test for *M. tuberculosis* infection; a chest radiograph; and microbiologic tests, including acid-fast stains and culture of clinical specimens, should be done.

TABLE 22. Interpretation of Tuberculin Skin Test Results

Criteria for Tuberculin Positivity by Risk Group		
≥5 mm Induration	≥10 mm Induration	≥15 mm Induration
HIV-positive persons Recent contacts of persons with active TB Persons with fibrotic changes on chest radiograph consistent with old TB Patients with organ transplants and other immunosuppressive conditions (receiving the equivalent of ≥15 mg/d of prednisone for >4 weeks)	Recent (<5 years) arrivals from high-prevalence countries Injection drug users Residents or employees of high-risk congregate settings: prisons and jails, nursing homes and other long-term facilities for the elderly, hospitals and other health care facilities, residential facilities for patients with AIDS, homeless shelters Mycobacteriology lab personnel; persons with clinical conditions that put them at high risk for active disease; children aged <4 years or exposed to adults in high-risk categories	All others with no risk factors for TB

TB = tuberculosis infection.

Tuberculin Skin Test

The Mantoux TST involves injecting purified protein derivative intradermally (usually into the volar aspect of the forearm) and assessing the skin response. Measurement of induration (not erythema) is determined 48 to 72 hours later and, when positive, indicates a delayed-type hypersensitivity response. To increase the specificity of the test, criteria for positivity are based on the patient's risk factors for infection with *M. tuberculosis* (**Table 22**). Patients with HIV infection or other serious immunocompromising conditions who are close contacts of persons with active tuberculosis should be treated for LTBI regardless of the results of a TST or IGRA once active disease has been excluded.

Causes of false-negative results of the TST (occurring in at least 20% of persons with known active tuberculosis) include recently acquired tuberculosis infection, age younger than 6 months, overwhelming tuberculosis, recent vaccination with a live virus (for example, measles), recent viral infection (for example, measles, varicella), and anergy. False-positive results can be due to BCG vaccination and infection with nontuberculous mycobacteria. For persons who undergo routine serial testing, a positive TST result is considered an increased induration of 10 mm or more within a 2-year interval. Interpretation of the TST in persons with a history of BCG vaccination is the same as for persons who never received the vaccine (unless BCG vaccination was very recent), although IGRA assays (discussed next) may be preferred for those who were vaccinated with BCG.

Remote exposure to tuberculosis may result in an initially negative TST result that can become positive several weeks later. This "booster effect" represents a true-positive result and is especially helpful in evaluating elderly patients with a remote history of LTBI or differentiating remote exposures from new exposures in patients who undergo serial testing. The booster effect is also more common in patients with a history of BCG vaccination and in those with nontuberculous mycobacterial infections.

Interferon-γ Release Assays

The Centers for Disease Control and Prevention endorses the use of IGRAs in all clinical settings in which the TST is recommended. Two types of IGRAs are increasingly being used. Both indicate sensitization to *M. tuberculosis* by measuring release of interferon-γ in the blood by T cells as a response to *M. tuberculosis*–associated antigens. IGRAs are generally thought to be as sensitive as but more specific than the TST in diagnosing tuberculosis. As with the TST, a more vigorous IGRA response is needed for a low-risk person to be considered infected. Similar to the TST, IGRAs are not recommended for testing individuals who are at low risk for LTBI and development of active disease if infected. The exception is testing individuals who will be at increased risk in the future.

IGRAs are preferred to the TST when persons have received BCG either as treatment for cancer or as a vaccine or when testing persons who often fail to return for a follow-up reading of the TST (for example, injection drug users or homeless persons). Conversely, the TST is preferred when testing children younger than 5 years of age. In this population, some experts have recommended testing with both the TST and an IGRA to increase the specificity of diagnosis. An IGRA or a TST may be used for testing recent contacts of someone with active tuberculosis or for periodic screening of persons who are at risk for occupational exposure (for example, health care workers).

Compared with TST, the initial costs of IGRA testing are higher and laboratory processing is required. However, unlike TST, IGRA testing does not require a follow-up visit and interpretation to complete the testing process. Thus, when deciding which test to use, the costs and availability of both of these tests, as well as patient reliability and convenience, should be considered.

Culture and Other Microbiologic Tests

Bacteriologic evaluation of clinical specimens is recommended when active tuberculosis is suspected. Histopathologic evidence of caseating granulomas is helpful but not diagnostic, and just the presence of acid-fast bacilli (AFB) does not confirm a diagnosis of tuberculosis. Cultures need to be performed for confirmation. Because acid-fast staining characteristics from clinical specimens depend on the concentration of mycobacteria (sensitivity of 45% to 80%), culture should be obtained even when smears for AFB are negative. Routine cultures done on solid media optimized for the growth of mycobacteria are slow: the median time to positivity is 3 to 4 weeks, and some specimens can still grow after 5 weeks. Liquid media techniques that do not rely on the presence of visible colonies but can detect microbial metabolism turn positive within a median time of about 1 week. The Centers for Disease Control and Prevention also recommends performing nucleic acid amplification (NAA) testing on a sputum specimen when the diagnosis of tuberculosis is suspected but not established. The positive predictive value of NAA testing is greater than 95% in patients with AFB-positive smears. Perhaps more importantly, these tests are positive in 50% to 80% of patients with AFB-negative, culture-positive smears. A positive NAA test in a patient with suspected tuberculosis should prompt initiation of treatment regardless of whether the sputum smear is AFB-positive or -negative. NAA tests for tuberculosis have the added advantage of providing results within 2 days. They should not be used when the suspicion for tuberculosis is low, because their positive predictive value is less than 50% in this setting. These tests are also expensive and may not be suitable for low-resource areas.

Bronchoscopy, including bronchoalveolar lavage and biopsy, can be considered in patients who are suspected of having tuberculosis but whose sputum studies are negative. Evaluation of patients with suspected pleural tuberculosis may include biopsy to detect granulomas because the yield from pleural fluid cultures in these patients is low (<25%); pleural biopsy yields granulomas in 75% of cases. Some experts recommend measurement of pleural fluid adenosine deaminase levels to establish the diagnosis of pleural tuberculosis in patients with exudative lymphocytic pleural effusions.

Analysis of cerebrospinal fluid from patients with suspected tuberculous meningitis classically reveals a lymphocytic pleocytosis, decreased glucose levels, and elevated protein levels. However, cerebrospinal fluid stains for AFB are usually negative (positivity generally <25%). Cultures are also negative in up to 25% of patients. Assays for polymerase chain reaction have a high specificity (98%) but an average sensitivity of only about 50% in diagnosing tuberculous meningitis.

Drug susceptibility testing of the initial isolate should be routinely performed.

Radiographic Imaging

Primary progressive tuberculosis may present as localized infiltrates or paratracheal and hilar lymphadenopathy on chest radiographs. Reactivation pulmonary tuberculosis typically appears as fibrocavitary disease in the superior segments of the lower lobes or apical-posterior segments of the upper lobes. Atypical radiographic findings such as miliary patterns, middle and lower lung zone involvement, mediastinal lymphadenopathy, and pleural involvement are especially likely in patients with AIDS. CT scans may be helpful for detecting subtle manifestations of pulmonary tuberculosis that are not seen on plain radiographic films or for evaluating tuberculous involvement in extrapulmonary locations.

KEY POINTS

- Measurement of induration (not erythema) is used to determine a positive or negative response to the tuberculin skin test.

- Remote exposure to tuberculosis may result in an initially negative tuberculin skin test that can become positive several weeks later.

- Interferon-γ release assays are generally as sensitive as but more specific than the tuberculin skin test in diagnosing tuberculosis.

- Patients with suspected active tuberculosis require a tuberculin skin test or interferon-γ release assay; a chest radiograph; and microbiologic tests, including acid-fast stains and culture of clinical specimens.

- When active tuberculosis is suspected, culture should always be obtained, even when smears for acid-fast bacilli are negative.

- Nucleic acid amplification testing on a sputum specimen is recommended when the diagnosis of tuberculosis is suspected but not established.

- Bronchoscopy, including bronchoalveolar lavage and biopsy, can be considered in patients who are suspected of having tuberculosis but whose sputum studies are negative.

Treatment

In patients with evidence of tuberculosis infection as documented by a positive TST or IGRA and in whom active tuberculosis has been excluded, treatment should be initiated for LTBI. Treatment of LTBI usually involves a 9-month course of isoniazid. Because peripheral neuropathy may be associated with isoniazid therapy, concurrent treatment with pyridoxine (vitamin B$_6$) should be considered, particularly in those with an increased risk of neuropathy (diabetes, uremia, alcoholism, HIV infection, malnutrition, seizure disorder, or pregnancy). An alternative therapy is rifampin daily for 4 months. Recently, the Centers for Disease Control and Prevention also included 3 months of directly observed, once-weekly rifapentine and isoniazid combination therapy for treatment of latent tuberculosis.

Active tuberculosis is treated with multiple drugs for at least 6 months and involves an initial treatment phase and a continuation phase. In patients who are not believed to be infected with drug-resistant mycobacteria, the initial phase usually consists of a 2-month course of isoniazid, rifampin, ethambutol, and pyrazinamide. Interruptions in treatment are not uncommon. Treatment guidelines recommend that an interruption of 2 or more weeks during the initial 2-month phase of therapy requires restarting the same regimen from the beginning. The continuation phase generally involves treatment with isoniazid and rifampin for either 4 or 7 months. The 7-month course is given when patients have cavitary pulmonary disease at diagnosis and positive sputum cultures after completing initial therapy. Treatment of extrapulmonary tuberculosis is similar to that of pulmonary disease except for patients with tuberculous meningitis for whom the ideal duration of therapy is unknown; these patients are usually treated for 9 to 12 months. An initial course of adjunctive corticosteroids should be given to patients with tuberculous pericarditis or tuberculous meningitis to decrease the potentially deleterious inflammatory effects of treatment.

Drugs used to treat tuberculosis have a toxicity profile that should be discussed with the patient before therapy is begun (**Table 23**). In addition, drugs such as the rifamycins (including rifampin, rifapentine, and rifabutin) are potent inducers of the cytochrome P-450 hepatic enzyme system, which results in reduced serum concentrations of many drugs, including warfarin. Before treatment is begun, the

TABLE 23.	Antituberculous Drugs	
Agent	**Side Effects**	**Notes**
First-Line Medications		
Isoniazid	Rash; liver enzyme elevation; hepatitis; peripheral neuropathy; lupus-like syndrome	Hepatitis risk increases with age and alcohol consumption. Pyridoxine may prevent peripheral neuropathy. Adjust for kidney injury.
Pyrazinamide	Hepatitis; rash; GI upset; hyperuricemia	May make glucose control more difficult in diabetic patients. Adjust for kidney injury.
Rifampin	Hepatitis; rash; GI upset	Contraindicated or should be used with caution when administered with protease inhibitors and non-nucleoside reverse transcriptase inhibitors. Do not administer to patients also taking saquinavir/ritonavir. Colors body fluids orange.
Rifabutin	Rash; hepatitis; thrombocytopenia; severe arthralgia; uveitis; leukopenia	Dose adjustment required if taken with protease inhibitors or non-nucleoside reverse transcriptase inhibitors. Monitor for decreased antiretroviral activity and for rifabutin toxicity.
Rifapentine	Similar to rifampin	Contraindicated in HIV-positive patients (unacceptable rate of failure/relapse).
Ethambutol	Optic neuritis; rash	Baseline and periodic tests of visual acuity and color vision. Patients are advised to call immediately if any change in visual acuity or color vision. Adjust for kidney injury.
Second-Line Medications[a]		
Streptomycin	Auditory, vestibular, and kidney toxicity	Avoid or reduce dose in adults >59 years. Monitor hearing and kidney function tests. Adjust for kidney injury.
Cycloserine	Psychosis; convulsions; depression; headaches; rash; drug interactions	Pyridoxine may decrease CNS side effects. Measure drug serum levels.
Capreomycin	Kidney, vestibular and auditory toxicity	Monitor hearing and kidney function tests. Adjust for kidney injury.
Ethionamide	GI upset; hepatotoxicity; hypersensitivity	May cause hypothyroidism.
Kanamycin and amikacin	Auditory, vestibular, and kidney toxicity	Not approved by the FDA for TB treatment. Monitor vestibular, hearing, and kidney function.
Levofloxacin, moxifloxacin, gatifloxacin	GI upset; dizziness; hypersensitivity; drug interactions	Not approved by the FDA for TB treatment. Should not be used in children.
Para-aminosalicylic acid	GI upset; hypersensitivity; hepatotoxicity	May cause hypothyroidism, especially if used with ethionamide. Measure liver enzymes.

CNS = central nervous system; FDA = U.S. Food and Drug Administration; GI = gastrointestinal; TB = tuberculosis.

[a]Use these drugs in consultation with a clinician experienced in the management of drug-resistant TB.

following studies should be performed: hepatitis B and C virus serologic tests for at-risk patients; platelet count; and measurement of serum aminotransferase, bilirubin, alkaline phosphatase, and creatinine levels. Color vision and visual acuity testing is also needed if ethambutol is to be used.

Directly observed therapy is preferred for patients in whom self-administered treatment cannot be assured because nonadherence can result in ongoing transmission of mycobacteria, drug-resistance, and relapsed infection. Otherwise, at a minimum, patients should undergo a monthly clinical evaluation for documentation of adherence and detection of any adverse medication reactions. In patients receiving first-line antituberculosis medications, routine laboratory tests for monitoring kidney and liver function and platelet count are not needed unless clinically indicated or if abnormalities were documented at baseline.

Treatment durations and recommendations are generally the same for patients with tuberculosis who are coinfected with HIV. Dose adjustments for antiretroviral therapy (ART) and rifamycin agents may be required because of drug interactions. Treatment of tuberculosis in patients with HIV infection should be started at or before the initiation of ART. Early initiation of ART in HIV-infected patients with tuberculosis appears to be most beneficial in those with advanced immunosuppression.

Multidrug-Resistant and Extensively Drug-Resistant Tuberculosis

Resistance to commonly used antituberculosis drugs is increasingly being recognized worldwide. Infection with potentially drug-resistant strains should be suspected in (1) patients who were previously treated for tuberculosis, especially if treatment was inadequate because of patient nonadherence or an inappropriate initial regimen; (2) patients who were infected in countries where high rates of drug resistance are present; (3) adherent patients who are not responding to standard empiric therapy; and (4) close contacts of patients with drug-resistant tuberculosis. Multidrug-resistant (MDR) tuberculosis strains are resistant to at least isoniazid and rifampin. Extensively drug-resistant (XDR) strains are MDR strains that are also resistant to fluoroquinolones and to at least one of the following three second-line injectable drugs: kanamycin, capreomycin, and amikacin. In the United States, 88 cases of primary MDR tuberculosis were reported in 2010; 82% involved foreign-born persons. Between 1993 and 2007, a total of 83 cases of XDR tuberculosis were reported in the United States.

Although the presence of MDR and XDR strains is thought to be associated with higher mortality rates, these strains are potentially curable when use of antituberculosis drugs is directed by comprehensive drug susceptibility testing. The drug regimen for treating MDR and XDR tuberculosis usually includes more medications, and the duration of treatment is much longer. Because of the delay in obtaining results from susceptibility testing, patients may initially receive an ineffective regimen. Development of more rapid diagnostic studies for susceptibility testing, including automated rapid liquid culture techniques and NAA assays, is needed. Surgery may be required for management of localized drug-resistant pulmonary tuberculosis, particularly XDR strains, when patients do not respond to appropriate medical therapy.

KEY POINTS

- Treatment for latent tuberculosis infection usually involves a 9-month course of isoniazid along with pyridoxine (vitamin B_6).
- Active tuberculosis treatment involves an initial phase (usually a 2-month course of isoniazid, rifampin, ethambutol, and pyrazinamide) and a continuation phase (usually a 4- or 7-month course of isoniazid and rifampin).
- Directly observed therapy is preferred when treating patients with tuberculosis because medication nonadherence can result in transmission of mycobacteria, drug-resistance, and relapsed infection.
- Multidrug-resistant tuberculosis strains are resistant to at least isoniazid and rifampin; extensively drug-resistant strains are also resistant to fluoroquinolones and to at least one of the following: kanamycin, capreomycin, and amikacin.

Prevention

BCG vaccine is derived from an attenuated strain of *Mycobacterium bovis*. Although the vaccine is widely used worldwide, it is not generally administered in the United States. BCG vaccine is most effective for preventing disseminated disease and tuberculous meningitis in children. Its protective effect in adults is variable. BCG vaccine should not be given to immunocompromised patients because it is a live vaccine and may cause disseminated disease.

KEY POINT

- Bacillus Calmette-Guérin vaccine is most effective for preventing disseminated tuberculosis and tuberculous meningitis in children.

Nontuberculous Mycobacterial Infections

The term "nontuberculous mycobacteria (NTM)" refers to a group of environmental mycobacteria that are found in soil and natural and treated water. Most identified species are nonpathogenic. NTM are also found as colonizers of medical equipment and surgical solutions, which may explain nosocomial transmission of pathogenic microorganisms.

NTM infections tend to affect young adults and elderly persons. The most common clinical manifestations are pulmonary,

TABLE 24. Diseases Caused by Common Nontuberculous Mycobacterial Species

Disease	*Mycobacterium* species
Pulmonary disease	*M. avium* complex, *M. kansasii*, *M. abscessus*, *M. xenopi*, *M. malmoense*
Lymphadenitis	*M. avium* complex, *M. malmoense*, *M. scrofulaceum*
Skin, soft tissue, and musculoskeletal diseases	*M. abscessus, M. chelonae, M. fortuitum, M. marinum, M. ulcerans*
Disseminated disease	*M. avium* complex, *M. kansasii*, *M. abscessus*, *M. xenopi*, *M. genavense, M. haemophilum, M. chelonae*
Health care–associated infections	*M. abscessus, M. chelonae, M. fortuitum*

lymphatic, cutaneous, soft tissue, and disseminated infection (**Table 24**). Host defenses, body morphotype, and immune status figure significantly in the clinical manifestations of NTM infection. Structural lung conditions (including COPD, bronchiectasis, cystic fibrosis, and pneumoconiosis) and esophageal motility disorders appear to be associated with NTM lung disease. The presence of a slender body habitus, pectus excavatum, scoliosis, and mitral valve prolapse may also be associated with NTM lung disease, especially in postmenopausal women. Abnormalities in interferon-γ and interleukin-12 pathways also predispose to developing severe NTM infections. Disseminated disease is observed most frequently in patients with advanced HIV infection and less often in patients who are immunocompromised. Whether tumor necrosis factor-α blocking agents also predispose to NTM infection is currently unknown.

The same techniques used in culture of *M. tuberculosis* are used in culture of NTM. Detecting NTM isolated from anatomic sites that are generally thought to be sterile suggests NTM infection. Because a single specific test to differentiate NTM colonization from active infection is not available, diagnostic criteria have been developed to aid in determining which patients require treatment (**Table 25**).

KEY POINTS

- Most infections caused by nontuberculous mycobacteria affect young adults and elderly persons.

- The most common clinical manifestations of nontuberculous mycobacterial infections are pulmonary, lymphatic, cutaneous, soft tissue, and disseminated infections.

- Because a single specific test to differentiate nontuberculous mycobacterial colonization from active infection is not available, diagnostic criteria have been developed to aid in determining which patients require treatment.

Mycobacterium avium Complex Infection

Mycobacterium avium complex (MAC) is the most common cause of NTM lung disease and is acquired by inhaling the

TABLE 25. Diagnostic Criteria for Nontuberculous Mycobacterial Lung Disease

Criteria	Findings
Clinical and imaging criteria	Evidence of pulmonary symptoms and abnormal chest imaging studies (nodular or cavitary lung lesions on radiographs and high-resolution CT scans), with exclusion of other possible causes
Laboratory (microbiologic) criteria	Positive isolation of NTM from at least two separate sputum samples
	or
	Positive isolation of NTM from at least one bronchoalveolar lavage sample
	or
	Histopathologic demonstration of AFB and/or granulomatous disease with a positive culture for NTM from lung tissue specimen; or histopathologic demonstration of AFB and/or granulomatous disease on lung tissue specimen with a positive culture for NTM from one or more sputum samples or bronchoalveolar lavage sample
Other considerations	The isolation of an unusual NTM species or of an NTM species that is usually a contaminant should prompt consultation with an infectious diseases specialist.
	The suspicion of NTM lung disease that does not fulfill the above diagnostic criteria should prompt follow-up until a definitive diagnosis is made or excluded.
	Whether to treat pulmonary infections due to NTM should be based on the potential benefits and risks for individual patients.

AFB = acid-fast bacilli; NTM = nontuberculous mycobacteria.

Data from Griffith DE, Aksamit T, Brown-Elliott BA, et al; the ATS Mycobacterial Diseases Subcommittee; American Thoracic Society; Infectious Disease Society of America. An official ATS/IDSA statement: diagnosis, treatment, and prevention of nontuberculous mycobacterial diseases. Am J Respir Crit Care Med. 2007;175(4):367-416. [Erratum in: Am J Respir Crit Care Med. 2007;175(7):744-745 (dosage error in article text)]. [PMID: 17277290] aerosolized microorganisms from colonized soil and water. Two distinct presentations of MAC lung infection are common. The first is a fibrocavitary disease (similar to tuberculosis) that often involves the upper lobes, occurs primarily in middle-aged men with a history of smoking or other chronic lung injury, and, if left untreated, progresses rapidly to cavitary lung destruction and respiratory failure. The second type of infection tends to occur in middle-aged or elderly women who have no history of smoking or underlying lung disease (Lady Windermere syndrome). Patients have a chronic cough and nodular infiltrates (nodular bronchiectatic disease) that frequently involve the right middle lobe or lingula. Although this disease generally has an indolent course, some patients may have aggressive disease with fever, weight loss, and progressive respiratory insufficiency.

Other presentations of MAC infection are less common. A hypersensitivity-like pneumonitis, referred to as "hot tub lung," is linked to inhalation of aerosolized household water colonized by MAC. The onset is subacute; patients present with dyspnea, cough, and fever, and resolution occurs following removal of the aerosol. Lymphadenitis, primarily of the head and neck, is the primary presentation of NTM infection in children, and MAC is isolated in about 80% of these patients. Disseminated MAC disease is one of the most common infections in patients with advanced HIV infection, particularly those with CD4 cell counts less than 50/microliter.

Antimicrobial therapy is indicated for most patients in whom MAC is determined to be an invasive pathogen. In vitro susceptibility testing is usually not indicated before therapy is begun. Treatment usually consists of a combination of a macrolide (clarithromycin, azithromycin), ethambutol, and a rifamycin (rifampin, rifabutin). Adding amikacin or streptomycin is recommended for the first 2 to 3 months of therapy for patients with severe or previously treated MAC infection. Surgical intervention may be indicated when disease is predominantly localized to one lung. Adding corticosteroids for treatment of MAC hypersensitivity-like pneumonitis may hasten recovery. Lymphadenitis caused by MAC should be treated with excisional surgery alone.

KEY POINTS

- *Mycobacterium avium* complex most often manifests as a tuberculosis-like infection in middle-aged men with a history of smoking and chronic lung disease and in middle-aged or elderly women with no history of smoking or underlying lung disease.
- Treatment of *Mycobacterium avium* complex infection generally includes a combination of a macrolide (clarithromycin, azithromycin), ethambutol, and a rifamycin (rifampin, rifabutin).

Mycobacterium kansasii

Mycobacterium kansasii is the second most common NTM species causing lung disease. Unlike other NTM species, *M. kansasii* is not normally found in natural environments but is commonly isolated from urban municipal water supplies. A single clinical isolate is therefore unlikely to represent colonization and should be considered diagnostic of disease. Patients with *M. kansasii* lung infection have symptoms and signs suggestive of tuberculosis. Treatment consists of isoniazid, rifampin, and ethambutol given daily for 18 months, and results of sputum cultures must be negative for at least 12 months before therapy is discontinued.

KEY POINTS

- Patients with *Mycobacterium kansasii* lung disease present with symptoms and signs suggestive of tuberculosis.
- Treatment of *Mycobacterium kansasii* lung disease consists of isoniazid, rifampin, and ethambutol.

Rapidly Growing Mycobacteria

Rapidly growing mycobacteria (RGM) are defined by their brief growing period in culture media (within 7 days). They are generally ubiquitous saprophytes that are widely distributed in nature. The three most clinically relevant species are *M. fortuitum*, *M. chelonae*, and *M. abscessus*. RGM have a wide spectrum of clinical manifestations, including pulmonary, skin, soft tissue, and musculoskeletal infections. They are sometimes acquired by direct inoculation such as with cosmetic procedures. Dissemination of RGM is rare and occurs only in patients who are severely immunocompromised. RGM, especially *M. fortuitum* and *M. abscessus*, may also be associated with health care–associated infections, including, but not limited to, surgical site, catheter-related bloodstream, and prosthetic device–related infections. The common factor in these infections is exposure to colonized liquid, usually tap water. Because drug susceptibility varies among the RGM species, in vitro susceptibility testing of all clinically significant RGM isolates is recommended before therapy is begun. Treatment with a multiple antibiotic regimen is required. **H**

KEY POINTS

- Rapidly growing mycobacteria have a wide spectrum of clinical manifestations, including pulmonary, skin, soft tissue, and musculoskeletal infections, and are sometimes acquired by direct inoculation.
- Treatment of infection due to rapidly growing mycobacteria requires in vitro susceptibility testing and combination antibiotic therapy.

Fungal Infections

Systemic Candidiasis

Systemic or invasive candidiasis includes candidemia, disseminated candidiasis, and focal organ involvement. *Candida* bloodstream infection, such as catheter-related candidemia, may initially be the primary disorder but may lead to disseminated or focal organ involvement as a result of hematogenous spread. In disseminated or focal organ involvement, candidemia may be present secondary to the primary infection, but in many circumstances, blood cultures are negative. Although *Candida albicans* is the most common pathogen, identification of non-*albicans* species is increasing. Any *Candida* species that is obtained from a blood culture should never be considered a contaminant but instead should initiate investigation for a cause.

Risk factors for systemic candidiasis include medications (broad-spectrum antibiotics, chemotherapeutic agents, immunosuppressive agents), catheter-related causes (central venous catheters, parenteral nutrition, hemodialysis), and hospitalization (especially a prolonged stay in an intensive care unit). Patients with malignancies, acute kidney injury, neutropenia, and severe acute pancreatitis are at increased risk as are transplant recipients and those recovering from recent surgery.

Clinical Manifestations and Diagnosis

Initial clinical manifestations of systemic candidiasis range from fever, hypotension, and leukocytosis to sepsis syndrome and septic shock, which are indistinguishable from severe bacterial infection. Characteristic eye and skin lesions may be present. Eye lesions are characterized by distinctive white exudates in the retina. Skin lesions are generally painless papules or pustules on an erythematous base. Tissue from the skin lesions contains yeast and can help determine the diagnosis rapidly. Other common sites of dissemination are the kidneys, liver, spleen, and brain. However, microabscesses in all organs have been described. Although *Candida* can infect any organ, the most frequent focal infections are urinary tract infections, peritonitis, bone and joint infections, endophthalmitis, and meningitis. Even though *Candida* is frequently isolated from the sputum, pneumonia from this pathogen is extremely rare. Chronic disseminated candidiasis (also called hepatosplenic candidiasis) occurs in patients with hematologic malignancies who are no longer neutropenic. Clinical manifestations include fever, right upper quadrant abdominal pain, nausea, and vomiting. The gold standard for diagnosing systemic candidiasis is a positive culture from the blood or a normally sterile body fluid or site. A negative culture does not exclude this diagnosis. If organ involvement is suspected, biopsy specimens should be obtained and sent for histopathologic studies and culture. Identification of the specific *Candida* species is important to guide appropriate antifungal therapy.

Treatment

Empiric therapy for suspected candidiasis is similar to that for proven infection. Fluconazole or an echinocandin (caspofungin, anidulafungin, or micafungin) is recommended as initial therapy for most non-neutropenic patients with candidemia. Fluconazole is preferred for patients who are less critically ill. An echinocandin is preferred for patients with moderate to severe illness who recently received an azole. Changing from an echinocandin to fluconazole is indicated if the *Candida* isolate is likely to be susceptible to fluconazole and if the patient is clinically stable. An echinocandin is initially preferred for infection due to *Candida glabrata*, and an oral azole agent may be substituted at a later date. However, fluconazole and voriconazole susceptibility testing is needed before changing to an azole in patients with *C. glabrata* infection. Susceptibility testing may also be indicated for other *Candida* species in which azole resistance is suspected.

Fluconazole is recommended for infection due to *Candida parapsilosis*. Voriconazole is used as step-down oral therapy for infection due to *Candida krusei* or voriconazole-susceptible *C. glabrata*. Treatment of uncomplicated candidemia should be continued for 2 weeks after clearance of the pathogen from the bloodstream and resolution of symptoms.

Removal of intravenous catheters is strongly recommended for non-neutropenic patients with candidemia because catheter removal has been associated with a shorter duration of infection and improved patient outcomes. Candidemia caused by *C. parapsilosis* is almost always catheter-related.

In neutropenic patients with proven *Candida* infection, an echinocandin or voriconazole (if coverage of molds is desired) may be used. Because neutropenic patients may develop candidemia if the pathogen enters the bloodstream from the gastrointestinal tract, the role of catheter removal is less clear. However, if candidemia persists for more than a few days in a neutropenic patient with a catheter, the catheter should be removed. Empiric therapy for suspected invasive candidiasis in neutropenic patients may include a lipid formulation of amphotericin B, an echinocandin, or voriconazole.

Therapy is not usually indicated for patients with asymptomatic cystitis caused by *Candida* species unless the patient is neutropenic or is undergoing a urologic procedure. The treatment of choice for symptomatic cystitis and pyelonephritis is fluconazole.

Treatment for most focal infections is consistent with the recommendations for the treatment of candidemia, except that echinocandins should not be used to treat meningitis or endophthalmitis because of poor penetration. ▇

- The gold standard for diagnosing systemic candidiasis is a positive culture from the blood or a normally sterile body fluid or site.
- Removal of intravenous catheters is strongly recommended for non-neutropenic patients with candidemia.
- Fluconazole or an echinocandin should be used as initial therapy for candidemia and other forms of invasive candidiasis.

Aspergillosis and Aspergilloma

Aspergillus species are ubiquitous in the environment. The primary route of acquisition is inhalation of aerosolized spores, and the principal site of disease is the lung. The most common *Aspergillus* species causing infection are *A. fumigatus, A. flavus, A. niger,* and *A. terreus*, and the most common forms of pulmonary infection are allergic bronchopulmonary aspergillosis, aspergilloma (fungus ball), and invasive aspergillosis.

Allergic bronchopulmonary aspergillosis most often occurs in patients with chronic asthma or cystic fibrosis. Diagnostic criteria include asthma, central bronchiectasis, fleeting pulmonary infiltrates on chest imaging studies, and laboratory studies showing eosinophilia, elevated serum IgE levels, cutaneous reactivity to *Aspergillus* antigens, and the presence of *Aspergillus*-precipitating antibodies. Recommended treatment is administration of oral corticosteroids during an acute phase or exacerbation. Adding the antifungal agent itraconazole has been shown to improve outcomes and have a corticosteroid-sparing effect.

Symptoms of aspergilloma (fungus ball) include cough, hemoptysis, dyspnea, weight loss, fatigue, fever, and chest pain. Hemoptysis can be life-threatening. Radiographic studies show a rounded mass in a preexisting pulmonary cavity or cyst or in areas of devitalized lung. Sputum culture is usually positive for *Aspergillus*. Surgical resection is considered the definitive therapy.

Invasive sinopulmonary aspergillosis and disseminated aspergillosis generally occur in immunocompromised patients. The lung is the most common site of invasive disease. The organism invades blood vessels and causes distal infarction of tissue. Patients may present with fever, cough, chest pain, hemoptysis, and pulmonary infiltrates or nodules on chest radiographs. Wedge-shaped densities resembling infarcts may also be seen on radiographs. CT scans may show a target lesion with a necrotic center surrounded by a ring of hemorrhage (the halo sign). Dissemination may occur to the central nervous system (CNS) and cause a brain abscess or to blood vessels in the heart, gastrointestinal tract, or skin. Diagnosis may be difficult, because *Aspergillus* is a frequent contaminant in sputum.

The diagnosis of invasive aspergillosis is established by tissue biopsy showing *Aspergillus* in histopathologic and culture specimens, especially specimens that were obtained from a normally sterile site. Blood cultures are rarely positive. The galactomannan antigen immunoassay is a useful diagnostic test for detecting fungi in serum, cerebrospinal fluid, and bronchoalveolar lavage fluid, and serial measurements can be used for monitoring therapy. The β-D-glucan assay and polymerase chain reaction are also promising diagnostic tests. Treatment of invasive aspergillosis includes conventional and lipid formulations of amphotericin B, voriconazole, itraconazole, posaconazole, or caspofungin. Voriconazole is superior to conventional amphotericin B for primary therapy. The lipid formulation of amphotericin B, echinocandins, or other triazole agents are indicated for patients who cannot tolerate voriconazole, have contraindications to its use, or have progressive infection. Combination therapy is not routinely recommended. H

- The most common forms of pulmonary aspergillosis are allergic bronchopulmonary aspergillosis, aspergilloma (fungus ball), and invasive aspergillosis.
- Treatment of allergic bronchopulmonary aspergillosis consists of oral corticosteroids during an acute phase or exacerbation with itraconazole added to achieve a corticosteroid-sparing effect.
- Voriconazole is superior to conventional amphotericin B for primary treatment of invasive aspergillosis.

Mucormycosis

Mucormycosis (formerly zygomycosis) is an acute and rapidly progressive infection that most commonly occurs in patients with hematologic malignancies associated with prolonged neutropenia, other disorders causing prolonged neutropenia or immunosuppression, severe burns or trauma, or poorly controlled diabetes mellitus. Patients taking corticosteroids, cytotoxic agents, or deferoxamine are also at increased risk. Rhinocerebral mucormycosis is the most common presentation; pulmonary, gastrointestinal, cutaneous, and disseminated infections rarely occur. Rhinocerebral mucormycosis is a rapidly fatal infection that spreads from the sinuses retroorbitally and to the CNS. Patients present with headache, epistaxis, and ocular findings, including proptosis, periorbital edema, and decreased vision. Examination of the nose or palate may show black necrotic tissue, which is usually pathognomonic. Pulmonary mucormycosis with thrombosis and infarction most frequently develops in patients with hematologic malignancies. Cutaneous mucormycosis is rare and develops most often in burn and trauma patients or as a result of dissemination from another site. Gastrointestinal mucormycosis is also rare, occurring primarily in patients with gastrointestinal tract abnormalities or severe malnutrition.

Isolated CNS mucormycosis may result from hematogenous spread and occurs in injection drug users.

The diagnosis of mucormycosis is confirmed by tissue biopsy and culture. Histopathologic studies show characteristic broad, irregular, ribbon-like, aseptate hyphae that exhibit broad right-angle branching. Blood cultures are usually negative. Therapy requires both medical and surgical interventions. High-dose conventional or lipid-based amphotericin B is the antifungal agent of choice. Immediate, aggressive surgical debridement is essential and may have to be repeated. **H**

KEY POINTS

- Rhinocerebral mucormycosis is a rapidly fatal infection; finding black necrotic tissue on examination of the nose or palate is pathognomonic.
- Treatment of mucormycosis requires a combination of high-dose conventional or lipid-based amphotericin B and immediate, aggressive surgical debridement.

Cryptococcosis

Cryptococcosis is an invasive mycosis that occurs worldwide. The lungs are the primary portal of entry for *Cryptococcus* species. Although immunocompetent hosts are generally able to contain the pathogen as a result of cell-mediated immunity, immunocompromised patients are at risk for pulmonary infection that can rapidly disseminate. Disseminated infection most often involves the CNS and causes subacute or chronic meningoencephalitis or meningitis. Headache and alterations in mental status are the most common symptoms. Fever and nuchal rigidity occur less often. Complications include hydrocephalus, encephalitis, brainstem vasculitis, involvement of the optic pathways, and mass lesions (cryptococcomas) of the brain. Other forms of disseminated cryptococcosis include skin, prostate, bone, eye, and urinary tract involvement. Whenever cryptococcosis occurs at a site outside the CNS, a lumbar puncture should be done to determine if CNS infection is also present.

The diagnosis is made initially by histopathologic studies showing cryptococci *or* cryptococcal antigen in serum or cerebrospinal fluid and is confirmed by isolation of cryptococci in culture. Pulmonary cryptococcosis found incidentally in an asymptomatic immunocompetent host may resolve without treatment. However, all patients with CNS cryptococcosis or extrapulmonary disease require therapy. Fluconazole is the antifungal agent of choice for primary cutaneous infection without evidence of dissemination and for isolated mildly symptomatic pulmonary disease. The preferred treatment for disseminated infection, infection in an immunocompromised patient, or cryptococcal meningoencephalitis or meningitis is amphotericin B plus flucytosine, given as induction therapy for 2 weeks; 4 weeks of induction therapy are recommended for non–HIV-infected, nontransplant patients. Consolidation therapy with fluconazole is then administered for at least

8 weeks. Maintenance therapy can be discontinued in HIV-positive patients who are receiving effective antiretroviral therapy, have a CD4 cell count of 100/microliter or greater for 3 or more months, and have been receiving antifungal therapy for at least 1 year. Organ transplant recipients who must remain on high-dose immunosuppressive agents may require lifelong maintenance therapy. An important part of treating patients with CNS cryptococcosis is management of elevated intracranial pressure (for example, frequent lumbar punctures and removal of cerebrospinal fluid) or placement of a ventriculoperitoneal shunt if the patient is receiving appropriate antifungal therapy and other measures to reduce elevated intracranial pressure have failed. **H**

KEY POINTS

- The diagnosis of cryptococcosis is made initially by histopathologic studies showing cryptococci or cryptococcal antigen in tissue, serum, or cerebrospinal fluid and is confirmed by isolation of cryptococci in culture.
- The preferred treatment of disseminated cryptococcosis, cryptococcal infection in an immunocompromised host, or cryptococcal meningoencephalitis or meningitis is amphotericin B plus flucytosine induction therapy followed by fluconazole consolidation therapy.

Blastomycosis **H**

Blastomycosis is a systemic pyogranulomatous disease caused by *Blastomyces dermatitidis,* a thermal dimorphic fungus that is endemic to states that border the Ohio and Mississippi river valleys as well as states and Canadian provinces that border the Great Lakes and St. Lawrence River. Infection occurs by inhalation of spores and primarily involves the lungs. The skin is the second most common site of infection, followed by the bones, joints, and prostate. The diagnosis of primary pulmonary blastomycosis is often difficult because patients may be asymptomatic or have only nonspecific symptoms such as fever, cough, and dyspnea. A presumptive diagnosis is based on finding characteristic yeast forms on histopathologic samples, and the definitive diagnosis is established by isolation of *B. dermatitidis* on culture.

Acute pulmonary blastomycosis may be mild and self-limited in the immunocompetent host and may not require treatment; however, therapy may prevent extrapulmonary dissemination. All immunocompromised patients and all patients with moderate to severe pneumonia or disseminated infection require treatment. Oral itraconazole is the agent of choice for patients with mild to moderate pulmonary blastomycosis and is given for 6 to 12 months. Patients with moderately severe to severe disease should receive a conventional or lipid formulation of amphotericin B for 1 to 2 weeks followed by oral itraconazole for 6 to 12 months.

Extrapulmonary blastomycosis can occur in the absence of lung disease. Cutaneous blastomycosis is most common and is frequently a marker for disseminated infection. Mild to moderate disseminated extrapulmonary blastomycosis is treated with oral itraconazole, and moderately severe to severe disease requires a conventional or lipid formulation of amphotericin B. **H**

KEY POINTS

- A presumptive diagnosis of pulmonary blastomycosis is based on the finding of characteristic yeast forms on histopathologic samples, and the definitive diagnosis is established by isolation of *Blastomyces dermatitidis* on culture.

- Patients with mild or moderate pulmonary blastomycosis are treated with oral itraconazole, and those with moderately severe to severe disease should receive a conventional or lipid formulation of amphotericin B followed by oral itraconazole.

Histoplasmosis

Histoplasmosis is caused by *Histoplasma capsulatum*, a thermal dimorphic fungus that is endemic to the midwestern states of the Ohio and Mississippi river valleys. Infection is usually asymptomatic but occasionally causes acute and chronic pulmonary disease, granulomatous mediastinitis, fibrosing mediastinitis, broncolithiasis, pulmonary nodules (histoplasmomas), and acute and chronic disseminated disease. The diagnosis is established by histopathologic studies, antigen determination, and isolation of *H. capsulatum* on culture. Because the sensitivity of these studies differs depending on the extent of infection and the time following exposure, a battery of tests is usually required to confirm the diagnosis.

In most symptomatic patients, disease is mild and resolves without therapy. Therapy is indicated for patients with moderately severe or severe infection, acute diffuse pulmonary involvement, and chronic cavitary pulmonary disease. Treatment should also be considered for patients with mild infection who are immunocompromised or have had symptoms for 4 or more weeks. Itraconazole is the antifungal agent of choice for mild to moderate histoplasmosis, and a conventional or lipid formulation of amphotericin B is used to treat moderately severe to severe infection. **H**

KEY POINTS

- The diagnosis of histoplasmosis is established by histopathologic studies, antigen determination, and isolation of *Histoplasma capsulatum* on culture.

- Itraconazole is the antifungal agent of choice for treating mild to moderate histoplasmosis, and a conventional or lipid formulation of amphotericin B is used to treat moderately severe to severe infection.

Coccidioidomycosis

Coccidioidomycosis is caused by the thermal dimorphic fungi *Coccidioides immitis* and *Coccidioides posadasii,* which are endemic to the deserts of the southwestern United States, parts of Mexico, and Central and South America. Most infections are caused by inhalation of spores and are asymptomatic. Primary infection most frequently presents as community-acquired pneumonia occurring 1 to 3 weeks following exposure. In endemic areas, up to one third of cases of community-acquired pneumonia are caused by *Coccidioides* species. Valley fever is a subacute infection with respiratory symptoms, fever, and erythema nodosum. Extrapulmonary infection most commonly involves the skin, bones, joints, and CNS. The diagnosis is established by isolation of *Coccidioides* species in culture. Serologic tests are useful both for diagnosis and for monitoring the course of therapy and are the preferred method for diagnosing primary coccidioidal infections. Serologic studies are more helpful than culture in establishing the cause of chronic coccidioidal meningitis because cultures of cerebrospinal fluid are frequently negative. Because a negative serologic test does not exclude infection, repeated tests are needed to improve sensitivity.

Treatment is indicated for patients with severe disease or those with an increased risk for disseminated infection. Ketoconazole, fluconazole, and itraconazole are all reasonable treatment options for uncomplicated primary coccidioidal infection. The duration of therapy generally ranges from 3 to 6 months. An amphotericin B–based regimen is indicated for patients with severe coccidioidal pneumonia. Oral fluconazole is the antifungal agent of choice for treatment of meningitis, and therapy should be continued for life because relapses are common after medication is discontinued. However, intrathecal amphotericin B is indicated for patients who fail to respond to azole agents and for women during the first trimester of pregnancy. **H**

KEY POINTS

- Primary coccidioidomycosis most frequently presents as community-acquired pneumonia occurring 1 to 3 weeks following exposure.

- Serologic tests are useful for diagnosing primary coccidioidal infection and monitoring the course of therapy; repeated testing may be needed to improve sensitivity.

- Treatment of uncomplicated primary coccidioidal infection is ketoconazole, fluconazole, or itraconazole for 3 to 6 months.

Sporotrichosis

Infections caused by *Sporothrix schenckii* are usually associated with inoculation of skin from contaminated soil that tends to occur while gardening. A papule appears days to weeks later at the site of inoculation and usually ulcerates. Similar lesions then occur along lymphatic channels proximal to the inoculation site. The diagnosis is established by culture. Itraconazole is the treatment of choice for cutaneous and osteoarticular *S. schenckii* infection.

KEY POINT

- Cutaneous and osteoarticular *Sporothrix schenckii* infections are treated with itraconazole.

Sexually Transmitted Infections

Introduction

Sexually transmitted infections can be categorized as those that cause cervicitis and urethritis (and resultant complications such as pelvic inflammatory disease and epididymitis-orchitis), genital ulcers, and external genital warts. The diagnosis and treatment of sexually transmitted infections are important not only in the care of individual patients but also for preventing transmission of infection to other persons.

Cervicitis and Urethritis

Cervicitis and urethritis are most commonly caused by *Chlamydia trachomatis* and *Neisseria gonorrhoeae*. In women, herpes simplex virus (HSV) may also cause cervicitis. In men, urethritis may be due to HSV, *Trichomonas vaginalis*, and *Mycoplasma genitalium*. *N. gonorrhoeae* and *C. trachomatis* may cause proctitis in both men and women who have receptive anal intercourse.

Women with cervicitis generally present with purulent vaginal discharge. Intermenstrual bleeding (especially after intercourse) and dysuria may also develop. On examination, the vulva and the vaginal mucosa appear normal, but the cervix is inflamed, and mucopurulent discharge may be seen from the endocervical canal. Bleeding may occur when a swab is passed through the cervical os. Men with urethritis present with dysuria and penile discharge. Purulent discharge may be noted at the urethral meatus or expressed by applying gentle pressure with the forefinger on the dorsum of the penis and the thumb on the ventral surface at the base and moving towards the meatus.

Patients with proctitis present with rectal pain, tenesmus, and rectal discharge. Anoscopy reveals erythematous, friable mucosa in the rectal vault. In addition to *N. gonorrhoeae* and *C. trachomatis*, the differential diagnosis of proctitis includes HSV and syphilis.

KEY POINTS

- Cervicitis and urethritis are most commonly caused by *Chlamydia trachomatis* and *Neisseria gonorrhoeae*.

- Women with cervicitis generally present with purulent vaginal discharge; intermenstrual bleeding (especially after intercourse) and dysuria may also develop.

- Men with urethritis present with dysuria and penile discharge.

Chlamydia trachomatis Infection

Risk factors for *C. trachomatis* infection include age 25 years or younger, new or multiple sexual partners, and engaging in unprotected sex. Infection may be asymptomatic. Sequelae of untreated infection in women include pelvic inflammatory disease, ectopic pregnancy, and infertility. Annual screening of sexually active young women (≤25 years of age) and of older women with other risk factors is recommended. Nucleic acid amplification tests are the most sensitive diagnostic modality and may be performed on an endocervical or urethral swab or a urine sample. In patients with documented infection, all sexual partners in the 60 days preceding the onset of symptoms (or the last sexual partner if more than 60 days have elapsed since symptom onset) should be referred for evaluation and treatment.

Treatment of *C. trachomatis* infection is discussed later in this section. Test of cure is recommended only for pregnant women.

KEY POINTS

- Risk factors for *Chlamydia trachomatis* infection include age 25 years or younger, new or multiple sexual partners, and engaging in unprotected sex; sexually active women aged 25 years or younger and older women with risk factors should be screened annually.

- Nucleic acid amplification tests are the most sensitive study to diagnose *Chlamydia trachomatis* infection and may be performed on an endocervical or urethral swab or a urine sample.

Neisseria gonorrhoeae Infection

The highest rates of *N. gonorrhoeae* infection occur in sexually active young women. However, more infections are diagnosed in men because of the high rates of infection in men who have sex with men and the greater ease of diagnosis in male patients. Although visualization of intracellular gram-negative diplococci on a cervical or urethral smear has a high specificity for *N. gonorrhoeae*, the absence of this finding is not sensitive enough to exclude infection. Nucleic acid amplification tests therefore are preferred.

N. gonorrhoeae may cause pharyngeal infection (most cases of which are asymptomatic) and disseminated gonococcal infection (DGI). DGI presents as a febrile arthritis-dermatitis syndrome with migratory polyarthralgia evolving into frank arthritis with or without tenosynovitis that involves one or more joints. *N. gonorrhoeae* infection should be considered in the differential diagnosis of monoarticular septic arthritis in a sexually active patient. Skin lesions occur in 75% of patients with DGI. The classic lesion is characterized by a small number of necrotic vesicopustules on an erythematous base. Blood and synovial fluid cultures are often negative. A high index of clinical suspicion for DGI should prompt the collection of specimens from the cervix or urethra, pharynx, and rectum for culture to make a presumptive diagnosis.

There is a high rate of coinfection with *C. trachomatis* in patients diagnosed with *N. gonorrhoeae*. Consequently, it is recommended that individuals diagnosed with *N. gonorrhoeae* be treated concurrently for both infections.

As described for sexual partners of patients with *C. trachomatis* infection, sexual partners of patients with *N. gonorrhoeae* infection should be referred for evaluation and treatment. Treatment is discussed later in this section.

KEY POINTS

- Patients with *Neisseria gonorrhoeae* infection should also be treated for *Chlamydia trachomatis* infection because of the high rate of coinfection.

- All recent sexual partners of patients with *Neisseria gonorrhoeae* or *Chlamydia trachomatis* infection should be referred for evaluation and treatment of possible infection.

Complications of Cervicitis and Urethritis

Pelvic Inflammatory Disease

Pelvic inflammatory disease (PID) is an ascending infection of the genital tract. Patients may present with endometritis, salpingitis, or both, and PID can be complicated by the development of a tubo-ovarian abscess. PID is considered a polymicrobial infection. *C. trachomatis* and *N. gonorrhoeae* cause most infections; other possible pathogens include enteric gram-negative organisms, organisms that originate from the normal vaginal flora (especially anaerobes), and streptococci. The risk of PID is particularly high in sexually active young women (especially adolescents). The possibility of PID should be considered in women who present with pelvic or lower abdominal pain, particularly if accompanied by vaginal discharge, intermenstrual bleeding, or dyspareunia. The presenting symptoms can be mild. However, a high index of suspicion for PID must be maintained, especially in sexually active young women because unrecognized and untreated infection can lead to fallopian tube scarring and infertility.

The clinical diagnosis of PID is imprecise. PID should be considered in sexually active women who present with lower abdominal or pelvic pain and one or more of the following findings: cervical motion tenderness, uterine tenderness, or adnexal tenderness. The presence of mucopurulent cervical discharge or numerous leukocytes in a wet mount of vaginal secretions increases the specificity of the diagnosis. Other findings that increase diagnostic specificity include fever (temperature >38.3 °C [100.9 °F]), an increased erythrocyte sedimentation rate or C-reactive protein concentration, and confirmation of infection caused by either *N. gonorrhoeae* or *C. trachomatis*. Patients in whom the diagnosis is suspected should be tested for these two pathogens, although recommended antimicrobial regimens for PID target all possible causative organisms. Many women with PID can be managed as outpatients with oral antibiotic therapy. Hospitalization is recommended for patients with the following criteria: (1) inability to exclude a surgical emergency as the cause of clinical findings; (2) pregnancy; (3) failure to respond to outpatient treatment with oral therapy; (4) inability to tolerate oral therapy; (5) severe signs of systemic toxicity, such as nausea, vomiting, and high fever; or (6) suspected tubo-ovarian abscess.

KEY POINTS

- The risk of pelvic inflammatory disease is particularly high in sexually active young women (especially adolescents).

- Pelvic inflammatory disease should be considered in sexually active women who present with lower abdominal or pelvic pain and one or more of the following findings: cervical motion tenderness, uterine tenderness, or adnexal tenderness.

Epididymitis

Acute epididymitis in sexually active men younger than age 35 years is most frequently due to *C. trachomatis*; *N. gonorrhoeae* also causes epididymitis in this age group. In older men, most infections occur in conjunction with urinary tract infection caused by enteric gram-negative organisms. Urinary obstruction secondary to benign prostatic hyperplasia is a common predisposing factor. Infection due to Enterobacteriaceae should also be considered in men who have sex with men who are the insertive partner in anal intercourse.

Patients with epididymitis present with unilateral pain and tenderness in the epididymis and testis (epididymitis-orchitis). The spermatic cord is enlarged and tender on palpation. The finding of leukocytes (≥10/hpf) on urine microscopic examination or positive leukocyte esterase on urine dipstick is supportive of the diagnosis. Patients with sudden onset of severe testicular pain or those without pyuria should be evaluated for possible testicular torsion. When *N. gonorrhoeae* or *C. trachomatis* infection is suspected, a urethral swab or urine sample should be obtained for nucleic acid amplification testing. Urine culture and susceptibility testing should also be done.

- Patients with epididymitis present with unilateral pain and tenderness in the epididymis and testis (epididymitis-orchitis) and an enlarged and tender spermatic cord.

Treatment

Recommendations for treatment of cervicitis, urethritis, proctitis, and associated complications are listed in **Table 26**. Antibiotic recommendations for the management of infections due to *N. gonorrhoeae* have changed significantly in the past several years because of increasing antimicrobial resistance among *N. gonorrhoeae* isolates in the United States. In 2010, the Centers for Disease Control and Prevention (CDC) recommended administration of ceftriaxone, 250 mg

intramuscularly as a single dose, for the treatment of all infections due to *N. gonorrhoeae* because of reports of decreased susceptibility of *N. gonorrhoeae* isolates to cephalosporins and increasing reports of clinical failures with lower doses of ceftriaxone (125 mg). Oral cefixime should be used only if ceftriaxone is unavailable. In addition, all patients treated for *N. gonorrhoeae* should receive azithromycin or doxycycline (azithromycin is preferred) not just because of the high rate of coinfection with *C. trachomatis*, but because of the additional activity of these agents against isolates with decreased susceptibility to cephalosporins.

Cervicitis and urethritis can be treated empirically or based on the results of diagnostic testing. Patients who are seen in the emergency department or urgent care clinic and those who are unlikely to follow up after diagnostic testing

TABLE 26. Treatment of *Chlamydia trachomatis* and *Neisseria gonorrhoeae* Infections and Their Complications

Clinical Syndrome	Preferred Regimen	Alternative Regimen
Cervicitis and urethritis (empiric therapy)	Ceftriaxone, 250 mg IM single dose **plus** azithromycin, 1 g PO single dose	Cefixime, 400 mg PO single dose **plus** doxycycline, 100 mg PO twice daily for 7 days
Chlamydia cervicitis, urethritis, or proctitis	Azithromycin, 1 g PO single dose **or** doxycycline, 100 mg PO twice daily for 7 days	Erythromycin base, 500 mg PO four times daily **or** erythromycin ethylsuccinate, 800 mg PO four times daily **or** levofloxacin, 500 mg PO daily **or** ofloxacin, 300 mg PO twice daily for 7 days
Gonococcal cervicitis, urethritis, or proctitis and pharyngeal infection[a]	Ceftriaxone, 250 mg IM single dose **plus** azithromycin, 1 g PO single dose (preferred) **or** doxycycline, 100 mg PO twice daily for 7 days	Cefixime, 400 mg PO single dose plus azithromycin, 1 g PO single dose (preferred) **or** doxycycline, 100 mg PO twice daily for 7 days; test of cure of *N. gonorrhoeae* 1 week following treatment
Disseminated gonococcal infection	Ceftriaxone, 1 g IM or IV every 24 h	Cefotaxime, 1 g IV every 8 h **or** ceftizoxime, 1 g IV every 8 h
Pelvic inflammatory disease		
Parenteral Therapy	Cefotetan, 2 g every 12 h; **or** cefoxitin, 2 g every 6 h **plus** doxycycline, 100 mg PO or IV every 12 h **or** Clindamycin, 900 mg every 8 h **plus** gentamicin, 2 mg/kg loading dose followed by 1.5 mg/kg every 8 hours or a single daily dose of 3-5 mg/kg/d	Ampicillin-sulbactam, 3 g every 6 h **plus** doxycycline, 100 mg PO or IV every 12 h
Oral/IM Therapy	Ceftriaxone, 250 mg IM single dose **plus** doxycycline, 100 mg PO twice daily for 14 days **with or without** metronidazole, 500 mg PO twice daily for 14 days **or** Cefoxitin, 2 g IM single dose, with probenecid, 1 g PO **plus** doxycycline, 100 mg PO every 12 h for 14 days **with or without** metronidazole, 500 mg PO twice daily for 14 days	
Epididymitis[b]	Ceftriaxone, 250 mg IM single dose **plus** doxycycline, 100 PO twice daily for 10 days	

IM = intramuscularly; IV = intravenously; PO = orally.

[a]Treatment for possible *Chlamydia* infection is recommended for all patients diagnosed with gonorrhea.

[b]The recommended regimen for acute epididymitis likely due to enteric gram-negative organisms is levofloxacin, 500 mg PO daily, or ofloxacin, 300 mg PO twice daily × 10 days.

should receive single-dose empiric therapy for both *N. gonorrhoeae* and *C. trachomatis* at the time of diagnosis. Patients diagnosed with any one sexually transmitted infection should be offered testing for other sexually transmitted infections, including HIV.

KEY POINTS

- Ceftriaxone, 250 mg intramuscularly as a single dose, plus azithromycin (preferred) or doxycycline is the currently recommended treatment for *Neisseria gonorrhoeae* infection.

- Patients with cervicitis and urethritis can be treated empirically, or therapy can be based on results of diagnostic testing.

- Patients diagnosed with any one sexually transmitted infection should be offered testing for other sexually transmitted infections, including HIV.

Genital Ulcers

Herpes Simplex Virus Infection

Herpes simplex virus (HSV) is the most common cause of genital ulcer disease in the United States. Up to 50% of primary genital infections are due to HSV-1, whereas recurrent genital and perianal ulcers caused by this virus are generally due to HSV-2. This distinction has clinical implications because subclinical viral shedding and recurrent ulcers are less likely in patients with HSV-1 infections. Although most patients with HSV-2 infection have mild or subclinical disease and have never been diagnosed with genital ulcers, they may still shed virus and serve as a source of transmission to others.

Patients with symptomatic primary infection have multiple genital lesions in various stages of evolution from vesicles to pustules to shallow ulcerations on an erythematous base (see MKSAP 16 Dermatology). Women may present with cervicitis, and both men and women may have urethritis. Patients often have tender inguinal lymphadenopathy and significant systemic symptoms. Patients with recurrent infection present with fewer lesions; many patients may experience a prodrome of burning or pruritus in the genital region before the appearance of ulcers. Systemic symptoms are absent. Atypical clinical presentations, including the presence of linear fissures, are well described.

The initial clinical diagnosis of genital HSV infection should always be confirmed by viral culture or nucleic acid amplification tests such as polymerase chain reaction (PCR). PCR has superior sensitivity. Confirming HSV-1 as the cause of a primary genital infection is particularly important because this information will significantly impact patient counseling regarding risk of transmission and recurrence. Serologic tests that are type specific (can reliably distinguish HSV-1 from HSV-2) can be used for patients with a negative culture or those who present with a history of genital HSV infection that was never confirmed by culture or PCR.

Antiviral medications can reduce symptoms in patients with primary and recurrent HSV infections (**Table 27**). Patients who experience frequent recurrences of genital HSV infection (six or more episodes per year) or those who have less frequent recurrences associated with severe symptoms may be offered long-term suppressive therapy (see Table 27). Because recurrences become less frequent over time, the need for ongoing suppressive therapy should be reviewed periodically. Daily suppressive therapy with valacyclovir has been shown to reduce the risk of transmission between heterosexual partners.

Patients diagnosed with genital HSV infection need to be counseled regarding the chronic nature of their infection and the risk of transmission as a result of asymptomatic viral shedding. Patients should inform sexual partners of their diagnosis, use condoms consistently, and avoid sexual activity when experiencing prodromal symptoms or ulcer outbreaks. Type-specific serologic testing of sexual partners can determine if they are at risk of acquiring infection. Pregnant women with genital HSV infection should inform their obstetrician, and later, their newborn's pediatrician, of their diagnosis.

TABLE 27. Treatment of Herpes Simplex Virus Genital Infections	
Clinical Syndrome	**Recommended Regimen**
Primary infection[a]	Acyclovir, 400 mg three times daily **or** acyclovir, 200 mg five times daily **or** famciclovir, 250 mg three times daily **or** valacyclovir, 1 g twice daily; all regimens for 7-10 days (all regimens to be given orally)
Recurrent infection	Acyclovir, 400 mg three times daily for 5 days **or** acyclovir, 800 mg twice daily for 5 days **or** acyclovir, 800 mg three times daily for 2 days **or** famciclovir, 125 mg twice daily for 5 days **or** famciclovir, 1 g twice daily for 1 day **or** famciclovir, 500 mg once followed by 250 mg twice daily for 2 days **or** valacyclovir, 500 mg twice daily for 3 days **or** valacyclovir, 1 g once daily for 5 days
Suppressive therapy	Acyclovir, 400 mg twice daily **or** famciclovir, 250 mg twice daily **or** valacyclovir, 500 mg daily[b] **or** valacyclovir, 1 g daily

[a]Therapy can be extended if healing is incomplete after 10 days of treatment.

[b]The 500-mg dose of valacyclovir may be less effective than the 1-g dose in patients who have very frequent recurrences (≥10 episodes per year).

- Although most patients with genital herpes simplex virus type 2 infections have mild or subclinical disease and have never been diagnosed with genital ulcers, they may still shed virus and serve as a source of transmission to others.

- The initial clinical diagnosis of genital herpes simplex virus infection should always be confirmed by viral culture or polymerase chain reaction.

- Patients with genital herpes simplex virus infection should be counseled to inform sexual partners of their diagnosis, use condoms consistently, and avoid sexual activity when experiencing prodromal symptoms or ulcer outbreaks.

Syphilis

In the past decade, many urban areas in the United States have reported an increase in the number of cases of syphilis, especially among men who have sex with men. Clinical manifestations are classified according to stage to assist in decisions regarding treatment and follow-up.

Primary syphilis presents as an ulcer (chancre) that appears at the site of inoculation and may occur on the mouth, external genitalia, perianal area, or anal canal. Chancres are usually single, but several lesions can develop. A typical chancre is a painless round lesion with a raised regular border that has a firm induration on palpation. Genital lesions are frequently associated with nontender inguinal lymphadenopathy. The clinical diagnosis of primary syphilis is usually confirmed by serologic testing, although very early treatment may abort the antibody response.

The most common clinical manifestation of secondary syphilis is a generalized rash that is typically nonpruritic and often involves the palms and soles. Lesions may be macular, papular, or pustular. Silvery gray erosions with an erythematous border may be visualized on mucosal surfaces (mucus patches). Patients with secondary syphilis frequently have systemic symptoms.

Patients with positive serologic tests for syphilis but no clinical manifestations of disease have latent infection. If previous positive serologic test results are available and the infection is known to have been present for 1 year or less, patients are classified as having early latent infection. All other patients are classified as having late latent infection or syphilis of unknown duration.

Tertiary syphilis includes neurologic manifestations, ocular manifestations, cardiovascular disease (aortitis), and gummas (which can occur in any organ). Tertiary neurologic manifestations include meningovascular disease and parenchymatous disease. However, patients with neurosyphilis may be asymptomatic. Cerebrospinal fluid (CSF) examination should be performed in patients with neurologic or ophthalmic symptoms or signs, evidence of active tertiary syphilis, and serologic treatment failure.

Penicillin is the treatment of choice for all stages of syphilis, and treatment recommendations are provided in **Table 28**. Serologic testing is performed to document response to therapy. A fourfold (two-dilution) change in titer is considered significant.

Patients with primary and secondary syphilis should have repeat serologic tests at 6 and 12 months after treatment. All patients diagnosed with syphilis should be tested for HIV infection. The sexual partners of patients diagnosed with any stage of syphilis should also be evaluated. Partners

TABLE 28.	Treatment of Syphilis	
Stage	**Recommended Regimen**[a]	**Alternative Regimen for Penicillin-Allergic Patients**
Primary and secondary	Benzathine penicillin G, 2.4 million units IM single dose	Doxycycline, 100 mg PO twice daily **or** tetracycline, 500 mg PO four times daily for 14 days
Early latent	Benzathine penicillin G, 2.4 million units IM single dose	Doxycycline, 100 mg PO twice daily **or** tetracycline, 500 mg PO four times daily for 14 days
Late latent or syphilis of unknown duration	Benzathine penicillin G, 2.4 million units IM at 1-week intervals for 3 doses	Doxycycline, 100 mg PO twice daily **or** tetracycline, 500 mg PO four times daily for 28 days
Neurosyphilis	Aqueous crystalline penicillin G, 18-24 million units daily given as 3-4 million units IV every 4 h or by continuous infusion for 10-14 days **or** procaine penicillin, 2.4 million units IM daily **plus** probenecid, 500 mg PO four times daily, both for 10-14 days	Ceftriaxone, 2 g IM **or** IV daily for 10-14 days[b]

IM = intramuscularly; IV = intravenously; PO = orally.

[a]Penicillin is the only effective antimicrobial agent for treatment of syphilis at any stage in pregnancy; therefore, pregnant penicillin-allergic patients should be desensitized and treated with the appropriate penicillin regimen as outlined above.

[b]Limited data are available to support the use of this alternative regimen, and the possibility of cross-reaction in penicillin-allergic patients must be considered.

exposed to a patient with primary, secondary, or early latent syphilis within the previous 3 months should be treated even if serologic test results are negative.

- Primary syphilis presents as an ulcer (chancre) at the site of inoculation; secondary syphilis is characterized by a generalized rash (especially on the palms and soles); and tertiary syphilis is associated with neurologic and ocular manifestations, cardiovascular disease, and gummas.

- Penicillin is the treatment of choice for all stages of syphilis.

- Partners exposed to a patient with primary, secondary, or early latent syphilis within the previous 3 months should also be treated for syphilis, even if serologic test results are negative.

Chancroid

Although chancroid is the most frequent cause of genital ulcer disease worldwide, it is uncommon in the United States where it is most often reported as an outbreak of infections in urban areas that typically occurs in association with trading sex for drugs, particularly crack cocaine.

Chancroid is caused by *Haemophilus ducreyi*. Lesions may be single or multiple and begin as tender, erythematous papules that become pustular and rupture to form a painful ulcer. Patients may have tender, enlarged inguinal lymph nodes that are frequently unilateral and may suppurate and drain.

The CDC recommends that a clinical diagnosis of chancroid be made in patients with all of the following criteria: (1) single or multiple painful genital ulcers, (2) no evidence to support a diagnosis of syphilis, (3) a typical clinical presentation and appearance of the ulcer, and (4) a negative test for the presence of HSV in the ulcer exudate.

Treatment of chancroid is outlined in **Table 29**. Patients must have a repeat evaluation within 1 week of treatment to document improvement. Failure to respond to therapy may indicate that the diagnosis is incorrect, and the patient should be referred to a clinician with expertise in the evaluation and management of genital ulcer disease.

- Chancroid lesions may be single or multiple and begin as tender, erythematous papules that become pustular and rupture to form a painful ulcer.

- Patients treated for chancroid must have a repeat evaluation within 1 week of beginning therapy because failure to document improvement may indicate an incorrect diagnosis.

Lymphogranuloma Venereum

Lymphogranuloma venereum (LGV) is caused by *C. trachomatis* (serovars L1, L2, and L3). Infection is only rarely reported in the United States. LGV presenting as proctitis and proctocolitis (sometimes with isolated perianal ulcers) among men who have sex with men has been recently reported in many countries in Western Europe. Classic LGV presents as a papule or ulcer at the site of inoculation that is painless and resolves without treatment. Painful unilateral inguinal lymphadenopathy then develops and is accompanied by fever and malaise. Lymph nodes may suppurate and drain. Genital specimens or lymph node drainage specimens can be tested for *C. trachomatis* using nucleic acid amplification techniques. Nucleic acid amplification testing can also be used in patients with proctitis, although these tests are not approved by the FDA for rectal specimens. Patients who have a compatible clinical presentation may be treated presumptively (see Table 29).

- Lymphogranuloma venereum typically presents as a papule or ulcer at the site of inoculation that is painless and resolves without treatment.

Genital Warts

Genital warts (condylomata acuminata) are most often due to human papillomavirus (HPV) serotypes 6 and 11, although many other serotypes can cause these lesions. HPV serotypes 16 and 18 are strongly associated with cervical cancer. Perianal warts are common in men who have sex with men and are associated with anal cancer. Warts most commonly are flesh-colored exophytic lesions that appear hyperkeratotic and are often pedunculated. Genital warts are asymptomatic in most persons. Diagnosis can be made based on the clinical appearance of the lesions.

Two HPV vaccines are currently licensed in the United States for the prevention of infection due to HPV serotypes associated with genital warts and cervical cancer. In 2011, the

TABLE 29. Treatment of Chancroid and Lymphogranuloma Venereum

Clinical Entity	Recommended Regimen
Chancroid	Azithromycin, 1 g PO single dose **or** ceftriaxone, 250 mg IM single dose **or** ciprofloxacin, 500 mg PO twice daily for 3 days **or** erythromycin base, 500 mg PO three times daily for 7 days
Lymphogranuloma venereum	Doxycycline, 100 mg PO twice daily for 21 days (preferred) **or** erythromycin base, 500 mg PO four times daily for 21 days (alternative)

IM = intramuscularly; PO = orally.

CDC's Advisory Committee on Immunization Practices (ACIP) recommended the routine vaccination of males 11 or 12 years old with three doses of the quadrivalent HPV vaccine for protection against HPV and HPV-related conditions and cancers in males. The vaccination of males with HPV may also provide indirect protection of women by reducing transmission of HPV. Catch-up vaccination is recommended for all men aged 19 to 21 years. Men aged 22 to 26 years should be vaccinated if they have underlying immunosuppression (including HIV infection) or if they are men who have sex with men. Women 19 to 26 years of age who were not previously vaccinated should also receive the HPV vaccine.

Treatment is only indicated for patients who have symptomatic lesions or who are concerned about the cosmetic appearance of the warts. However, treatment does not eliminate the possibility of HPV transmission. Patient-applied topical agents and physician-administered treatments are available.

KEY POINTS

- Genital warts most commonly present as asymptomatic, flesh-colored, exophytic lesions that appear hyperkeratotic and are often pedunculated.
- Treatment of genital warts is only indicated for patients who have symptomatic lesions or are concerned about the cosmetic appearance of the warts.

Osteomyelitis

Pathophysiology and Classification

Although normal bone is resistant to infection because it is not exposed to microbes, pathogens may reach the bone through hematogenous spread, direct inoculation following trauma or surgery, or by contiguous spread from colonized or infected adjacent soft tissues. Pathologic hallmarks of acute osteomyelitis include the presence of polymorphonuclear leukocytes, thrombosis of small vessels, and bone necrosis. The subsequent accompanying separated pieces of dead bone are known as the sequestrum. Once the sequestrum has formed and new bone formation has begun, the infection is considered chronic. Lymphocytes, histiocytes, and plasma cells are observed histologically, and sinus tracts and local bone loss are seen clinically.

Hematogenous osteomyelitis is generally a disease of children, but it also accounts for approximately 20% of cases in adults. Unlike in children in whom the most frequent sites of infection are the growing ends or metaphyses of long bones where rapid bone turnover occurs, the vertebral column is the most common location for hematogenous osteomyelitis in adults. The sternoclavicular and sacroiliac bones may be involved, especially in injection drug users. The bacteremic events responsible for hematogenous osteomyelitis may be related to intravascular catheters, distant foci of infection, or

infective endocarditis. Except in patients with endocarditis, the bacteremia is often not apparent. Typically, a single (monomicrobial) bacterial species is responsible for hematogenous osteomyelitic infection. Although most cases are caused by *Staphylococcus aureus*, aerobic gram-negative bacilli cause disease in many patients. *Pseudomonas aeruginosa* and *Salmonella* species are associated with infections in injection drug users and patients with sickle cell disease, respectively.

Osteomyelitis associated with a contiguous focus of infection, vascular insufficiency, or decubitus ulcers may be polymicrobial or monomicrobial, with *S. aureus* as the most common organism. The presence of a foreign body and weak host defenses predispose to infection with less pathogenic organisms. Pathogens found alone or in combination in patients with contiguous osteomyelitis include gram-negative bacilli, enterococci, anaerobes, and fungi.

KEY POINTS

- Although most cases of hematogenous osteomyelitis are caused by *Staphylococcus aureus*, aerobic gram-negative bacilli such as *Pseudomonas aeruginosa* and *Salmonella* species are associated with infections in injection drug users and patients with sickle cell disease, respectively.
- *Staphylococcus aureus* is the most common causative organism of contiguous osteomyelitis, vascular insufficiency, or decubitus ulcers, and infection may be polymicrobial or monomicrobial.

Clinical Manifestations

The clinical manifestations of acute osteomyelitis customarily present subacutely, usually with dull pain from the infected bone. Local erythema, warmth, edema, and palpable tenderness often follow. Pus may spread into joints, presenting as septic arthritis. Fever may or may not be present. Patients with infection of the spine or pelvic joints may have constant pain exacerbated by movement. Chronic pain following the placement of a prosthetic joint or loosening of its components should be considered suspicious for prosthetic joint infection. The clinical features of chronic osteomyelitis are similar to those of acute osteomyelitis, but the presence of a draining sinus tract is somewhat pathognomonic of chronic osteomyelitis.

KEY POINTS

- The clinical manifestations of acute osteomyelitis customarily present subacutely, usually with dull pain from the infected bone, followed by local erythema, warmth, edema, and palpable tenderness; fever may or may not be present.
- The clinical features of chronic osteomyelitis are similar to those of acute osteomyelitis, but the presence of a draining sinus tract is pathognomonic of chronic osteomyelitis.

Diagnosis

Imaging Studies

In patients with osteomyelitis, conventional plain radiographs are limited by their poor sensitivity and specificity. Soft tissue swelling may be an early finding, but osseous abnormalities can take 2 weeks to become visible.

Nuclear imaging modalities include the three-phase bone scan, gallium scanning, and tagged leukocyte scanning. A three-phase bone scan uses a radionuclide tracer (usually technetium-99m) that is injected; γ images of the area of interest are taken at specific times following injection. Osteomyelitis shows enhancement in all three phases, whereas overlying soft tissue infections do not. Gallium-67 has an affinity for acute phase reactants and will accumulate in areas of infection following injection. Tagged leukocyte scanning involves use of a radiotracer to label autologous leukocytes, which are reinjected; they will accumulate at sites of infection or inflammation. All three nuclear imaging studies have high sensitivity (>90%) for osteomyelitis. However, specificity is more variable because these studies tend to be falsely positive in patients with conditions involving inflammation or bone turnover, such as degenerative joint disease, trauma, surgery, or cancer. The specificity of these tests is significantly improved when there is no evidence of another process involving the area of interest as documented by normal plain radiography.

MRI has generally become the preferred imaging technique for diagnosing osteomyelitis. It is readily available, quickly obtained, has a high sensitivity for bone infection, and can help exclude disease in the setting of a negative study. It may show evidence of bone infection within several days of onset, can delineate bone anatomy and changes in the surrounding soft tissues, and tends to be more effective than nuclear imaging in detecting osteomyelitis in specific anatomic locations such as the feet and vertebrae. However, the specificity of MRI is limited because the bone marrow edema changes seen in patients with osteomyelitis may be from other causes and may persist for months after effective therapy. Because follow-up MRIs can be confusing and lead to additional unwarranted therapy, they are generally not necessary. However, if an MRI is obtained, findings that are most worrisome will show new areas of bone involvement.

CT scanning is a reasonable choice when MRI is contraindicated, such as in patients with cardiac pacemakers, defibrillators, metallic artifacts, or kidney failure (gadolinium contraindicated).

Laboratory Studies

Blood tests lack specificity to assist in the initial diagnosis of osteomyelitis. The leukocyte count may not be elevated, but inflammatory markers, such as the erythrocyte sedimentation rate and C-reactive protein level, are generally increased; however, normal values do not exclude the diagnosis. Blood cultures may identify bacteremia in a small fraction of cases (almost all are acute osteomyelitis). In such cases, the infecting organism is likely to be identified. Nevertheless, blood cultures are recommended in all cases of suspected osteomyelitis because identifying a microorganism may eliminate the need for more extensive testing.

Bone Biopsy

Bone biopsy is considered the gold standard for diagnosing osteomyelitis and can be done by open surgical biopsy or needle aspiration. Bone biopsies showing microorganism inflammation and osteonecrosis can corroborate the diagnosis.

With the exception of *S. aureus*, collection of microorganisms isolated from culture specimens of superficial wounds or sinus tracts correlates poorly with deep cultures from bone; therefore, this approach is of limited value. Collection of surface swab cultures should be discouraged because it can misdirect therapy.

KEY POINTS

- In patients with osteomyelitis, conventional plain radiographs are limited by their poor sensitivity and specificity because osseous abnormalities can take 2 weeks to become visible.
- MRI is the preferred imaging modality for detecting osteomyelitis and has reliable sensitivity.
- Bone biopsy can be done in patients with osteomyelitis by open surgical biopsy or needle aspiration and is diagnostic when results demonstrate microorganism inflammation and osteonecrosis.

Treatment

Treatment is initiated once the diagnosis of osteomyelitis is established and the inciting pathogen identified. Successful treatment generally requires a combination of surgical debridement, removal of orthopedic hardware (if present and feasible), and administration of appropriate antibiotics for a prolonged period (see MKSAP 16 Rheumatology). The application of vacuum-assisted closure devices and use of hyperbaric oxygen exposure are adjunctive therapies, which may offer benefit for a selective group of patients. Prognosis depends on factors such as the chronicity of disease, organisms involved, comorbidities, and physiologic state of the infected individual, as well as the ability to remove all infected hardware or prosthetic devices. In patients in whom cure cannot be achieved, chronic suppressive antibiotic treatment is warranted. Similarly, in patients with no systemic or severe local signs of infection and in whom a prosthesis is not loose or in whom surgery is not possible or desired, lifelong oral antimicrobial therapy may be considered in an attempt to suppress the infection and retain usefulness of the total joint replacement.

- Successful treatment of osteomyelitis generally requires a combination of surgical debridement, removal of orthopedic hardware (if present and feasible), and administration of appropriate antibiotics for a prolonged period.

- In patients with osteomyelitis in whom cure cannot be achieved, chronic suppressive antibiotic treatment is warranted.

Evaluation and Management of Diabetes Mellitus–Associated Osteomyelitis

In patients with diabetes mellitus, skin and soft tissue infections and subsequent ulcer formation, particularly on the feet, may progress unrecognized, eventually resulting in contiguous osteomyelitis. Therefore, patients with diabetes must be vigilant to any signs of soft tissue disease and seek evaluation expeditiously, before a potentially limb-threatening condition develops.

Important clinical signs suggestive of a deeper infectious process in patients with diabetic foot ulcers are tenderness, erythema, warmth, and the presence of purulent material in the ulcer or from a sinus tract. Gas in the soft tissues, suggested by crepitus, bullous formation, and skin color changes, may indicate necrotizing fasciitis. Severe ischemia with gangrene may also occur.

Many patients with diabetes and complex foot infection lack classic systemic signs of infection, including fever. In general, ulcers that are greater than 2 cm, are present for 2 weeks or longer, and are characterized by visible bone or a positive probe-to-bone test, are predictive of contiguous osteomyelitis.

The approach to imaging and laboratory studies in patients with diabetes-associated osteomyelitis is the same as that for patients with osteomyelitis; however, the presence of visualized bone or palpation of bone by a sterile, blunt, stainless steel probe in the depth of a foot ulcer should obviate the need for diagnostic imaging.

Combined medical and surgical therapy, wound management, glucose control, and administration of antibiotics are recommended to increase the likelihood for a successful outcome. Debridement and culture before institution of antimicrobial therapy are recommended. Early surgical intervention for debridement and drainage decreases the risk for amputations. Revascularization procedures, if indicated, improve the arterial blood supply, promoting healing and preventing further ischemic necrosis.

Broad-spectrum antimicrobial treatment is usually required as initial therapy owing to the polymicrobial nature of diabetic foot infections. Patients with severe infections or those with suspected or proven osteomyelitis generally require parenteral therapy. Oral antimicrobial therapy may be adequate for patients with milder infections involving pathogens sensitive to agents demonstrating good oral bioavailability. Although not supported by good comparative data, standard treatment regimens include monotherapy or combination therapy with agents possessing good activity against staphylococci, streptococci, aerobic gram-negative bacilli, and anaerobes. Vancomycin combined with an agent active against gram-negative organisms would be appropriate empiric therapy. Advanced-generation cephalosporins (for example, ceftriaxone and cefepime) or fluoroquinolones (for example, ciprofloxacin or levofloxacin), combined with an agent with anaerobic activity, such as metronidazole or clindamycin, are also acceptable choices. In addition, a β-lactam/β-lactamase inhibitor combination drug and a carbapenem agent such as meropenem would provide appropriate coverage. The increasing prevalence of methicillin-resistant *S. aureus* emphasizes the importance of establishing a microbiologic diagnosis. The initial empiric antimicrobial regimen should be narrowed after culture and sensitivity information becomes available, with the understanding that not every isolate from these polymicrobial infections requires treatment. The duration of antimicrobial therapy should be individualized based on the clinical circumstances. Generally, therapy should be given until the wound and the signs of infection have resolved. In patients with osteomyelitis, antimicrobial therapy is usually given for 6 weeks following surgical debridement unless the infected bone has been totally removed, in which case the medication can be stopped once the wound has adequately healed. ▪

- Diabetic foot ulcers that are generally greater than 2 cm, are present for 2 weeks or longer, and are characterized by visible bone or a positive probe-to-bone test are predictive of contiguous osteomyelitis.

- Debridement and culture before institution of antimicrobial therapy are recommended in patients with diabetes mellitus and osteomyelitis.

- In patients with osteomyelitis, antimicrobial therapy is usually given for 6 weeks following surgical debridement unless the infected bone has been totally removed, in which case the medication can be stopped after the wound has adequately healed.

Evaluation and Management of Vertebral Osteomyelitis

Infection of the vertebral bones and contiguous disk space, termed spondylodiskitis, most often occurs as a consequence of bacteremia. The segmental arteries that supply the vertebral column bifurcate, thereby permitting the infecting organism to simultaneously reach two adjacent vertebral bodies, with subsequent bony destruction. The intervertebral disk space becomes secondarily involved by direct invasion from the adjacent bones. Alternatively, these anatomic areas can become infected following spinal surgery or as a rare complication from injection or catheter placement. The lumbar spine is involved most frequently, followed by the thoracic and cervical vertebrae. *S. aureus* (including methicillin-resistant *S. aureus*) is the most commonly involved pathogen, although, coagulase-negative staphylococci may also be a cause of infection in the spine. Gram-negative bacilli, streptococci, *Candida* species, and unusual organisms (for example, *Brucella* species) may also be involved.

Progressively worsening back or neck pain over several weeks without an alternative explanation should prompt an evaluation for possible vertebral osteomyelitis. Tenderness localized over the spinal site of infection is common, and neurologic deficits may occur.

Although fever and elevated leukocyte counts are present in only half of patients, an increased erythrocyte sedimentation rate (often >100 mm/h) and C-reactive protein level are present in more than 80% of patients. Obtaining blood cultures, which are positive in more than 50% of patients, is essential, because isolation of a probable pathogen can minimize the extent of the evaluation and facilitate focused antibiotic therapy.

The lack of sensitivity of plain radiographs limits their utility in patients with vertebral osteomyelitis. MRI offers the best sensitivity, but false-positive scans may occur in patients with uninfected fractures. Radionuclide scans may be helpful diagnostic aids but, with the exception of gallium scans, lack sufficient specificity. A CT-guided percutaneous needle aspiration biopsy and culture are needed to confirm the diagnosis when blood cultures are negative. Even in patients in whom the first sample is nondiagnostic, a second biopsy attempt can help to determine the microbial cause. Ideally, biopsy attempts should be performed before antibiotics are given, but biopsy should not be avoided in patients already receiving therapy.

The mainstay of vertebral osteomyelitis treatment includes prolonged pathogen-directed, or occasionally, empiric parenteral antimicrobial therapy. In patients in whom a pathogen is not isolated, an empiric regimen including a reliable agent aimed at gram-positive cocci, such as vancomycin, with a broad-spectrum antibiotic against gram-negative bacilli, such as cefepime or ceftriaxone, would be reasonable. Oral antimicrobial agents are generally not used for treatment of vertebral osteomyelitis except in specific situations, such as when a fluoroquinolone (ciprofloxacin)-sensitive gram-negative bacillus proves to be the infecting pathogen, or possibly, when long-term chronic antimicrobial suppression is warranted, such as in patients with retained orthopedic hardware.

Antimicrobial therapy is generally given for 6 to 8 weeks, but prolonged therapy may be necessary in patients with extensive or advanced disease. Surgical intervention is rarely required except when it is necessary to stabilize the spine, drain an abscess, or pursue the diagnosis in patients in whom empiric treatment is not effective. **H**

Follow-up MRI is usually not warranted except for patients in whom improvement is expected but not achieved, when complications develop, or when inflammatory markers remain elevated without explanation.

KEY POINTS

- Progressively worsening back or neck pain over several weeks without an alternative explanation and localized tenderness over the spinal site of infection should prompt an evaluation for possible vertebral osteomyelitis.

- An increased erythrocyte sedimentation rate (often >100 mm/h) and C-reactive protein level are present in more than 80% of patients with vertebral osteomyelitis.

- Obtaining blood cultures, which are positive in more than 50% of patients, is essential in diagnosing patients with vertebral osteomyelitis.

- A CT-guided percutaneous needle aspirate biopsy and culture are needed to confirm the diagnosis of vertebral osteomyelitis when blood cultures are negative.

Fever of Unknown Origin

Introduction

Fever is a complex cytokine-mediated response of the body to many infectious and noninfectious causes. Although the source of fever is often determined by a thorough history, physical examination, and basic laboratory studies, the cause cannot be established in a subgroup of patients who are said to have fever of unknown origin (FUO). FUO is classically defined as an illness that lasts at least 3 weeks in a patient with a temperature greater than 38.3 °C (101.0 °F) on several occasions and whose diagnosis remains uncertain despite having been evaluated in a hospital for at least 1 week.

However, because of improved diagnostic methods, it has been suggested that the classic definition of FUO should be changed, with a particular focus on specific risk groups:

- Classic FUO: temperature higher than 38.0 °C (100.4 °F) for more than 3 weeks and either more than 3 days of hospital investigation or more than two outpatient visits without determination of the cause.

- Health care–associated FUO: temperature higher than 38.0 °C (100.4 °F) for more than 3 days in a hospitalized patient receiving acute care with infection not present or incubating on admission.

- Immune-deficient FUO: temperature higher than 38.0 °C (100.4 °F) in a patient in whom the diagnosis remains uncertain after more than 3 days despite appropriate investigation, including at least 48 hours' incubation of microbiologic cultures.

- HIV-related FUO: temperature higher than 38.0 °C (100.4 °F) in a patient with confirmed HIV infection for more than 3 weeks in outpatients or more than 3 days in inpatients. ◫

Causes

Although some FUOs are due to infections, other broad diagnostic categories include noninfectious inflammatory disorders (connective tissue diseases, vasculitis syndromes, and granulomatous diseases), malignancies, and other specific disorders. Historically, infections were considered the most likely cause of fever, followed by noninfectious inflammatory disorders and malignancies. More recently, infections and malignancies have become less commonly associated with FUO, and undetermined causes are increasing in prevalence. However, even with current diagnostic methods, the cause remains undetermined in a significant number of patients.

The patient's age may provide a clue to diagnosis. Infections and malignancies are responsible for most FUOs in adults; however, malignancy is an uncommon cause in children. Noninfectious multisystemic inflammatory disorders (polymyalgia rheumatica, temporal arteritis, and rheumatoid arthritis) are most frequently associated with FUO in older patients.

The duration of fever is also important in diagnosing FUOs. For example, factitious fever and granulomatous diseases should be strongly considered in patients with a history of unexplained fever of more than 6 months.

Immune status should also be considered because this may alter the differential diagnosis of potential causes. The number of immunocompromised persons (transplant recipients and patients receiving cancer therapy) and patients with stable AIDS infection has increased in recent years. In patients with neutropenia and fever, the initial diagnostic consideration should include bacterial infection, particularly because an impaired immune response may change the typical presentation of many infections. Persistent fever may also be due to fungi, including infections caused by *Aspergillus* and *Candida* species. In patients with AIDS and a low CD4 cell count, the most common causes of FUO are infections (particularly mycobacterial infections), followed by malignancies such as non-Hodgkin lymphoma.

In all patients with FUO, the response to empiric antimicrobial therapy may provide a clue as to whether a bacterial infection may be the underlying cause. An initial response with relapse may suggest a localized infection, such as an abscess. No response may be associated with an atypical infection or a noninfectious cause.

Occult abscesses in the kidneys, liver, and spleen may not always have well-defined localizing features, especially in elderly or immunocompromised patients. Blood culture results are not always positive, and other serologic test results may be insensitive in these patients. Similarly, patients with vertebral osteomyelitis may not have localizing symptoms.

Infective endocarditis was once a common cause of FUO. However, modern microbiologic techniques are effective in identifying causative pathogens, including the HACEK organisms (*Haemophilus aphrophilus*, *Actinobacillus actinomycetemcomitans*, *Cardiobacterium hominis*, *Eikenella corrodens*, and *Kingella kingae*). Exceptions are pathogens associated with culture-negative infective endocarditis, including *Coxiella burnetii*, *Tropheryma whipplei*, and *Brucella*, *Bartonella*, *Chlamydia*, *Histoplasma*, and *Legionella* species. Tuberculosis may not always be suspected as a cause of FUO, particularly in patients without a clear exposure history and without pulmonary symptoms or findings. This is particularly true in immunocompromised patients with atypical clinical manifestations, such as those with extrapulmonary involvement.

Patients with acute HIV infection may present with fever and various other findings. Enzyme-linked immunosorbent assays (ELISA) for HIV can be negative during early infection; a repeat ELISA or a viral load determination may be necessary for diagnosis. Because fever is an integral part of the mononucleosis syndromes, Epstein-Barr virus and cytomegalovirus infections should always be considered. Results of mononucleosis testing may be negative in up to 15% of younger patients, and the presentation of Epstein-Barr virus infection in older adults may differ from that seen in younger individuals. Toxoplasmosis can cause fever and lymphadenopathy, but the acute illness is seldom diagnosed or treated except in the setting of pregnancy.

Neoplastic-associated causes of FUO include lymphoma, posttransplant lymphoproliferative disorders, leukemia, myelodysplastic syndromes, renal cell carcinoma, hepatocellular carcinoma, liver metastases, colon cancer, and atrial myxoma. A clue to cancer-related fever is that patients often appear less toxic and may not be aware of having fever. Noninfectious inflammatory disorders to be considered include systemic lupus erythematosus, cryoglobulinemia, polyarteritis nodosa, and granulomatosis with polyangiitis (also known as Wegener granulomatosis). Adult-onset Still disease should be considered in a patient with arthritis, evanescent rash, fever, neutrophilic leukocytosis, pharyngitis, lymphadenopathy, hepatosplenomegaly, and abnormal liver chemistry test results. Giant cell arteritis should be suspected in patients over 50 years of age who present with jaw claudication, headache, visual disturbances, a significantly elevated erythrocyte sedimentation rate, and polymyalgia rheumatica.

Medications may be associated with FUO. Drug fever may cause rash and eosinophilia and can be diagnosed when fever resolves after discontinuation of the causative agent.

Hereditary periodic fever syndromes are rare but should be considered when fever-free intervals of at least 14 days occur in patients with recurrent FUO. These include hyper-immunoglobulin D syndrome (HIDS), tumor-necrosis factor receptor-1–associated periodic syndrome (TRAPS), Muckle-Wells syndrome, and familial Mediterranean fever.

Familial Mediterranean fever is an autosomal recessive disease occurring in certain ethnic groups, including persons of Jewish, Armenian, Arab, and Turkish descent, and is characterized by serositis, arthritis, chest and abdominal pain, and rarely, a distal lower extremity rash. Patients with the Muckle-Wells syndrome, an autosomal dominant disorder resulting from a defective gene that encodes the cryopyrin protein, exhibit progressive sensorineural hearing loss; episodic urticarial rash, fever, abdominal pain, and arthralgia/arthritis; and possibly, eventual amyloidosis. HIDS, an autosomal recessive disease, presents at a very young age and manifests as recurrent episodes of fever, abdominal pain, diarrhea, lymphadenopathy, maculopapular rash, and joint pain; elevated serum IgD and IgA levels are characteristic. TRAPS is an autosomal dominant syndrome characterized by recurrent presentations of fever; tender, erythematous patches; periorbital edema; conjunctivitis; abdominal pain; arthritis; and testicular pain.

Miscellaneous causes of FUO include subacute thyroiditis or hyperthyroidism, sarcoidosis, pulmonary embolism, retroperitoneal or abdominal hematoma, pheochromocytoma, factitious fever, and habitual hyperthermia.

KEY POINTS

- Fever of unknown origin may be due to infections, noninfectious inflammatory disorders, malignancies, and many other disorders.

- Infections that commonly cause fever of unknown origin include tuberculosis, infective endocarditis, and intra-abdominal and pelvic abscesses.

- Hereditary periodic fever syndromes, such as hyper-immunoglobulin D syndrome, tumor-necrosis factor receptor-1–associated periodic syndrome, Muckle-Wells syndrome, and familial Mediterranean fever, should be considered when fever-free intervals of at least 14 days occur in patients with recurrent fever of unknown origin.

Evaluation

A comprehensive history and thorough physical examination, which should be repeated as the illness evolves, are essential in the evaluation of patients with FUO. The history should determine the presence of immunocompromising conditions or a predisposition to infective endocarditis (including injection drug use and valvular abnormalities), as well as medications, immunizations, hobbies, travel, sexual activity (including a history of sexually transmitted infections), and recent contacts with domestic or farm animals, insects, and ill persons. The physical examination should include pelvic, rectal, and temporal artery evaluation. The presence of rash, lymphadenopathy, cardiac murmurs, hepatosplenomegaly, and arthritic changes can provide valuable clues to the diagnosis.

Initial laboratory studies may include a complete blood count, erythrocyte sedimentation rate, measurement of C-reactive protein, peripheral blood smear, complete metabolic profile with liver chemistry studies, urinalysis with microscopic evaluation, and urine and blood cultures. Further testing should be done based on potential causes as assessed during the history and physical examination and may include an antinuclear antibody assay, measurement of rheumatoid factor, serum and urine protein electrophoresis, and serologic studies for hepatitis, syphilis, HIV, cytomegalovirus, Epstein-Barr virus, and *C. burnetii* (Q fever); tuberculosis testing (skin and interferon-γ release assays) may also be appropriate. Imaging should be directed by the potential cause of the FUO, and extensive studies based solely on the presence of an FUO should not be done. Based on the history and physical examination, a chest radiograph, echocardiogram, and CT scans of the abdomen, chest, and pelvis may be appropriate, depending on clinical considerations. Nuclear imaging studies are considered useful by some clinicians in identifying an inflammatory source of fever when initial imaging studies are normal. Further evaluation, including biopsies, is dictated by results of abnormal tests. Bone marrow examination may be useful in patients with anemia and thrombocytopenia.

Up to 50% of patients with FUO will not have an identified cause despite an extensive evaluation. The prognosis is generally good for these patients because symptoms tend to resolve within months of development. Although empiric antibiotics with or without corticosteroids are often considered, their use should be discouraged if the patient is stable and has no localizing signs. **H**

KEY POINTS

- A comprehensive history and thorough physical examination, which often needs to be repeated as the illness evolves, are essential in the evaluation of a patient with fever of unknown origin.

- Laboratory testing and imaging studies of patients with fever of unknown origin should be directed by the potential cause and findings on history and physical examination.

- Up to 50% of patients with fever of unknown origin will not have an identified cause despite an extensive evaluation.

Primary Immunodeficiencies

Introduction

Although uncommon, primary immunodeficiency syndromes should be considered in patients with frequent, multiple, or prolonged infections caused by certain pathogens such as *Streptococcus pneumoniae*, *Neisseria* species, and *Haemophilus influenzae*. Primary immunodeficiency syndromes are relatively rare and generally manifest in children.

Selective IgA Deficiency

Selective absence of serum and secretory IgA, inherited as an incompletely penetrant autosomal dominant or autosomal recessive trait, is the most common primary immunodeficiency and has a worldwide prevalence of approximately 1 in 300 to 700 persons. IgA is the major immunoglobulin in external secretions (for example, saliva, tears, nasal secretions) and blocks the binding of antigens (pathogens and toxins) to cell receptors. It binds antigens and facilitates their clearance by ciliated epithelium. Most patients with selective IgA deficiency develop few or no recurrent infections, although some have chronic or recurrent respiratory tract infections, atopic disorders, and an increased frequency of autoimmune disorders. Gastrointestinal and urogenital tract infections may also occur. Other immunoglobulin concentrations are usually normal, although an IgG_2 subclass deficiency has been reported in patients with the most morbidity, and IgM concentrations may be abnormal. Serum autoantibodies to IgA are found in up to 40% of patients with recurrent infections. Some patients have severe anaphylactic reactions to administration of intravenous immune globulin or blood products.

Common Variable Immunodeficiency

Common variable immunodeficiency (CVID) occurs in both adults and children. Most patients present before age 30 years. Approximately 1 in 25,000 persons is affected worldwide, and the disorder is more prevalent among those of northern European descent. CVID is caused by impaired B cell differentiation and defective immunoglobulin production. Serum IgG levels are markedly reduced, and serum IgA or IgM levels (or both) are frequently low.

Patients with CVID frequently develop chronic lung diseases, autoimmune disorders, malabsorption, recurrent infections, and lymphoma, and their response to vaccination is poor or absent. Sinopulmonary infections, ear infections, and conjunctivitis are common and are most often caused by pneumococci, *Mycoplasma* species, and *Haemophilus influenzae*. Some patients are also susceptible to infection with enteroviruses, *Candida* species, and *Giardia lamblia*. Septic arthritis and chronic pulmonary diseases (bronchiectasis, restrictive or obstructive lung disease) have also been reported. Gastrointestinal diseases occur in approximately 20% of patients with CVID and include inflammatory bowel disease, sprue-like disorders, and pernicious anemia. Approximately 25% of patients have an autoimmune disorder, such as rheumatoid arthritis or hemolytic anemia and thrombocytopenia. Up to 20% of patients have evidence of granulomatous disease associated with noncaseating granulomas in lymphoid or solid organs.

Patients with CVID usually show impaired responses to vaccines. If CVID is suspected, quantitative serum IgG, IgA, and IgM levels should be measured. If levels are low, antibody response to vaccination should be tested by determining the response to protein- and polysaccharide-based vaccines. Such testing is not needed in patients with very low (<200 mg/dL [2.0 g/L]) or undetectable serum IgG levels because these patients will most likely not respond to vaccines.

Use of immune globulin replacement therapy has reduced the number of recurrent infections in patients with CVID. Prophylactic antibiotics should not be routinely administered to all patients but should be reserved for those with chronic lung disease and those who require oral corticosteroids or immunosuppressive agents for more than 1 month.

Abnormalities in the Complement System

Complement deficiency states may be inherited or acquired. Complement deficiencies predispose to bacterial infections and autoimmune disorders. The frequency of inherited complement deficiencies in the general population is about 0.03%. Most complement deficiencies are inherited as autosomal recessive traits. However, C1 inhibitor deficiency is inherited as an autosomal dominant trait, and properdin deficiency is an X-linked disorder. Deficiencies of C3, factor H, factor I, and properdin are associated with severe recurrent infections caused by encapsulated organisms such as *Streptococcus pneumoniae*. Deficiency of the terminal complement components C5, C6, C7, and C8 increases susceptibility to disseminated neisserial infections (primarily due to meningococci but also to gonococci), which tend to be recurrent and have mild to moderate clinical manifestations. Inherited defects of the alternative complement pathway, including factor D and properdin, are rare. Patients with properdin deficiency are at risk for neisserial infections. Recurrent pneumonia and otitis media have also been reported in these patients. Systemic lupus erythematosus (SLE) is the most common autoimmune disorder in patients with complement deficiencies. Autoimmune disease (most commonly SLE) is more common in those with inherited complement deficiencies, especially those with C1, C4, C2, or C3 deficiency.

When a complement pathway defect is suspected, patients should be tested for total hemolytic complement (CH_{50}). If the serum CH_{50} concentration is very low or undetectable, specific complement components should be measured.

Vaccination is the most effective way to prevent infections in patients with complement deficiencies. All routine vaccinations (especially meningococcal, pneumococcal, and *Haemophilus influenzae* vaccines) should be administered. Conjugate vaccines are preferred to polysaccharide vaccines in these patients.

KEY POINTS

- Patients with common variable immunodeficiency frequently develop chronic lung diseases, autoimmune disorders, malabsorption, recurrent infections, and lymphoma, and their response to vaccination is poor or absent.

- In patients with suspected chronic variable immunodeficiency and low serum immunoglobulin levels, the antibody response to vaccination should be tested to help establish the diagnosis.

- When a complement pathway defect is suspected, patients should be tested for total hemolytic complement (CH_{50}).

- Vaccination is the most effective way to prevent infections in patients with complement deficiency.

Bioterrorism

Introduction

Bioterrorism is defined as the intentional release of bacteria, viruses, or toxins for the purpose of harming or killing civilians.

A bioterrorism attack results in an increased incidence of a disease (epidemic) above its usual rate in a population (endemic), which occurs suddenly and within a relatively confined geographic area (outbreak). Biologic agents that can potentially be used are prioritized into three classes (A, B, and C), based on their ability to cause illness and death, capacity for dissemination, public perception as related to plausible civil disruption, and special needs required for effective public health intervention. Class A agents have the greatest potential for causing a major public health impact associated with a high mortality rate and are discussed in this chapter (**Table 30**).

In general, class B agents (for example, *Coxiella burnetii*, *Brucella* species, *Salmonella* species, *Vibrio cholerae*) are disseminated less easily, result in less morbidity and lower mortality rates, and would be expected to have a lower medical and public health impact. Class C agents include emerging pathogens (for example, Nipah virus, hantavirus) that are currently not believed to have a high risk for use as bioterrorism agents but could have the potential for wide dissemination in the future.

Except for smallpox (eradicated by vaccine), all of the major bioterrorism agents are naturally occurring. Epidemiologic features may help distinguish a bioterrorism attack from a naturally occurring disease. Illness due to bioterrorism is more likely to be associated with suddenness of onset, a large number of cases, increased severity or an uncommon clinical presentation, and an unusual geographic, temporal, or demographic clustering of cases. Syndromic surveillance refers to using health-related data to signal the probability that a case or an outbreak of illness is related to bioterrorism and therefore warrants a further public health response.

TABLE 30. Class A Bioterrorism Agents

Disease - Agent	Incubation Period	Clinical Features	Treatment	Prophylaxis
Anthrax – *Bacillus anthracis*	1 to 60 days	Inhalational (febrile respiratory distress); cutaneous (necrotic eschar); gastrointestinal (distention, peritonitis)	Ciprofloxacin or doxycycline plus 1 or 2 additional agents[a]	Ciprofloxacin or doxycycline
Smallpox virus – variola virus	7 to 17 days	Fever followed by pustular cutaneous rash	Supportive care	Vaccine if exposure was in the past 3 days
Plague – *Yersinia pestis*	1 to 6 days	Fulminant pneumonia and sepsis	Streptomycin or gentamicin	Doxycycline or ciprofloxacin
Botulism – *Clostridium botulinum*	2 hours to 8 days	Cranial nerve palsies and descending flaccid paralysis	Antitoxin and supportive care	Antibotulinum antitoxin
Tularemia – *Francisella tularensis*	3 to 5 days	Fever, respiratory distress, and sepsis	Streptomycin or gentamicin (severe disease); doxycycline or ciprofloxacin (nonsevere disease)	Doxycycline or ciprofloxacin
Viral hemorrhagic fever – various viruses	Variable	Hemorrhage and multiorgan failure	Supportive care	None available

[a]Penicillin, ampicillin, imipenem, meropenem, clindamycin, rifampin, vancomycin, or clarithromycin.

- Bioterrorism is defined as the intentional release of bacteria, viruses, or toxins for the purpose of harming or killing civilians.
- Biologic agents that can potentially be used for bioterrorism are prioritized into three classes (A, B, and C), with class A agents having the greatest potential for causing a major public health impact associated with a high mortality rate.

Anthrax

Anthrax infection is caused by the bacterium *Bacillus anthracis* ("coal" in Greek) to describe the distinctive black eschar associated with cutaneous disease. This gram-positive, "box-car"–shaped, aerobic, nonmotile bacillus is found in soil worldwide, predominantly in agricultural areas (**Figure 9A**). Under favorable environmental conditions, it transforms into 1- to 5-micron spores that may remain viable for decades (**Figure 9B**). Spores may be acquired by inhalation, cutaneous contact, or ingestion. Cutaneous anthrax is most common, but inhalational anthrax is most likely to be lethal. Gastrointestinal anthrax is uncommon in humans.

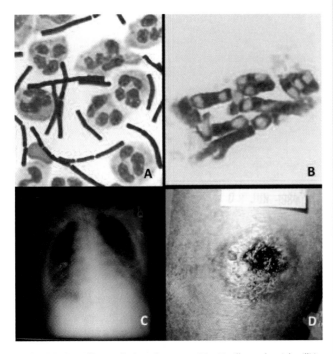

FIGURE 9. *A,* "box-car"–shaped, gram-positive *Bacillus anthracis* bacilli in the cerebrospinal fluid of the index case of inhalational anthrax due to bioterrorism in the United States; *B,* terminal and subterminal spores of *B. anthracis; C,* widened mediastinum on chest radiograph due to hemorrhagic lymphadenopathy in a patient with anthrax; *D,* black eschar lesion of cutaneous anthrax.

Because spores are easily dispersed by aerosolization and infective spores can be sent by mail (for example, the October 2001 occurrence of bioterrorism-related anthrax in the United States), even a single case of inhalational anthrax should raise the possibility of deliberate spread. Inhaled spores are transported to draining mediastinal lymph nodes. After an incubation period of 1 to 6 days (potentially up to 60 days), a prodromal "flu-like" illness characterized by low-grade fever, malaise, fatigue, myalgia, and headache occurs. Cough, dyspnea, and chest pain are rapidly followed by fulminant septic shock and death.

B. anthracis is diagnosed by culture or polymerase chain reaction (PCR) of blood, tissue, or fluid samples. The presence of mediastinal widening on a chest radiograph or CT scan is suggestive of inhalational anthrax in the right clinical setting (**Figure 9C**).

Inhalational anthrax is initially treated with intravenous ciprofloxacin or doxycycline combined with one or two additional antibiotics (see Table 30); total treatment course is 60 days, although oral antibiotics may be substituted for intravenous agents after the first 10 to 14 days. Postexposure prophylaxis with ciprofloxacin or doxycycline should be started as soon as possible following an actual or suspected anthrax attack. Although not licensed by the FDA for this purpose, a cell-free anthrax vaccine is available for postexposure immunization and is administered intramuscularly as a three-dose series in conjunction with the postexposure antibiotic regimen.

Cutaneous anthrax develops on exposed areas of the body after contact with infective spores and may occur even when skin is intact. A small pruritic papule forms at the inoculation site 1 to 7 days after exposure, followed by a vesicle and then an ulcer that evolves into a flat black eschar (**Figure 9D**). Most lesions occur on the head, neck, or extremities. Vesicular fluid and biopsy samples should be sent for culture and PCR, preferably before beginning antibiotic therapy. Unless there is definite evidence that the infection was naturally acquired, a 60-day course of ciprofloxacin or doxycycline is recommended as first-line therapy. Antibiotics do not affect the evolution of skin lesions. However, if cutaneous anthrax is not treated, the mortality rate is estimated to be 10% to 20% because of secondary bacteremic spread.

Gastrointestinal anthrax is uncommon in humans and usually results from the ingestion of undercooked meat contaminated with spores of *B. anthracis* from an infected animal. A high mortality rate (25% to 60%) is reported and is probably the result of late diagnosis and delay in treatment.

Although meningitis or meningoencephalitis may develop in patients with all three forms of anthrax, most central nervous system involvement occurs in patients with inhalational disease. It is often hemorrhagic and may rarely be the presenting manifestation of anthrax. However, the cerebrospinal fluid is not the initial site of infection. Prognosis is extremely poor.

- Because anthrax spores are easily dispersed by aerosolization and infective spores can be sent by mail, even a single case of inhalational anthrax should raise the possibility of a bioterrorism attack.

- Clinical manifestations of inhalational anthrax include low-grade fever, malaise, fatigue, myalgia, headache, cough, dyspnea, and chest pain, which are rapidly followed by fulminant septic shock and death.

- Inhalational anthrax is treated with a 60-day course of ciprofloxacin or doxycycline combined with one or two additional antibiotics.

- Cutaneous anthrax is characterized by a small pruritic papule followed by a vesicle and then an ulcer that evolves into a flat black eschar; most lesions occur on the head, neck, or extremities.

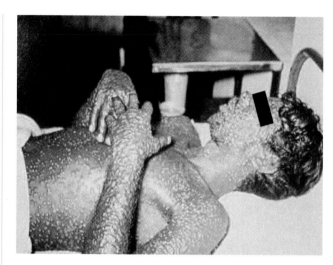

FIGURE 10. Diffuse synchronous skin lesions of smallpox.

Smallpox (Variola)

Smallpox is caused by variola, a selective human-only virus. Although it was once the leading cause of death due to an infectious agent, smallpox has been eradicated worldwide. The virus now exists in only a few laboratory repositories, and routine civilian vaccination against smallpox was suspended in the United States in 1971. The disease is easily acquired, because inhaling only a few virions carried on airborne droplets from an infected patient is sufficient to cause infection. Aerosol infectivity, the high degree of contagion, and widespread susceptibility because of a large nonimmunized population make smallpox a serious bioterrorism threat.

An initially asymptomatic respiratory tract infection and subsequent viremia develop during a 7- to 17-day incubation period. High fever, headache, vomiting, and backache then occur and last for 2 to 4 days, during which time the patient is extremely ill. The rash first appears on the buccal and pharyngeal mucosa and most often spreads to the hands and face and then to the arms, legs, and feet. The centrifugally distributed skin lesions evolve synchronously (same stage of maturation on any one area of the body) from macules to papules to vesicles to pustules and eventually become crusted (**Figure 10**). Patients remain contagious until all scabs and crusts are shed. Blindness due to keratitis or corneal ulceration is a serious complication. The overall mortality rate is about 30%.

Smallpox should be differentiated from varicella (chickenpox) (see Viral Infections), in which the rash starts centrally on the trunk and spreads toward the periphery, although the greatest number of lesions remain concentrated on the trunk (centripetal distribution). Unlike smallpox lesions, varicella lesions show differing stages of maturation on any one area of the body. A much milder form of smallpox, also known as variola minor or alastrim, has a typical febrile prodrome and rash, but is associated with a mortality rate of less than 1%.

The diagnosis of smallpox is primarily clinical, although PCR assays are available. The Centers for Disease Control and Prevention (CDC) provides a useful diagnostic tool (http://emergency.cdc.gov/agent/smallpox/diagnosis/#diagnosis). There is currently no established treatment for smallpox, although the antiviral agent cidofovir may have some therapeutic efficacy. Postexposure vaccination with vaccinia virus should be performed, with attention to its known potential adverse complications. One strategy, referred to as "ring vaccination," targets vaccination of close contacts of patients with smallpox who will be at greatest risk of contracting the disease. When given within 3 days of exposure, this active immunization can prevent or significantly lessen the severity of smallpox symptoms in most people.

- The smallpox rash first appears on the buccal and pharyngeal mucosa and spreads to the hands and face and then to the arms, legs, and feet; lesions evolve synchronously from macules to papules to vesicles to pustules and eventually become crusted.

- There is currently no established treatment for smallpox, although the antiviral agent cidofovir may have some therapeutic efficacy.

Plague

Plague, also known as the "Black Death," has been responsible for several pandemics. The infection is caused by the bacterium *Yersinia pestis*, a gram-negative coccobacillus that generally infects rodents and is transmitted to humans by the bite of an infected flea.

Bubonic plague is characterized by purulent lymphadenitis near the inoculation site and is more common in the naturally occurring zoonotic form of infection. Septicemic plague refers to the syndrome of overwhelming *Y. pestis* bacteremia, which is often characterized by disseminated intravascular coagulation and multiorgan dysfunction usually following primary cutaneous exposure. Primary pneumonic plague is caused by direct inhalation of respiratory droplets from infected humans or animals (particularly domestic cats) or potentially as a result of intentional aerosol release of pathogens. Since primary lung infection and human-to-human spread with *Y. pestis* are extremely rare, a case of pneumonic plague should suggest bioterrorism. Secondary pneumonic plague refers to hematogenous spread of *Y. pestis* to the lungs in patients with untreated bubonic or septicemic disease.

After a short incubation period of 1 to 6 days, patients with pneumonic plague present with sudden fever, chest discomfort, a productive cough, hemoptysis, and radiographic evidence of bronchopneumonia. Sputum Gram stain (and possibly blood smear) may identify gram-negative bacilli demonstrating the classic bipolar staining or "safety pin" shape.

Without rapid treatment, the mortality rate approaches 100%. Streptomycin and gentamicin are the antibiotics of choice, and doxycycline and fluoroquinolones are alternative agents. The antibiotics are continued for 10 days. Respiratory droplet isolation precautions must be instituted for at least 48 hours after starting antibiotic therapy. Postexposure prophylactic antibiotics (doxycycline or a fluoroquinolone for 7 days) should be given to asymptomatic persons known to have been exposed to aerosolized *Y. pestis* or to those who have had close contact with an infected patient. No effective vaccine for prevention of primary pneumonic plague is currently available. **H**

KEY POINTS

- Because primary pneumonic plague is extremely rare, an identified case should suggest the possibility of bioterrorism.

- Patients with pneumonic plague present with sudden fever, chest discomfort, a productive cough, hemoptysis, and radiographic evidence of bronchopneumonia.

- Streptomycin and gentamicin are the antibiotics of choice for treating pneumonic plague.

- Postexposure prophylactic antibiotics (doxycycline or a fluoroquinolone for 7 days) should be given to asymptomatic persons known to have been exposed to aerosolized *Y. pestis* or to those who have had close contact with an infected patient.

Botulism

Botulinum toxin is the most lethal biologic substance known. The toxin is produced by the anaerobic, gram-positive, spore-forming bacillus *Clostridium botulinum*. After the toxin enters the systemic circulation, it is transported to sites of acetylcholine-mediated neurotransmission. Because the toxin prevents release of acetylcholine, muscular contractions cannot occur and flaccid paralysis results.

Of the seven distinct antigenic forms of botulinum toxin, almost all human cases of botulism have been caused by serotypes A, B, and E. Ingestion of preformed toxin from exposure to home-canned foods or in vivo toxin production after spore germination following ingestion (infant botulism with honey) or wound contamination are the most common forms of botulism illness.

Aerosol-disseminated botulism (lethal inhaled toxin dose, 0.70 to 0.90 micrograms) and foodborne botulism would be the most likely types identified in a bioterrorism attack. Contaminating the water supply with botulinum toxin is believed to be an impractical and unlikely scenario. Clinical manifestations develop within 24 to 72 hours of toxin exposure (possibly more quickly following inhalation) and consist of a classic triad of (1) descending flaccid paralysis with prominent bulbar signs, (2) normal body temperature, and (3) normal mental status. Bulbar signs include the "4 Ds": Diplopia, Dysarthria, Dysphonia, and Dysphagia. Paralysis may progress to involve the respiratory muscles. The differential diagnosis includes the Guillain-Barré syndrome and myasthenia gravis, which are the two disorders that most closely mimic the clinical syndrome of botulism.

The presumptive diagnosis is based on the clinical presentation. Confirmation depends on identifying botulinum toxin from samples of the patient's blood, stool, gastric contents, and wound swabs, as well as from suspected foods. The standard method of identification is a mouse bioassay conducted at the CDC laboratories. Treatment includes supportive care and early administration of an equine-derived trivalent antitoxin available from the CDC through state and local health departments. However, the antitoxin will not reverse existing paralysis. **H**

KEY POINTS

- Clinical manifestations of botulism consist of a classic triad of (1) descending flaccid paralysis with prominent bulbar signs [diplopia, dysarthria, dysphonia, and dysphagia], (2) normal body temperature, and (3) normal mental status.

- Treatment of botulism includes supportive care and the early administration of an equine-derived trivalent antitoxin.

Tularemia

Tularemia is a widespread zoonotic disease caused by a small, fastidious, gram-negative coccobacillus, *Francisella tularensis*. The organism occurs naturally throughout North America and Eurasia and has been isolated from over 250 species of wildlife. Humans become infected via arthropod bites (predominantly ticks), ingestion of contaminated food or water, handling of infectious animal tissue, and inhalation of aerosols. Exposure to very few organisms is sufficient to produce disease. No human-to-human transmission occurs.

Tularemia is characterized by several distinct presentations. A bioterrorism attack would probably involve aerosolized *F. tularensis,* with the principal presentations being pneumonic, typhoidal, septicemic, and potentially, oropharyngeal. Following a usual incubation period of 3 to 5 days, all patients develop the abrupt onset of fever, chills, myalgia, and anorexia. A dry cough is common in all forms of the disease, and a sore throat, abdominal pain, and diarrhea may be present. Relative bradycardia (pulse-temperature dissociation) may be noted.

Patients with pneumonic tularemia from either hematogenous spread or direct inhalation have no or minimal sputum production, substernal tightness, and pleuritic chest pain. Severe respiratory failure may develop. Chest radiograph findings show subsegmental or lobar infiltrates (including ovoid densities) and pleural effusions. Hilar lymphadenopathy is common. All forms of tularemia may spread to various organs and be associated with septic shock.

The diagnosis relies on a high index of clinical suspicion. Samples of blood, tissue, sputum, or fluid aspirates should be collected. Because *F. tularensis* is highly infectious, samples should only be sent to Biosafety Level 3 laboratories, and laboratory personnel must be notified in advance to take necessary precautions. *F. tularensis* does not grow readily on routine culture media, and serologic studies are generally needed to confirm the diagnosis. However, the natural delay in the development of antibody titers makes serologic studies impractical for rapid diagnosis after an intentional release. PCR and immunofluorescence testing may be performed directly on tissue specimens. A granulomatous infiltrate in tissue samples resulting from a cell-mediated immune response to infection with *F. tularensis* may be misdiagnosed as tuberculosis if the granulomas are caseating.

The treatment of choice for pneumonic, septicemic, or typhoidal tularemia is streptomycin or gentamicin for 7 to 14 days. Treatment following a mass exposure or postexposure prophylaxis after intentional release of *F. tularensis* is a 14-day course of doxycycline or ciprofloxacin. Mortality rates may be as high as 30% in untreated patients with pneumonic or typhoidal tularemia. The *F. tularensis* vaccine once approved for laboratory workers is no longer available for use. **H**

KEY POINTS

- Patients with all forms of tularemia experience abrupt-onset fever, chills, myalgia, and anorexia.
- Serologic studies are impractical for rapid diagnosis of tularemia after a bioterrorism attack.
- The treatment of choice for pneumonic, typhoidal, or septicemic tularemia is streptomycin or gentamicin for 7 to 14 days.

Viral Hemorrhagic Fever

Viral hemorrhagic fevers (VHFs) are a group of febrile illnesses caused by RNA viruses from four families (**Table 31**). These viruses are considered likely candidates for use as biologic weapons because of their high infectivity and virulence after low-dose exposure, their capacity for causing significant morbidity and mortality, and the few, if any, treatment options available. The viruses are widely distributed in nature and, with the exception of dengue virus, are both stable and infectious by airborne dissemination.

The pathogenesis of VHF is poorly understood. Because the target organ is the vascular bed, the dominant clinical features are usually due to microvascular damage and changes in vascular permeability. After a variable incubation period of 2 to 21 days, all of the VHF pathogens cause a febrile prodrome, myalgia, and prostration. Early signs of infection often include conjunctival injection, mild hypotension, and petechial hemorrhages. Patients with advanced VHF develop shock and generalized bleeding from the mucous membranes, skin, and gastrointestinal tract, which are frequently accompanied by neurologic, hematopoietic, and pulmonary involvement.

In naturally occurring VHF, an appropriate epidemiologic exposure history would aid in the diagnosis. In a bioterrorism attack, however, deliberate aerosolization would be the most likely route of dissemination and would result in the simultaneous presentation of multiple patients. Specific diagnostic studies are available at the CDC laboratories that detect viral RNA by reverse transcription PCR, presence of viral protein antigens, development of IgM antibodies, or isolation of the virus.

Intensive supportive care is the mainstay of treatment. Potentially effective antiviral agents are limited (for example, ribavirin for Arenaviridae and Bunyaviridae viruses). Because of the potential for person-to-person transmission of some VHF pathogens, such as Ebola virus, appropriate isolation measures

TABLE 31.	Families of Viral Hemorrhagic Fever
Virus Family	**Disease**
Flaviviridae	Yellow fever
	Dengue fever
	Various tick-borne flavivirus hemorrhagic fevers
Filoviridae	Ebola hemorrhagic fever
	Marburg hemorrhagic fever
Arenaviridae	Lassa fever
	Various South American hemorrhagic fevers
Bunyaviridae	Rift Valley fever
	Crimean Congo hemorrhagic fever
	Hantavirus pulmonary syndrome
	Hemorrhagic fever with renal syndrome

for individuals with suspected or confirmed VHF include a combination of airborne and contact precautions. **H**

KEY POINTS

- Patients with viral hemorrhagic fever present with a febrile prodrome, myalgia, and prostration.
- Patients with advanced viral hemorrhagic fever experience shock and generalized bleeding from the mucous membranes, skin, and gastrointestinal tract.
- Intensive supportive care is the mainstay of treatment of viral hemorrhagic fever.

Travel Medicine

The practice of travel medicine encompasses both prevention (pre-travel advice about preventable infections, appropriate prophylaxis and immunizations, and behavioral practices to avoid exposure to infective agents) and treatment of returning travelers who have symptoms of infection. The most common travel-associated infections are listed in **Table 32**.

TABLE 32. Common Travel-Associated Infections

Febrile illnesses

Malaria

Dengue fever

Typhoid fever

Rickettsial infection

Yellow fever

Mononucleosis syndrome
(cytomegalovirus and Epstein-Barr virus)

Brucellosis

Travelers' diarrhea

Bacterial agents: *Escherichia coli, Campylobacter, Salmonella,* and *Shigella* species

Viral agents: rotavirus

Protozoa: *Cryptosporidium,* microsporidia, *Giardia,* and *Isospora* species

Malaria

H

Malaria is caused by infection with various *Plasmodium* species parasites that are transmitted by the bite of the female *Anopheles* mosquito. Malaria can be prevented by use of bed nets, insect repellents containing about 30% *N,N*-diethyl-3-methylbenzamide (DEET), and adherence to an appropriate chemoprophylaxis regimen. Yet, despite all precautions, infection can occur. The most common symptoms are fever (occurring in characteristic paroxysms of 48- or 72-hour cycles), headache, myalgia, nausea, vomiting, abdominal pain, and diarrhea. Patients found to have hyperparasitemia, defined as 5% to 10% or more of parasitized erythrocytes, may develop more severe signs and symptoms collectively referred to as complicated malaria because of the parasitized erythrocytes' adherence to and sequestration in small blood vessels. Generally more often associated with *Plasmodium falciparum* infection, this form of disease may be characterized by alteration in mentation with seizures, hepatic failure, disseminated intravascular coagulation, brisk intravascular hemolysis, metabolic acidosis, kidney insufficiency, and hypoglycemia. Patients with long-standing infection may present with anemia and splenomegaly. Thrombocytopenia and abnormal liver chemistry test results are also frequent findings.

The diagnosis of malaria relies on examination of peripheral blood smears. In some patients, the precise identification of the malarial species requires laboratory molecular techniques. The characteristics of the different malarial species are summarized in **Table 33**. *P. falciparum,* more so than other malaria species, and *Plasmodium knowlesi* may cause severe and potentially lethal infection.

Plasmodium knowlesi, the recently described species infecting macaque monkeys in Southeast Asia and now also known to infect humans, completes its blood stage cycle every 24 hours. Consequently, very high parasite loads develop, and a potentially severe and fatal infection can occur. On peripheral blood smear examination, *P. knowlesi* mimics *Plasmodium malariae,* with demonstration of all stages of the parasite in the circulation. Owing to the absence of its specific macaque reservoir hosts, this fifth *Plasmodium* species is not encountered in Africa.

TABLE 33. Characteristics of *Plasmodium* species

Characteristics	*P. vivax*	*P. ovale*	*P. malariae*	*P. falciparum*	*P. knowlesi*
Incubation period	10-30 days	10-20 days	15-35 days	8-25 days	Indeterminate
Geographic distribution	Tropical and temperate zones	West Africa and Southeast Asia	Tropical zones	Tropical and temperate zones	South and Southeast Asia
Parasitemia level	Low	Low	Very low	High	Can be high
Risk of disease severity	Low risk	Low risk	Very low risk	High risk	High risk
Disease relapse risk	Yes	Yes	Yes	None	None
Chloroquine resistance	Yes	No	Rare	Yes	No

CONT.

Clues to the diagnosis of falciparum malaria include travel to Africa, early onset of infection after returning from an endemic area, a peripheral blood smear showing a high level of parasitemia invading both young and old erythrocytes, and typically, the presence of thin, often multiple, "ring forms" lining the inner surface of the erythrocytes. Moreover, with *P. falciparum* infection, there is an absence of trophozoites and schizonts, although banana-shaped gametocytes may be detected in the smear.

The risk of exposure to malaria, presence of antimalarial drug resistance in endemic areas, and recommendations for chemoprophylaxis depend on the travel destination. Antimalarial chemoprophylaxis regimens are listed in **Table 34**. Unless travel is absolutely necessary, pregnant women are advised against entering malarial areas of the world. Chloroquine chemoprophylaxis can be safely administered during pregnancy. For travel to areas where chloroquine-resistant malaria is present, mefloquine is recommended for all travelers, although its safety is less well studied.

Information about malaria prophylaxis and treatment is frequently updated in the "Yellow Book" publication from the Centers for Disease Control and Prevention; the 2012 guidelines are now available (http://wwwnc.cdc.gov/travel/yellowbook/2012/chapter-3-infectious-diseases-related-to-travel/malaria.htm). ⓗ

KEY POINTS

- The most common symptoms of malaria are fever (occurring in characteristic paroxysms of 48- or 72-hour cycles), headache, myalgia, nausea, vomiting, abdominal pain, and diarrhea.
- *Plasmodium falciparum* and *Plasmodium knowlesi* may cause severe and potentially lethal malaria.
- The risk of exposure to malaria, presence of antimalarial drug resistance in endemic areas, and recommendations for chemoprophylaxis depend on the travel destination.

TABLE 34.	Antimalarial Chemoprophylaxis Regimens		
Drug	**Dose**	**Time of Prophylaxis Initiation**	**Time of Prophylaxis Discontinuation**
For endemic areas with chloroquine-resistant *Plasmodium falciparum*			
Mefloquine	250 mg once weekly	1-2 weeks before travel	4 weeks after returning
Atovaquone/proguanil	250 mg/100 mg once daily	1-2 days before travel	7 days after returning
Doxycycline	100 mg once daily	1-2 days before travel	4 weeks after returning
For endemic areas with chloroquine-sensitive *Plasmodium falciparum*			
Chloroquine	500 mg once weekly	1-2 weeks	4 weeks
Hydroxychloroquine	400 mg once weekly	1-2 weeks	4 weeks
Atovaquone/proguanil	250/100 mg once daily	1-2 days	7 days
Mefloquine	250 mg once weekly	2 weeks	4 weeks
Doxycycline	100 mg once daily	1-2 days	4 weeks
Primaquine[a]	26.3 mg once daily	1-2 days	1 week
For endemic areas with *Plasmodium vivax*			
Primaquine[a]	52.6 mg once daily	1-2 days	1 week
Chloroquine	500 mg once weekly	1-2 days	4 weeks
Hydroxychloroquine	400 mg once weekly	1-2 days	4 weeks
Atovaquone/proguanil	250/100 mg once daily	1-2 days	7 days
Mefloquine	250 mg once weekly	2 weeks	4 weeks
Doxycycline	100 mg once daily	1-2 days	4 weeks
Prophylaxis for relapse due to *Plasmodium vivax* or *Plasmodium ovale*			
Primaquine[a]	52.6 mg once daily	As soon as possible	2 weeks

[a]Contraindicated in persons with severe forms of glucose-6-phosphate dehydrogenase deficiency or methemoglobin reductase deficiency; should not be administered to pregnant women.

Reprinted with permission from Freedman, DO. Clinical practice. Malaria prevention in short-term travelers. N Engl J Med. 2008;359(6):603-612. [PMID: 18687641] Copyright 2008 Massachusetts Medical Society.

Typhoid Fever

Typhoid fever is a potentially life-threatening febrile illness caused by the bacterium *Salmonella enterica* serotype Typhi (formerly *Salmonella typhi*). Nontyphoidal *Salmonella* infection is discussed elsewhere in this syllabus (see Infectious Gastrointestinal Syndromes). Typhoid fever most often occurs in travelers who recently returned from endemic areas and is caused by consumption of water or food contaminated by human feces. Unlike other salmonellae, *S. enterica* serotype Typhi causes disease only in humans. Travelers to South, East, and Southeast Asia are at especially increased risk for infection.

Symptoms include fatigue, fever ("enteric fever" daily for 4 to 8 weeks in untreated patients), headache, cough, anorexia, hepatosplenomegaly, and, at times, a macular rash on the trunk (rose spots) that appears after an incubation period of 6 to 30 days. Diarrhea may be present early and resolve spontaneously. However, many patients with typhoid fever have constipation at diagnosis. Serious complications, such as intestinal hemorrhage or perforation, may occur 2 to 3 weeks after infection develops. Invasion of the gallbladder by typhoid bacilli may result in the long-term typhoid carrier state, especially in patients with gallstones.

The diagnosis of typhoid fever often relies on isolation of the organism in the blood, bone marrow, stool, and/or urine. Serologic studies may also be used. The classic Widal test, which measures anti-O and H antigen titers, has been widely substituted with newer, more sensitive and specific assays developed to detect antibodies to lipopolysaccharide or outer membrane proteins of *S. enterica* serotype *Typhi*. Fluoroquinolones, most often ciprofloxacin, are generally used for empiric therapy. However, because fluoroquinolone resistance is becoming high in South Asia and increasing in other areas, a third-generation cephalosporin (for example, ceftriaxone) is becoming the empiric antibiotic of choice pending in vitro susceptibility testing. Typhoid vaccine is recommended for travelers to areas at risk for infection. Either an oral live-attenuated vaccine or an intramuscular cell-free Vi capsular polysaccharide vaccine may be used. Both vaccines protect approximately 50% to 80% of recipients. 🄷

KEY POINTS

- Symptoms of typhoid fever include fatigue, fever ("enteric fever" daily for 4 to 8 weeks in untreated patients), headache, cough, anorexia, hepatosplenomegaly, and, at times, a macular rash.
- Although fluoroquinolones are frequently used for empiric treatment of typhoid fever, a third-generation cephalosporin is becoming the drug of choice because of increasing fluoroquinolone resistance.
- An oral live-attenuated typhoid vaccine and an intramuscular cell-free Vi capsular polysaccharide typhoid vaccine are available, and both vaccines are equally effective.

Travelers' Diarrhea

Travelers' diarrhea is the most common infection in travelers to developing countries and is estimated to affect 40% to 60% of travelers. It is usually a self-limited condition but may occasionally induce life-threatening volume depletion. This food- and waterborne illness is caused by various pathogens (see Table 32). The risk of transmission may be reduced by appropriate selection of food and water sources. It is advisable to avoid consuming water and drinks and ice made from tap water and to avoid brushing teeth with tap water. It is also prudent to not eat undercooked meats and poultry, unpasteurized dairy products, and fruits that are not peeled just prior to eating. Carbonated drinks and beer and wine are thought to be safe. Water may be purified by adding sodium hypochlorite (2 drops/1.89 L) or tincture of iodine (5 drops/0.95 L) to local water sources or boiling water for 3 minutes before allowing it to cool. Antibiotic prophylaxis for travelers' diarrhea is not recommended for most patients; however, it may be considered for patients with coexisting inflammatory bowel disease. The Infectious Diseases Society of America has published guidelines for the use of oral agents for prophylaxis and for treatment of travelers' diarrhea with a prolonged clinical course (**Table 35**). Bismuth subsalicylate can be used to prevent or treat diarrhea, but excessive doses are required that are inconvenient and can lead to salicylate toxicity. Rifaximin, a nonabsorbed antibiotic, is effective and safe when prescribed at doses of 200 mg, once or twice daily for 2 weeks, particularly when *Escherichia coli* will be the most likely acquired pathogen during travel.

TABLE 35. Treatment and Prophylaxis for Travelers' Diarrhea

Agent	Treatment Regimen (oral)
Bismuth subsalicylate	1 oz every 30 min for 8 doses
Norfloxacin	400 mg twice daily for 3 days
Ciprofloxacin	500 mg twice daily for 3 days
Ofloxacin	200 mg twice daily for 3 days
Levofloxacin	500 mg once daily for 3 days
Azithromycin	1000 mg, single dose
Rifaximin	200 mg three times daily for 3 days
Agent	**Prophylaxis Regimen (oral)**
Bismuth subsalicylate	Two tablets chewed 4 times daily
Norfloxacin	400 mg daily[a]
Ciprofloxacin	500 mg daily[a]
Rifaximin	200 mg once or twice daily[a]

[a]Chemoprophylaxis is recommended for no more than 2 to 3 weeks (the period studied in trials and a period short enough to minimize the risk of antimicrobial-associated adverse effects).

Reprinted with permission from Hill DR, Ericsson CD, Pearson RD, et al; Infectious Diseases Society of America. The practice of travel medicine: guidelines by the Infectious Diseases Society of America. Clin Infect Dis. 2006;43(12):1499-1539. [PMID: 17109284] Copyright 2006 Oxford University Press.

Antimotility agents such as diphenoxylate and loperamide may relieve symptoms but should be given only with antibiotic diarrhea treatment. These agents should not be used when dysenteric disease or bloody diarrhea is present.

Dengue Fever

Dengue fever is caused by four serotypes of viruses belonging to the family Flaviviridae (DENV-1 through DENV-4) and is transmitted by a mosquito vector (*Aedes aegypti*) with prominent diurnal activity. Although dengue fever is becoming ubiquitous in many parts of the world, geographic areas with the highest endemicity include the Caribbean, South and Central America, and Asia.

Infection may be asymptomatic or may cause an acute febrile illness associated with frontal headache, myalgia, and retro-orbital pain, with or without minor spontaneous bleeding manifestations (purpura, melena, conjunctival injection). Because prominent lumbosacral pain is a frequent manifestation, the term "breakbone fever" has been used to describe infection with the dengue virus. Some patients develop a macular or scarlatiniform rash as the fever abates. The rash spares the palms and soles and evolves into areas of petechiae on extensor surfaces. A second febrile period ("saddleback" pattern) may occur. In patients with severe infection, a life-threatening hemorrhagic or shock syndrome may develop that includes liver failure and encephalopathy. This entity appears to be related to previous dengue viral infection, often of a different type. Laboratory findings may include leukopenia, thrombocytopenia, and elevated serum aminotransferase levels.

The diagnosis is often made based on clinical findings and is sometimes confirmed by enzyme-linked immunosorbent assay or reverse transcriptase polymerase chain reaction. Since there is no specific antiviral agent for treatment of dengue fever, therapy is supportive. No effective vaccine is currently available. H

Hepatitis A Virus Infection

Hepatitis A virus (HAV) infection is acquired by ingesting contaminated water or food. Travelers to developing countries should be given HAV vaccine 1 month before going to an endemic area, provided they have not been previously immunized or have not contracted HAV infection in the past. A second booster dose is given 6 to 12 months after the initial vaccination. Serum immune globulin, once widely used for pre-exposure passive protection, is rarely indicated except perhaps for the very young (<12 months), for immunocompromised persons (who are less responsive to HAV vaccine), and for persons who choose not to be vaccinated. If HAV infection does occur, therapy is symptomatic, as no antiviral agent is currently available for treatment.

Rickettsial Infection

Rickettsioses are caused by obligate intracellular gram-negative bacteria that are transmitted by small vectors (fleas, lice, mites, and ticks). *Rickettsia typhi*, which causes endemic or murine typhus, is transmitted by fleas from a rodent reservoir, and *Rickettsia prowazekii*, which causes epidemic or louse-borne typhus, is transmitted by human body lice. Outbreaks of rickettsial infection have been reported during periods of war and natural disasters and are associated with poor hygienic conditions and tick infestation. The clinical presentation is usually vague and includes fever, headache, and malaise, which are often accompanied by a maculopapular, vesicular, or petechial rash. An eschar at the site of the insect bite often develops after infection with *Rickettsia africae* (African tick typhus), *Rickettsia conorii* (Mediterranean spotted fever), and *Orientia tsutsugamushi* (previously *Rickettsia tsutsugamushi* [scrub typhus]). Infection with *R. africae* is a very common cause of fever in travelers to South Africa.

When clinically suspected, the diagnosis may be confirmed by polymerase chain reaction, immunohistochemical analysis of tissue samples, or culture during the acute stage of illness before antibiotic therapy is begun. The treatment of choice is doxycycline. No vaccine or antimicrobial prophylaxis is available. Prevention therefore relies on minimizing exposure to vectors (for example, by use of repellents) when traveling in endemic areas. H

- Doxycycline is the antibiotic of choice for treating rickettsial infections; no vaccine or antimicrobial prophylaxis is available.

Brucellosis

Infection by human pathogenic species of the gram-negative coccobacillus *Brucella* (*B. abortus*, *B. melitensis*, *B. suis*, and *B. canis*) is acquired by ingestion of contaminated milk, by direct inoculation through skin wounds and mucous membranes, or by inhalation after exposure to domestic animals giving birth. Since this is a zoonotic infection with reservoirs in cattle and other animals, travelers usually become infected after consuming unpasteurized milk, other dairy products, or undercooked meat in countries where brucellosis is endemic. The Mediterranean basin, Indian subcontinent, Arabian Peninsula, and parts of Central and South America, Mexico, Asia, and Africa are high-prevalence areas. After a variable incubation period of usually weeks, patients develop fever, myalgia, fatigue, headache, and night sweats. Some patients may develop endocarditis and neuropsychiatric symptoms.

The diagnosis is established by isolating the organism in blood or bone marrow cultures or by specific serologic testing. The treatment of choice for brucellosis is a combination of doxycycline, rifampin, and streptomycin (or gentamicin). Antimicrobial prophylaxis is not recommended. Infection prevention relies on avoiding the ingestion of unpasteurized products or exposure to cattle or other animals in endemic areas. **H**

KEY POINTS

- Clinical manifestations of brucellosis include fever, myalgia, fatigue, headache, and night sweats and, less often, endocarditis and neuropsychiatric symptoms.
- The treatment of choice for brucellosis is a combination of doxycycline, rifampin, and streptomycin (or gentamicin).

Travel-Associated Fungal Infections

Most pathogenic fungi are endemic to the soil of certain geographic areas (**Table 36**) and are acquired either by inhalation of airborne mycelial organisms or by direct inoculation through cutaneous wounds or abrasions (see Fungal Infections). Although most of these infections are asymptomatic in immunocompetent hosts, immunocompromised patients are at risk of developing serious, often systemic, clinical manifestations. *Histoplasma capsulatum*, a dimorphic fungal organism that is particularly endemic to the southeastern United States, is found in high concentrations in soil contaminated with bird or bat droppings. The infection is acquired through inhalation of the fungus in its mold form.

TABLE 36. Common Travel-Associated Acquired Fungal Infections

Organism	Geographic Distribution
Coccidioides species	Southwest United States
	Mexico
	Central and South America
Histoplasma species	Ohio River Valley
	Mexico
	Central America
Penicillium marneffei	Southeast Asia
	China

Infection due to *Penicillium marneffei* is a rapidly growing problem among HIV-infected or generally immunocompromised persons living in or traveling to Southeast Asia. In this subset of persons, *P. marneffei* infection causes serious systemic manifestations associated with a high mortality rate. Survival depends on early diagnosis and institution of appropriate antifungal therapy, often for life, because of the propensity for relapses.

Since prophylaxis with antimycotic agents is not recommended and vaccines are not available, travelers to endemic areas may decrease their risk of contracting a fungal infection by limiting their exposure to outdoor dust and/or wearing well-fitted dust masks. **H**

KEY POINTS

- Infection due to *Penicillium marneffei* is a rapidly growing problem among HIV-infected or generally immunocompromised persons living in or traveling to Southeast Asia.
- Since prophylaxis with antimycotic agents is not recommended and vaccines are not available, travelers to endemic areas may decrease their risk of contracting a fungal infection by limiting their exposure to outdoor dust and/or wearing well-fitted dust masks.

Infectious Gastrointestinal Syndromes

Diarrhea is the most common clinical presentation of gastroenteritis but may also be caused by extraintestinal infections (Legionnaires disease, toxic shock syndrome), medications (amoxicillin-clavulanate), or noninfectious diseases (ischemic colitis, inflammatory bowel disease, celiac disease). Noninfectious causes of diarrhea are discussed elsewhere (see MKSAP 16 Gastroenterology and Hepatology).

Classification schema for infectious diarrhea have been developed to maximize judicious testing and aid empiric therapy, recognizing that the yield of stool culture for all patients with diarrhea is low. Infectious diarrhea can be broadly categorized as community acquired (including travelers' diarrhea), health care associated, or persistent (lasting >7 days). Most episodes of diarrhea caused by bacteria and viruses are brief, with symptoms persisting for less than 1 week even in the absence of treatment. Diarrhea in an otherwise healthy person lasting for more than 7 days suggests a parasitic or noninfectious origin.

The diagnostic yield of bacterial stool culture is low (less than 3%); however, identification of a pathogen has important treatment and public health implications and may be useful in identifying and tracking a foodborne outbreak. Because most cases of community-acquired diarrhea are self-limited, stool cultures are not required in all cases; cultures are generally indicated for symptoms lasting longer than 72 hours, particularly in patients with associated fever, tenesmus, or bloody or mucoid stools. Stool cultures are rarely positive if gastrointestinal symptoms have been present for more than 1 week's duration or if diarrhea develops in a hospitalized patient more than 3 days after admission. Routine bacterial stool cultures detect infection with *Salmonella*, *Shigella*, and *Campylobacter* species. Directed testing for Shiga toxin–producing *Escherichia coli* (STEC) may be reflexively performed in some laboratories when stool cultures are ordered. When not done automatically, STEC testing should be performed on all samples with visible or occult blood. Assays for *Clostridium difficile* are indicated for patients with recent antibiotic use, hospitalization, or comorbid disease. A focused history may elucidate epidemiologic features that may further guide diagnostic testing and empiric treatment (**Table 37**).

Infectious diarrhea is frequently transmitted by consumption of infected food products. Although knowing the type of food ingested is rarely useful in identifying a causative agent, the time from ingestion to development of symptoms may be helpful. Onset of gastrointestinal symptoms within 6 hours of ingestion is suggestive of a preformed toxin, such as *Staphylococcus aureus* or *Bacillus cereus* food poisoning, which are associated with nausea and vomiting rather than diarrhea. Symptoms due to most infections caused by ingesting viable bacteria develop 24 to 72 hours following ingestion. Person-to-person transmission can occur by fecal-oral spread and is particularly common for pathogens that cause infection with low inoculums (for example, *Shigella* species) and in preschools or health care settings where fecal soilage leads to environmental contamination.

The physical examination is important to assess the severity of illness but rarely provides clues to the causative organism. In contrast, laboratory findings may suggest specific pathogens. Grossly bloody stools are associated with infection caused by *Escherichia coli* O157:H7 or other

TABLE 37. Epidemiologic and Clinical Features Suggestive of Specific Pathogens in Patients with Diarrhea

Exposure, Symptom, or Risk Factor	Pathogen
Raw or undercooked eggs	*Salmonella*
Reptiles (turtles, snakes, lizards)	*Salmonella*
Puppy or kitten with diarrhea	*Campylobacter*
Travel to developing countries	≤7 days: bacterial (ETEC, EAEC, Enterobacteriaceae); >7 days: parasites
Recent antibiotics or hospitalization	*Clostridium difficile*
Chitterlings (pork intestines)	*Yersinia*
Seafood or seawater exposure	*Vibrio*
Cruise ship	Norovirus
Drinking from untreated natural bodies of water	*Giardia lamblia*
Ingestion of untreated fresh water or contaminated shellfish	*Aeromonas* or *Plesiomonas*
Day care centers	*Shigella, G. lamblia*, norovirus, rotavirus
Bloody stools (gross blood or heme-positive)	STEC, *Shigella, Salmonella Campylobacter, Entamoeba*
Mimic of acute appendicitis	*Yersinia*

EAEC = enteroaggregative *Escherichia coli*; ETEC = enterotoxigenic *E. coli*; STEC = Shiga toxin–producing *E. coli*.

STEC. Invasive pathogens such as *Salmonella*, *Shigella*, and *Campylobacter* species may also cause bloody stools. Fecal leukocytes, when present, suggest an invasive pathogen, but the sensitivity of this finding is low.

All patients should be evaluated for evidence of volume depletion, and fluid resuscitation is a cornerstone of treatment. Use of antimotility agents such as loperamide is reserved for patients with mild diarrhea and is discouraged for patients with fever, significant abdominal pain, or bloody stools. Decisions regarding empiric antibiotic therapy must be individualized based on suspicion for a particular pathogen and should be carefully considered because treatment of some types of infectious diarrhea may prolong bacterial shedding or increase the risk for complications (see later discussion of specific causes of diarrhea). Viral infections, noninvasive bacterial infections, and many parasitic infections generally resolve without antimicrobial therapy.

KEY POINTS

- Most episodes of diarrhea caused by bacteria and viruses are brief, with symptoms persisting for less than 1 week; diarrhea in an otherwise healthy person lasting more than 7 days suggests a parasitic or noninfectious origin.

- Onset of gastrointestinal symptoms within 6 hours of ingestion suggests a pre-formed toxin, such as *Staphylococcus aureus* or *Bacillus cereus* food poisoning, whereas symptoms due to most infections caused by ingesting viable bacteria develop 24 to 72 hours following ingestion.

Campylobacter Infection

Several *Campylobacter* species are capable of causing human disease, with *Campylobacter jejuni* most frequently associated with gastroenteritis. *Campylobacter* are normal bowel flora in many animals, including livestock. Foodborne transmission as a result of inadequate cooking or preparation of poultry is the most common route of infection. Diarrhea, fever, and abdominal pain are frequently present, and onset occurs several days after ingestion of bacteria. Grossly bloody stools are noted in fewer than 10% of patients; however, occult blood is found in a significantly higher percentage. Fecal leukocytes are variably present. The diagnosis is established by isolation of bacteria on stool culture. Late complications of *Campylobacter* infection include a reactive arthritis and Guillain-Barré syndrome.

Campylobacter infection typically resolves spontaneously even without antibiotic treatment. Treatment is indicated for patients with severe symptoms (high fever, frequent or bloody stools), or symptoms lasting longer than 7 days. Treatment should also be considered for patients at highest risk for complications, including those at extremes of age and patients who have a comorbid illness or are severely immunocompromised. Fluoroquinolone resistance among *Campylobacter* isolates approaches 20% in the United States and may be higher when infections are acquired during travel abroad. In contrast, most isolates are susceptible to macrolides, and recommended treatment for *Campylobacter* gastroenteritis is azithromycin or erythromycin.

KEY POINTS

- The most frequent symptoms of *Campylobacter* infection are diarrhea, fever, and abdominal pain, with onset several days after ingestion of bacteria.
- Recommended treatment for *Campylobacter* gastroenteritis is azithromycin or erythromycin.

Shigella Infection

There are four species of *Shigella* (*S. dysenteriae*, *S. boydii*, *S. flexneri*, and *S. sonnei*), all of which have been associated with diarrheal illness. Because shigellosis can be caused by very low infectious inoculums (<100 organisms), both foodborne and fecal-oral transmission can occur. Outbreaks of shigellosis in day-care centers and residential institutions typically occur through the fecal-oral route of infection.

Shigellosis most frequently presents as dysentery, characterized by bloody or mucoid stools, abdominal cramps, tenesmus, and high fever. The bacteria invade colonic tissue and cause inflammation. Fecal leukocytes are found in many patients. The diagnosis is established by bacterial stool culture. Reactive arthritis has been reported as a rare complication following resolution of infection.

Empiric therapy should be considered for patients with clinical evidence of dysentery pending culture confirmation of infection. Treatment is recommended for all patients with a positive culture for *Shigella* to decrease the duration of bacterial shedding and limit secondary spread of infection, even if symptoms have resolved by the time culture results are available. Most isolates remain susceptible to fluoroquinolones, and treatment with one of these agents for 5 days is recommended.

KEY POINTS

- Shigellosis most frequently presents as dysentery, characterized by bloody or mucoid stools, abdominal cramps, tenesmus, and high fever.
- Treatment with a fluoroquinolone is recommended for all patients with a positive culture for *Shigella*, even if symptoms have resolved by the time culture results are available.

Salmonella Infection

Salmonella infections are caused by several closely related bacteria belonging to a single species, *Salmonella enterica*. Organisms may be further characterized microbiologically by serotype. Isolates are often referred to by the genus and serotype (for example, *Salmonella enteritidis*) rather than the taxonomically correct, but lengthier, designation (*S. enterica* serotype Enteritidis).

Clinically, infections may be broadly categorized as typhoidal (associated with *S. enterica* serotype Typhi or *S. enterica* subtype paratyphi) or nontyphoidal. Although typhoid fever is endemic to developing countries, infection in the United States is usually limited to travelers returning from endemic areas (see Travel Medicine). In contrast, nontyphoidal serotypes of *Salmonella* are common causes of gastroenteritis in the United States. *Salmonella* organisms are most frequently transmitted by consumption of contaminated food, especially undercooked or raw eggs. Contaminated chicken and other meat products, milk, fruits, and vegetables have also caused outbreaks. Approximately 5% of patients develop infection after being exposed to reptiles, including turtles, snakes, and lizards.

Symptomatic disease typically occurs within 72 hours of ingestion and even without treatment resolves in 7 to 10 days in most patients. Clinically, *Salmonella* gastroenteritis is indistinguishable from other forms of invasive diarrhea. Associated symptoms include fever and abdominal pain, with gross or occult blood variably present in stool specimens. The diagnosis is established by bacterial stool culture.

Bacteremia occurs in 5% of patients and may cause endovascular infections, particularly aortitis. This uncommon complication of *Salmonella* infection should be considered in patients with known atherosclerotic vascular disease and persistent bacteremia despite antibiotic therapy; diagnosis is established by abdominal CT scan. Risk factors for salmonellosis include age greater than 65 years, use of agents that decrease stomach acid production (antacids, proton pump inhibitors), or impaired cellular immunity (HIV/AIDS, corticosteroid use, transplant recipients). Patients with sickle cell diseases are also at increased risk for disseminated salmonellosis, and osteomyelitis is a reported complication in these patients.

Several studies have found that antibiotic therapy for *Salmonella* gastroenteritis does not decrease the duration of symptoms and may actually prolong fecal shedding of bacteria. Consequently, treatment is discouraged for patients younger than 50 years of age who have relatively mild disease. Antibiotic therapy is indicated for patients with severe infection who require hospitalization in whom bacteremia or other disseminated infection is a concern. Treatment is also recommended for milder disease in the following groups of patients, who are most susceptible to complications of salmonellosis: (1) patients younger than 6 months or older than 50 years of age; (2) presence of prosthetic heart valves or joints; (3) comorbidities (malignancy, uremia, sickle cell disease); (4) significant atherosclerotic disease (because of risk of infectious arteritis); and (5) impaired cellular immunity.

Antibiotic treatment should be based on individual susceptibility patterns when these are known. Most isolates are susceptible to fluoroquinolones, which offer the advantage of oral dosing and are recommended for empiric therapy. Treatment is continued for 5 to 7 days for patients with severe disease or those at risk for complications due to bacteremia (groups 1 to 4). Treatment should be continued for at least 14 days for patients with cellular immune defects (group 5), in whom relapsing infection is common. The median duration of fecal shedding of bacteria after symptomatic infection is 5 weeks; however, surveillance cultures to document clearance are generally not recommended. Strict attention to hand hygiene should be emphasized to prevent secondary infection by person-to-person transmission.

KEY POINTS

- *Salmonella* gastroenteritis is indistinguishable from other forms of invasive diarrhea.
- Treatment of *Salmonella* gastroenteritis is discouraged for healthy patients younger than 50 years of age who have relatively mild disease.

Escherichia coli Infection

Escherichia coli are considered normal intestinal flora; however, specific strains are associated with various diarrheal syndromes (**Table 38**). Most diarrheagenic *E. coli* strains cause a self-limited and nonspecific gastroenteritis. Routine bacterial stool cultures do not distinguish between normal colonic and diarrheagenic *E. coli*, and diagnostic testing is generally restricted to epidemiologic studies or outbreak investigations. The exception is Shiga toxin–producing *E. coli* (STEC), which causes hemorrhagic gastroenteritis. The first reported outbreak of STEC was associated with ingestion of contaminated hamburger meat, and subsequent investigations have confirmed the role of transmission through ingestion of contaminated food products and water. A large European outbreak of hemorrhagic colitis in 2011 caused by *E. coli* O104:H4 was linked to consumption of raw sprouts. Person-to-person transmission may also occur by fecal-oral contamination and contact with animals at farms or petting zoos.

STEC causes diarrhea by production of Shiga toxin. *E. coli* O157:H7 is the most commonly identified STEC, but other strains, including the newly identified *E. coli* O104:H4, may cause a clinically identical hemorrhagic colitis, characterized by bloody diarrhea and abdominal pain in the absence of fever. Approximately 10% of patients with *E. coli* O157:H7 infection develop hemolytic uremic syndrome associated with kidney failure, hemolysis, and thrombocytopenia. Children are more susceptible than adults to this syndrome.

Routine stool cultures are not useful for isolating STEC. The Centers for Disease Control and Prevention (CDC)

TABLE 38. Diarrheagenic Strains of *Escherichia coli*		
Strain	**Epidemiology**	**Clinical Findings**
Enteroaggregative *E. coli* (EAEC)	Diarrhea in travelers, young children, and patients with HIV infection	Watery diarrhea, fever typically absent
Enteroinvasive *E. coli* (EIEC)	All ages, primarily in developing countries	Inflammatory diarrhea (dysentery) with fever, abdominal pain
Enteropathogenic *E. coli* (EPEC)	Sporadic, occasionally persistent diarrhea in young children	Nausea, vomiting, malnutrition (when chronic)
Enterotoxigenic *E. coli* (ETEC)	Diarrhea in travelers, foodborne outbreaks	Watery diarrhea, fever typically absent
Shiga-toxin producing *E. coli* (STEC)	Foodborne outbreaks (associated with beef and other contaminated food), person-to-person, and zoonotic transmission	Bloody stools, progression to hemolytic uremic syndrome

recommends that specific testing for *E. coli* O157:H7 be performed automatically by the laboratory on all stool specimens in patients with suspected community-acquired bacterial enteritis. *E. coli* O157:H7 can be cultured on a selective medium such as sorbitol-MacConkey agar. Culture-based techniques do not identify other strains of STEC; however, immunoassays to detect Shiga toxin are available and may have public health implications in identifying non-O157:H7 STEC-associated outbreaks.

Treatment of STEC infection is supportive. Antibiotics do not decrease the duration of symptoms and may increase the risk of developing hemolytic uremic syndrome. Empiric antibiotics should generally be withheld in patients presenting with bloody diarrhea unless there is supporting evidence for a cause other than STEC infection, and antibiotics should be discontinued if cultures confirm *E. coli* O157:H7 infection.

KEY POINTS

- Although most diarrheagenic *Escherichia coli* strains cause a self-limited and nonspecific gastroenteritis, Shiga toxin–producing *E. coli* (STEC) causes hemorrhagic gastroenteritis.
- *Escherichia coli* O157:H7 is the most commonly identified Shiga toxin–producing *E. coli*.
- *Escherichia coli* O157:H7 cannot be cultured on routine media but can be isolated on specialized sorbitol-MacConkey agar.
- Treatment of Shiga toxin–producing *Escherichia coli* infection is supportive.

Yersinia Infection

Yersiniosis refers to infection caused by *Yersinia enterocolitica* or *Y. pseudotuberculosis* but does not include infection caused by *Y. pestis*, the etiologic agent of plague (see Bioterrorism). Yersiniosis typically occurs following ingestion of contaminated food or water. Outbreaks of *Y. enterocolitica* have been traced to consumption of chitterlings (pork intestines). *Yersinia* gastroenteritis is clinically indistinguishable from other forms of inflammatory diarrhea and is most commonly identified in young children. In some cases, diarrhea may be absent with bacteria localizing to lymphoid tissue in Peyer patches and associated mesenteric lymph nodes. This presentation may mimic appendicitis clinically, leading to unnecessary appendectomy. Postinfectious complications occurring in yersiniosis include erythema nodosum and reactive arthritis.

Diagnosis is made by bacterial culture. *Yersinia* organisms grow poorly in routine stool cultures and, even on nonselective media, may be slow growing at normal temperatures. When yersiniosis is suspected, the laboratory should be notified to allow for plating onto specific media and

cold-enrichment, which may increase the yield of the culture. Whether antibiotic treatment of infection limited to the gastrointestinal tract is beneficial is unknown, and delays in diagnosis often result in symptom resolution before infection is confirmed by culture. Treatment with fluoroquinolones may be indicated for patients with severe or prolonged symptoms. **H**

Vibrio Infection

Vibrio species is a relatively uncommon cause of gastroenteritis in the United States. Conversely, *V. cholerae* is endemic throughout the developing world and is a significant cause of life-threatening diarrhea related to inadequate sanitation. Imported disease may occur in returning travelers as was the case with the recent cholera epidemic in Haiti following the devastating earthquake in 2010.

V. parahaemolyticus is the most common species causing diarrhea in the United States. The organism is widely distributed in salt water, with human infection associated with ingestion of contaminated seafood, particularly raw shellfish. Most infections are characterized by a relatively mild diarrhea, although this can be variably accompanied by nausea and vomiting, fever, and, occasionally, bloody stools. Infection may be particularly severe in patients with pre-existing liver disease, and this is a risk factor for secondary sepsis. In contrast, *V. vulnificus*, also found in saline environments, tends to cause bloodstream infections following ingestion, with diarrhea an uncommon manifestation.

Diarrhea caused by *Vibrio* species is likely underdiagnosed, because the organism requires specific media for culture from stool. The laboratory should be notified when *Vibrio*-associated diarrhea is suspected based on ingestion of raw or undercooked seafood or travel to a coastal region. Antibiotic treatment is indicated for severe illness, particularly in patients with liver disease. Doxycycline and the fluoroquinolones are both active against these organisms.

Clostridium difficile Infection **H**

Clostridium difficile infection (CDI) is the most common cause of health care–associated diarrhea. Risk factors for CDI include use of antibiotics or chemotherapeutic agents in the 8 weeks preceding infection because this causes alterations in enteric flora that allow bacterial overgrowth and toxin production. Although some studies have identified an epidemiologic association between the use of proton pump inhibitors and CDI, other well-controlled studies have suggested that this may be the result of confounding by underlying severity of illness and duration of hospital stay. Asymptomatic *C. difficile* colonization is common in hospitalized patients, and secondary environmental contamination occurs when fecal continence is impaired. *C. difficile* spores are resistant to many disinfectants, including alcohol-based hand sanitizers,

CONT.

and appropriate infection control measures (gowns, gloves, washing hands with soap and water) are recommended to reduce the risk of person-to-person transmission in the health care setting. In recent years, increasingly severe cases of CDI have been reported throughout North America. These infections may occur without previous antibiotic use or health care exposure and have been attributed to a more virulent strain of *C. difficile* termed NAP1/BI/027.

The hallmark of CDI is watery diarrhea that is frequently associated with fever and abdominal pain or cramps. Diarrhea may be absent in patients with significant ileus or toxic megacolon (maximum colonic diameter greater than 7 cm on radiography), leading to a delay in diagnosis. Grossly bloody stools are rare, although fecal occult blood testing may be positive. A pronounced peripheral leukocytosis is common and is a poor prognostic sign. In one study, 25% of hospitalized patients with a leukocyte count greater than 30,000/microliter (30×10^9/L) had CDI, suggesting that this diagnosis should be considered in all hospitalized patients who develop an unexplained leukemoid reaction.

Diagnosis of CDI requires laboratory confirmation of infection in a patient with diarrhea. Testing formed stools is not recommended because a positive result suggests *C. difficile* colonization that does not require treatment. Similarly, serial testing of stool specimens to document clearance of *C. difficile* is not indicated. When test results obtained on an initial appropriately collected stool sample are negative, the yield of sequential tests is low. Sequential testing should therefore be reserved for patients with ongoing symptoms in the absence of an alternative cause.

Stool culture for *C. difficile* with subsequent cytotoxicity testing is the most sensitive test for CDI. However, this study is time consuming and work intensive and is only done in research laboratories. Most commercial laboratories use an enzyme-linked immunosorbent assay to detect toxins A and

B. The sensitivity of this assay on a single diarrheal stool sample ranges from 63% to 94%. One strategy to improve sensitivity is through a two-step method that uses enzyme immunoassay detection of glutamate dehydrogenase (GDH) as an initial screen, followed by cell cytotoxicity assay or toxigenic culture as the confirmatory test for GDH-positive specimens. Polymerase chain reaction (PCR) testing to detect toxin-producing genes is also commercially available and is a highly sensitive and rapid means of diagnosis. Endoscopic examination showing colonic ulcerations with overlying pseudomembrane formation is suggestive of CDI, but these findings are seen in only 50% of patients.

Recently published treatment guidelines reflect the evolving epidemiology of CDI (**Table 39**), with vancomycin increasingly being preferred for treatment of severe or refractory infections. Both the type of antibiotic and the route of administration are important in ensuring that adequate drug levels are present at the luminal site of infection. Enteral administration of metronidazole is preferred except when significant ileus prevents transit of the drug, in which case intravenous administration is indicated. Vancomycin remains in the colonic lumen with minimal systemic absorption. Intravenous vancomycin does not penetrate into the colon and is therefore ineffective for treating CDI. When beginning antibiotic treatment of CDI, any other nonessential systemic antibiotics that may promote colonic overgrowth of *C. difficile* should be discontinued. Despite appropriate initial treatment, CDI recurs in approximately 20% of patients. The role of ancillary therapy (for example, rifampin, cholestyramine, probiotic agents) or alternative agents (for example, nitazoxanide, rifaximin) for treating recurrent infections has not been established. Fidaxomicin has recently been approved by the FDA for treatment of mild to moderate CDI and appears to be as effective as vancomycin but is associated with a lower

TABLE 39. Treatment Recommendations for *Clostridium difficile* Infection		
Presentation	**Severity**	**Antibiotic Regimen**
Initial episode	Mild to moderate	Metronidazole, 500 mg orally every 8 hours for 10-14 days
Initial episode	Severe	Vancomycin, 125 mg orally every 6 hours for 10-14 days
Initial episode	Severe with multiorgan system failure or hypotension	Vancomycin, 500 mg orally or by nasogastric tube every 6 hours for 10-14 days **plus** metronidazole, 500 mg intravenously every 8 hours for 10-14 days
Initial episode	Severe with ileus or toxic megacolon	Same as for severe infection with multiorgan system failure with the addition of vancomycin by rectal tube
First recurrence		Treatment regimen based on severity, as in initial episode
Second recurrence		Vancomycin taper: vancomycin, 125 mg orally four times daily for 10-14 days, then 125 mg orally twice daily for 7 days, then 125 mg orally daily for 7 days, then 125 mg orally every 2 to 3 days for 2-8 weeks

Adapted with permission from Cohen SH, Gerding DN, Johnson S, et al; Society for Healthcare Epidemiology of America; Infectious Diseases Society of America. Clinical practice guidelines for Clostridium difficile infection in adults: 2010 update by the society for healthcare epidemiology of America (SHEA) and the infectious diseases society of America (IDSA). Infect Control Hosp Epidemiol. 2010;31(5):431-455. [PMID: 20307191] Copyright 2010 The University of Chicago Press.

relapse rate; it is very expensive, and its role as initial therapy or for treatment of relapsing disease has not yet been defined. 🔲

KEY POINTS

- The hallmark of *Clostridium difficile* infection is watery diarrhea that is frequently associated with fever and abdominal pain or cramps, although diarrhea may be absent in patients with significant ileus or toxic megacolon.

- Detection of cytotoxins A and B in a patient with diarrhea is considered diagnostic of *Clostridium difficile* infection.

Viral Gastroenteritis

Viral gastroenteritis remains a significant cause of death among young children in developing countries. Although viral infections are the leading cause of gastroenteritis in the United States, they typically result in a relatively mild, self-limited illness. The two most common causes of viral gastroenteritis are rotavirus, which occurs almost exclusively in children under the age of 5 years, and noroviruses. Large outbreaks of gastroenteritis due to noroviruses have been documented in health care institutions, schools, cruise ships, and other settings where many people are housed in close proximity. Noroviruses are almost ideally suited for person-to-person transmission, as illness occurs with ingestion of fewer than 100 viral particles and fecal shedding of several million viral copies continues for prolonged periods following resolution of symptoms. In addition to fecal-oral transmission, infection can occur by ingestion of contaminated food or water, environmental contamination, or airborne inhalation of the virus.

Norovirus infection causes the abrupt onset of nausea, vomiting, and diarrhea, either singly or in combination, with fever noted in at least 50% of patients. The stool is typically watery without blood or leukocytes. Symptoms develop within 48 hours of infection and typically resolve after 72 hours, although findings may persist for longer periods in elderly or immunocompromised patients. Laboratory diagnosis is not routinely done because of the self-limited nature of the infection but may be important for public health investigations. If laboratory studies are indicated, PCR may be diagnostic. Antiviral agents are not available, and treatment, even in patients with severe infection, is supportive.

KEY POINTS

- Norovirus infection causes the abrupt onset of nausea, vomiting, and diarrhea, either singly or in combination, with fever noted in at least 50% of patients.

- Antiviral agents are not available for treatment of norovirus infection, and treatment, even in patients with severe infection, is supportive.

Parasitic Infections

Parasitic infection should be considered as a potential cause for diarrhea lasting for more than 7 days. In the United States, *Blastocystis* species are the most common parasites detected microscopically; however, whether this parasite is pathogenic is controversial. Reports have suggested resolution of gastrointestinal symptoms following treatment with metronidazole or other antimicrobial agents, but whether this is due to eradication of *Blastocystis* organisms or to treatment of other undiagnosed pathogens is unknown. Most authorities recommend reserving treatment only for patients with diarrhea lasting longer than 7 days in whom other infectious or noninfectious causes have been excluded. *Giardia lamblia* and *Cryptosporidium parvum* are the most commonly identified parasitic agents definitively known to cause diarrhea in the United States. Amebiasis is relatively uncommon in the United States but can cause hemorrhagic colitis in travelers and may occur several years after return from an endemic area.

Giardia Infection

G. lamblia is an environmental protozoal parasite that exists in fresh water sources throughout the United States and abroad. Cysts enter natural water supplies through excretion in animal feces, and ingestion of untreated water from contaminated streams or rivers is the major route of human infection. Hikers, campers, and outdoor enthusiasts are at highest risk of infection. Less commonly, infection is transmitted person-to-person by fecal-oral contamination.

Infection is asymptomatic in more than 50% of patients, and the protozoa clear spontaneously. In the remaining patients, symptoms typically occur 1 to 2 weeks after infection and include watery, foul-smelling diarrhea; bloating; flatulence; and belching. Significant weight loss is common because of anorexia and malabsorption, but fever is distinctly unusual. Gastrointestinal symptoms can persist for several weeks to months in the absence of treatment. Patients with hypogammaglobulinemia are at increased risk of developing severe or chronic infection.

Giardiasis can be diagnosed by examination of stool specimens for ova and parasites. Because protozoa may be shed sporadically in stool, examination of at least three specimens is suggested. Antigen testing of stool using immunoassays is more sensitive than microscopy for the diagnosis of *Giardia*, and is the preferred diagnostic test. Treatment is indicated for all symptomatic patients. First-line therapy is metronidazole for 7 to 10 days. Other active agents include tinidazole, nitazoxanide, mebendazole, and albendazole. Lactose intolerance is common following giardiasis and may persist for several weeks after completion of antibiotic therapy.

Cryptosporidium Infection

Cryptosporidium species, including *Cryptosporidium parvum*, are ubiquitous protozoal water parasites and have been responsible for large infectious outbreaks associated with contamination of municipal water supplies. Cryptosporidiosis is often asymptomatic, and infection in healthy persons is characterized by a relatively mild and self-limited diarrheal illness. In contrast, infection in patients with AIDS may result in prolonged diarrhea associated with significant weight loss and wasting. Patients with advanced HIV infection and low CD4 cell counts may also develop infection of the biliary tree causing acalculous cholecystitis

Cryptosporidia are not detected on routine examination of stool specimens for ova and parasites, but protozoa can be visualized with partial acid-fast staining of stools. Serologic assays directed against antigens in the stool have increased sensitivity compared with microscopic examination. Treatment in immunocompetent patients is often unnecessary, as cryptosporidiosis typically resolves spontaneously. Nitazoxanide may hasten resolution of symptoms in patients with severe infection. Treatment is challenging in patients with HIV infection because symptoms are often refractory to nitazoxanide and other antimicrobial agents. Reconstitution of cellular immunity may be curative in these patients, and optimization of antiretroviral therapy is indicated. Repletion of fluid losses and nutritional supplementation are important ancillary treatments.

Amebiasis

Amebiasis refers to infection with the protozoa *Entamoeba histolytica*, which is spread primarily through ingestion of contaminated food or water. Therefore, infection is more frequent in developing countries where sanitation may be suboptimal or in institutional settings owing to environmental contamination. Most infections are subclinical, with asymptomatic shedding of cysts over prolonged periods. In a minority of patients, invasive disease causes an inflammatory colitis characterized by bloody stools. Invasive disease is more common at the extremes of age and in immunocompromised patients. Amebic liver abscess is a well-described complication occurring when trophozoites enter the portal vein circulation and may occur in the absence of colitis.

Definitive diagnosis is established by stool antigen detection of *E. histolytica*. Serologic tests may support the diagnosis, particularly in patients with amebic liver abscess, because stool tests may be negative when disease is localized to the liver. Microscopy can identify trophozoites and cysts, but fecal shedding may be intermittent. *E. histolytica* is morphologically indistinguishable from other nonpathogenic entamoebae, potentially leading to misdiagnosis. Treatment of symptomatic patients is with metronidazole, followed by a luminally active agent such as paromomycin or iodoquinol to eradicate intestinal reservoirs. Asymptomatic patients with confirmed *E. histolytica* in stool should also receive a luminal amebicide.

KEY POINTS

- Signs and symptoms of giardiasis include watery, foul-smelling diarrhea; bloating; flatulence; belching; and often significant weight loss; however, fever is distinctly uncommon.
- First-line treatment of giardiasis is metronidazole for 7 to 10 days.
- Cryptosporidiosis is often asymptomatic in healthy persons or causes a relatively mild and self-limited diarrheal illness; infection in patients with advanced HIV infection may be associated with severe diarrhea, weight loss, and wasting.
- Although treatment of cryptosporidiosis in immunocompetent patients is often unnecessary, nitazoxanide may hasten resolution of symptoms in patients with severe infection.
- Amebiasis (*Entamoeba histolytica* infection) is spread primarily through ingestion of contaminated food or water and occurs more frequently in developing countries where sanitation may be suboptimal or in institutional settings owing to environmental contamination.

Infections in Transplant Recipients

Introduction

Transplantation of solid organs or hematopoietic stem cells continues to become more common as both the indications and the range of acceptable candidates increase. Advances in surgical techniques have reduced the rate of postoperative infections, and better immunosuppressive regimens have reduced the incidence of acute rejection. Despite these advances, infection remains common after transplantation and is responsible for up to 50% of deaths in solid-organ transplant recipients.

Antirejection Drugs in Transplant Recipients

A classification of the most commonly used agents to prevent or treat rejection in solid-organ transplant recipients is shown in **Table 40**. Different classes, and to some extent, even different agents within a class, have different risks for infectious complications. Most transplant centers use a three-drug regimen consisting of prednisone, a calcineurin inhibitor, and an antimetabolite (usually mycophenolate mofetil). Regimens that minimize use of corticosteroids are associated with

TABLE 40.	Immunosuppressive Agents Used in Transplant Recipients
Class	**Agents**
Corticosteroids	Prednisone, others
Cytotoxic agents (DNA synthesis inhibitors, antimetabolites)	Mycophenolate mofetil
	Azathioprine
	Methotrexate
	Cyclophosphamide
Calcineurin pathway inhibitors	Cyclosporine
	Tacrolimus
mTOR inhibitors	Sirolimus (rapamycin)
	Everolimus
Lymphocyte-depleting antibodies	
Polyclonal	Antithymocyte globulins
Monoclonal	Muromonab (anti-CD3 antibody)
	Basiliximab (anti-IL-2 receptor)
	Daclizumab (anti-IL-2 receptor)
	Rituximab (anti-CD20 antibody)
	Alemtuzumab (anti-CD52 antibody)

IL-2 = interleukin 2; mTOR = mammalian target of rapamycin.

reduced rates of *Pneumocystis jirovecii* and other fungal infections. Cyclosporine-based regimens are associated with reduced rates of infections compared with regimens that utilize high doses of cytotoxic agents.

Immunosuppression prior to allogeneic hematopoietic stem cell transplantation (HSCT) involves a conditioning regimen of whole-body irradiation and myeloablative high-dose chemotherapy. Posttransplant treatment, including treatment of graft-versus-host disease (GVHD), may include corticosteroids, cytotoxic agents, and/or antilymphocyte antibodies. The lymphocyte-depleting agents are primarily used for early induction therapy or for treatment of acute rejection or GVHD and can have a prolonged effect that lasts for months. However, lymphocyte depletion, especially of T cells, is associated with an increased risk for infection with cytomegalovirus (CMV), polyoma BK virus, *P. jirovecii* and other fungi and for development of Epstein-Barr virus (EBV)–associated posttransplant lymphoproliferative disease (PTLD).

Many of the immunosuppressive agents have significant drug interactions that must be considered before starting any agent. Overlapping toxicities must also be considered, especially nephrotoxicity, cytopenias, and a prolonged QT interval. Interactions affecting drug metabolism and levels are also common. Important examples are the interactions of cyclosporine, tacrolimus, and sirolimus with macrolide antibiotics and with azole antifungal agents, which result in increased levels of one or both drugs. H

KEY POINTS

- Most transplant centers use a three-drug regimen consisting of prednisone, a calcineurin inhibitor, and an antimetabolite (usually mycophenolate mofetil) to prevent or treat rejection in solid-organ transplant recipients.

- Immunosuppression prior to allogeneic hematopoietic stem cell transplantation involves a conditioning regimen of whole-body irradiation and myeloablative high-dose chemotherapy; posttransplant treatment may include corticosteroids, cytotoxic agents, and/or antilymphocyte antibodies.

- Many of the immunosuppressive agents have significant drug interactions that must be considered before starting any new drug in transplant recipients.

Posttransplantation Infections
Timeline and Type of Transplant

The risk for infections after transplantation depends on a number of factors, including the organ transplanted, immunosuppressive regimen used, development of rejection or GVHD and the treatment used, characteristics of both donor and recipient, and time since transplantation. Because some pathogens can be transmitted in the transplanted organ, donors are usually screened for active bacterial or fungal infections, various viruses (CMV, EBV, hepatitis B and C viruses, HIV), and tuberculosis.

In the early period (first month after solid-organ transplantation), patients are at risk for surgical site and wound infections, which are usually bacterial, as well as for other nosocomial infections, such as central line infections, pneumonia, and *Clostridium difficile* infection. Specific sites of likely bacterial infection are related in part to the organ transplanted (for example, urinary tract infection in kidney transplant recipients).

In the middle period (after 1 month), the consequences of immunosuppression on cell-mediated immunity predominate, and CMV reactivation and infection are common. Other viruses can also reactivate and cause disease during this period, including EBV, polyoma BK virus, and hepatitis B and C viruses. Infections with intracellular bacteria such as

Legionella species and with opportunistic pathogens such as *P. jirovecii* and other fungi may also occur.

In the late period (more than a few months posttransplantation), depletion of cell-mediated immunity continues at a reduced level, and opportunistic infections are less common. CMV infection may still occur, particularly in patients requiring more intense immunosuppression, and EBV-associated PTLD may develop. Polyomavirus infections more commonly present in this time period. Certain bacterial infections (such as *Listeria* and *Nocardia* infections) and fungal infections also become relatively more frequent, as do severe episodes of community-acquired infections.

The relationship between risk for different infections and time period after HSCT is depicted in **Figure 11**. Risk for

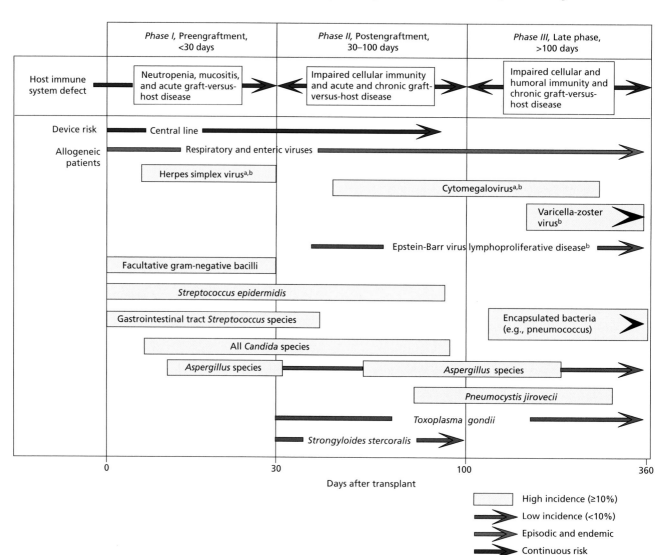

FIGURE 11. Phases of opportunistic infections in allogeneic hematopoietic stem cell transplant recipients. a = without standard prophylaxis; b = primarily among persons who are seropositive before transplant.

Reprinted with permission from CDC, Infectious Disease Society of America, and the American Society of Blood and Marrow Transplantation. Centers for Disease Control and Prevention. Guidelines for preventing opportunistic infections among hematopoietic stem cell transplant recipients. Recommendations of CDC, the Infectious Disease Society of America, and the American Society of Blood and Marrow Transplantation. Cytotherapy. 2001;3(1):41-54. [PMID: 12028843] infection is affected by the recipient's underlying disease, how well matched the donor and recipient are, and the presence of GVHD and consequent need for immunosuppression. Risk for infection following HSCT differs from that after solid-organ transplantation because of the profound neutropenia that follows HSCT, which increases the risk for bacterial and invasive fungal infections. [H]

KEY POINTS

- The risk for infection after transplantation depends on the organ transplanted, immunosuppressive regimen used, development of rejection or graft-versus-host disease and the treatment used, characteristics of both donor and recipient, and time since transplantation.

- The risk for infection after hematopoietic stem cell transplantation (HSCT) differs from that following solid-organ transplantation because of the profound neutropenia that follows HSCT, which increases the risk for bacterial and invasive fungal infections.

Specific Posttransplantation Infections
Viral Infections

CMV is the most important viral infection that occurs after transplantation. Reactivation and disease are most likely in CMV seronegative recipients of an organ from a seropositive donor. Onset usually occurs between 2 weeks and 4 months posttransplant, but may occur later because of prophylaxis. Reactivation is more likely to occur in the transplanted organ, and this may affect the clinical presentation. Patients may have a nonspecific febrile illness, often with leukopenia or thrombocytopenia. CMV can also cause a pneumonitis associated with high mortality rates or gastrointestinal tract or liver disease, including colitis, esophagitis, and hepatitis. As opposed to CMV infection in patients with AIDS, retinitis or central nervous system infection is rare in transplant recipients.

The most important consequence of EBV infection is B-lymphocyte proliferation leading to PTLD, which is more common following solid-organ transplantation than after HSCT. Patients usually present with fever and an extranodal mass or lymphadenopathy. Polyoma BK virus may cause nephropathy and ureteral strictures in kidney transplant recipients and may cause hemorrhagic cystitis in HSCT recipients. Hepatitis B and C may recur, especially after liver transplantation.

Bacterial Infections

Bacterial infections are common in the early period after transplantation, although prophylaxis has reduced this risk. The site of infection after solid-organ transplantation is often related to the surgical site and the transplanted organ. Examples are cholangitis and peritonitis after liver transplantation and pneumonia after lung transplantation. Pathogens include gram-negative bacilli (such as *Escherichia coli* and *Klebsiella* species) and staphylococci. Multidrug-resistant organisms, including *Pseudomonas aeruginosa* and

methicillin-resistant *Staphylococcus aureus*, are common, and organisms "carried over" from pretransplantation colonization (such as *Burkholderia cepacia* in patients receiving a lung transplant for cystic fibrosis) may cause infection.

The early period after HSCT is characterized by infections due to bacteria that are typically associated with neutropenia, including gram-negative bacilli and streptococci. During the late period after HSCT, an increase in infection by encapsulated organisms such as *Streptococcus pneumoniae* occurs. Because antibiotic regimens are likely to be given after any type of transplantation, *Clostridium difficile* infection must be considered in a patient presenting with diarrhea, fever, or leukocytosis.

Legionella infection tends to cause a severe, rapidly progressive, multilobar pneumonia in transplant recipients. *Listeria monocytogenes* causes bacteremia and meningoencephalitis, which may include cranial nerve and brainstem involvement manifesting as rhombencephalitis. Patients with *Nocardia* infection usually present with lung nodules, but dissemination occurs in about 25% of these patients and most often leads to brain abscesses. Tuberculosis usually occurs as reactivation disease in the first year after transplantation. Although tuberculosis may cause classic fever, cough, and focal lung lesions, about 50% of patients will have disseminated or extrapulmonary disease and may present with only sweats and weight loss.

Fungal Infections

Aspergillus species is the most common cause of invasive fungal infection after transplantation, especially following lung transplantation and during the neutropenic phase after HSCT. Invasive aspergillosis involves the lungs more often than the sinuses, and patients typically present with fever and possibly dry cough and chest pain. Dissemination to the brain is most common and is characterized by headache, focal deficits, and/or mental status changes. Non-*Aspergillus* molds, including the agents of mucormycosis, are increasingly being seen, including *Mucor* species and *Rhizopus* species, and have presentations indistinguishable from invasive aspergillosis.

Invasive *Candida* infections are common after transplantation, especially following liver transplantation and HSCT (particularly during the neutropenic phase). Fluconazole prophylaxis has reduced the overall incidence of these infections, but has also shifted the distribution of isolates to drug-resistant *Candida albicans* and *Candida glabrata*. Mucocutaneous infections, such as thrush and esophagitis, more commonly develop later after transplantation in patients who require ongoing immunosuppression.

Cryptococcus neoformans infection may develop in the late period after solid-organ transplantation but is uncommon following HSCT. Most patients have a subacute onset of fever, headache, and mental status changes (the latter two findings suggesting meningitis). Histoplasmosis and coccidioidomycosis can occur late after solid-organ transplantation in the Midwest and Southwest United States, respectively, but

CONT.

are rare following HSCT. Patients present with fever and respiratory signs and symptoms and possibly localized signs related to dissemination.

The incidence of *Pneumocystis* pneumonia after transplantation has been reduced significantly as a result of prophylaxis with trimethoprim-sulfamethoxazole and is usually a mid- to late-period posttransplantation opportunistic infection. Compared with *Pneumocystis* pneumonia in AIDS patients, pneumonia in transplant recipients has a more acute onset and is a more rapidly progressive illness.

Protozoa and Helminths

Toxoplasma gondii can reactivate after transplantation and usually causes central nervous system disease presenting as fever, headache, and focal neurologic changes. Imaging studies of the brain show multiple ring-enhancing lesions. Cardiac toxoplasmosis is a special problem in heart transplant recipients and may be caused by an infected transplanted heart.

Infection with *Strongyloides stercoralis* is more common in tropical and subtropical areas and can persist for many years in a subclinical state. Immunosuppression can then result in a hyperinfection syndrome; migration of *S. stercoralis* organisms in the lung and gastrointestinal tract can be associated with bacterial seeding, resulting in pneumonia and gram-negative bacteremia associated with a high mortality rate. **H**

KEY POINTS

- The most common viral infections in transplant recipients are caused by cytomegalovirus, Epstein-Barr virus, polyoma BK virus, and hepatitis B and C viruses.

- Bacterial infections are common in the early period after transplantation, although prophylaxis has reduced this risk.

- Multidrug-resistant organisms, including *Pseudomonas* species and methicillin-resistant *Staphylococcus aureus*, are common in transplant recipients.

- *Aspergillus* species is the most common cause of invasive fungal infection in transplant recipients, especially following lung transplantation and during the neutropenic phase after hematopoietic stem cell transplantation.

- *Toxoplasma gondii* infection following transplantation can cause central nervous system disease and cardiac toxoplasmosis.

Prevention of Infections in Transplant Recipients

Prevention of infections after transplantation relies on reducing exposures and administering prophylactic agents and immunizations. Prophylactic antibiotics are usually given

after solid-organ transplantation and HSCT. Prophylaxis reduces the incidence of postoperative infections after solid-organ transplantation and may include fluconazole for *Candida* prophylaxis, especially for liver transplant recipients. During the neutropenic phase after HSCT, bacterial prophylaxis with a fluoroquinolone is usually given along with fluconazole or another antifungal agent.

Considerable attention has been given to reducing CMV disease after transplantation. True prophylaxis requires giving an agent broadly to every recipient at risk, whereas preemptive therapy targets those who show signs of early infection (such as a positive polymerase chain reaction) before development of disease. Both approaches are used for prevention, and the preferred agent is intravenous ganciclovir or oral valganciclovir, administered for the first 3 to 4 months after transplantation.

Trimethoprim-sulfamethoxazole is used to prevent *Pneumocystis* pneumonia and also provides activity against some gram-negative bacteria and *Listeria*, *Nocardia*, and *Toxoplasma* species. It is often continued for 12 months or more. Patients with latent tuberculosis infection should be given preventive isoniazid, preferably before transplantation. Antiviral therapy can be given to reduce recurrence of hepatitis B virus infection after liver transplantation.

Recommendations for immunizations in transplant recipients are shown in **Table 41**. Generally, solid-organ transplant recipients receive all vaccinations before transplantation, and HSCT recipients are revaccinated after immune system reconstitution. Because of the risk due to immunosuppression, live attenuated vaccines are usually contraindicated after solid-organ transplantation or HSCT.

KEY POINTS

- Prophylactic antibiotics are usually given after solid-organ transplantation and hematopoietic stem cell transplantation.

- Solid-organ transplant recipients generally receive all recommended vaccinations before transplantation, and hematopoietic stem cell transplant recipients are revaccinated after immune system reconstitution.

Hospital-Acquired Infections

Epidemiology

Nosocomial, or hospital-acquired infections (HAIs), are one of the 10 leading causes of death and the most common complication in hospitalized patients in the United States. HAIs are defined as infections that develop after 48 hours of hospitalization, with no evidence that the infection was present or incubating at the time of admission. Between 5% and 10% of patients admitted to acute care hospitals (approximately 2 million patients per year) acquire one or more HAIs, resulting in

TABLE 41. Immunization Recommendations for Adult Transplant Recipients

Immunization	SOT Recipients	HSCT Recipients[a]
Pneumococcal	Polysaccharide vaccine pretransplant; repeat at 5 years	Conjugate vaccine, three to four doses starting 3-6 months posttransplant
Influenza (inactivated only)	Annually	Annually
Tetanus, diphtheria, and acellular pertussis (Tdap)	Complete series pretransplant, including Tdap booster	Tdap, three doses starting 6-12 months posttransplant
Measles-mumps-rubella	Contraindicated after transplantation	One dose 24 months posttransplant, only if no GVHD or immunosuppression
Inactivated polio	Complete series pretransplant	Three doses starting 6-12 months posttransplant
Haemophilus influenzae type b	No recommendations	Three doses starting 6-12 months posttransplant
Meningococcal	As per general recommendations	As per general recommendations
Hepatitis A virus	Complete series pretransplant if not already immune	As per general recommendations
Hepatitis B virus	Complete series pretransplant if not already immune	Three doses starting 6-12 months posttransplant if otherwise indicated
Varicella -zoster virus	Varicella pretransplant if not already immune; zoster pretransplant if meets general recommendations; both are contraindicated posttransplant	Not recommended; absolutely contraindicated before 24 months and in presence of GVHD or immunosuppression
Human papillomavirus	As per general recommendations; give pretransplant	As per general recommendations

GVHD = graft-versus-host disease; HSCT = hematopoietic stem cell transplantation; SOT = solid-organ transplantation.

[a]For multiple-dose immunizations, the period between doses is generally 1 to 2 months.

90,000 deaths and accounting for costs of 4.5 to 6.5 billion dollars annually.

Health care–associated infections have a more expansive definition. These include HAIs as well as infections in patients who were recently hospitalized, attend infusion centers, or reside in long-term-care facilities. This chapter will focus only on HAIs.

Health care organizations, professional associations, government and accrediting agencies, and third-party payers have all developed initiatives related to the prevention or reduction of HAIs. In 2008, the Centers for Medicare and Medicaid Services stopped reimbursing hospitals for some costs associated with certain HAIs, and this policy will be broadened in the near future. Hospitals are required to report their rates of HAIs to selected organizations and sometimes to the general public. Although prevention of infections primarily focuses on patient safety, prevention may also potentially reduce hospital costs and enhance institutions' reputations.

Prevention

Preventing HAIs requires a multifaceted and multidisciplinary approach. A stable infection control infrastructure is of paramount importance. One of the most important components of HAI prevention is hand hygiene compliance. Hand hygiene, enacted before and after patient contact, consists of hand washing with soap and water for at least 15 to 30 seconds; alcohol-based hand disinfectants are acceptable alternatives to soap and water. Standardization of cleaning practices and immunization of health care workers are additional measures. Many successful HAI prevention initiatives involve "bundles" of processes. Often, the individual impact of each component of a bundle on HAIs is not clearly defined, but when all components of the "entire" bundle are practiced together, infection rates decrease. **H**

KEY POINTS

- Hospital-acquired infections are defined as infections that develop after 48 hours of hospitalization, with no evidence that the infection was present or incubating at the time of admission.

- Hospital-acquired infections are one of the 10 leading causes of death and the most common complication in hospitalized patients in the United States.

- Hand hygiene is the single most important measure to prevent hospital-acquired infections.

Catheter-Associated Urinary Tract Infections   **H**

Catheter-associated urinary tract infection (CAUTI) is defined as a UTI occurring in a catheterized patient and accounts for more than 97% of UTIs acquired in the hospital. CAUTI is the

CONT.

most common type of HAI, with an average of 16.8 cases per 1000 catheter days.

Risk factors for CAUTI are listed in **Table 42**.

Diagnosis

The diagnosis of CAUTI is challenging. In patients with indwelling urethral, indwelling suprapubic, or intermittent catheterization, CAUTI is defined by the presence of symptoms or signs compatible with UTI with no other identified source of infection, along with 10^3 or more colony-forming units (cfu)/mL of one or more bacterial species in a single catheter urine specimen or in a midstream voided urine specimen from a patient whose catheter had been removed within the previous 48 hours. Symptoms and signs of a UTI may include new-onset or worsening fever, rigors, altered mental status, malaise or lethargy with no other identified cause, flank pain, costovertebral angle tenderness, acute hematuria, pelvic discomfort, and, in those whose catheters have been removed, dysuria, urgent or frequent urination, or suprapubic pain or tenderness. Because pyuria is not a reliable indicator of a UTI in a catheterized patient, systemic symptoms of infection may be the only indicators, especially in patients who have spinal cord injuries or who cannot provide a reliable history.

Treatment

Before initiating treatment for presumed CAUTI, a urine specimen for culture should be obtained to guide therapy and to account for the wide spectrum of potential organisms and the increased likelihood of antimicrobial resistance. If the catheter cannot be discontinued and has been in place for more than 2 weeks, the urine culture specimen should be obtained from a freshly placed catheter. The duration of treatment is 7 days for patients in whom symptoms resolve promptly and 10 to 14 days for those in whom response is delayed, regardless of whether the catheter remains in place.

Prevention

Measures and interventions to prevent CAUTI are shown in **Table 43**. Factors that have no role in the prevention of CAUTI include (1) screening for asymptomatic bacteriuria in catheterized patients; (2) treatment of asymptomatic bacteriuria, except in pregnant women and before invasive urologic procedures; (3) catheter irrigation; (4) routine changes of catheters; and (5) cleaning the meatal area with antiseptics before or during catheterization. The effect of using catheters coated with antiseptics (silver alloy or antibiotic) on the incidence of CAUTI remains unclear. Studies have demonstrated that antiseptic-coated catheters decrease the incidence

TABLE 42. Risk Factors for Catheter-Associated Urinary Tract Infection
Unmodifiable Risk Factors
Female sex
Age >50 years
Presence of a rapidly fatal underlying illness
Presence of diabetes mellitus
Serum creatinine >2.0 mg/dL (176.8 µmol/L) at time of catheterization
Modifiable Risk Factors
Prolonged duration of catheterization
Nonadherence to appropriate catheter care
Catheter insertion after day 6 of hospitalization
Catheter insertion performed outside the operating room
µmol = micromoles.

TABLE 43. Prevention of Catheter-Associated Urinary Tract Infection	
Period	**Preventive Measures**
Prior to catheterization	Avoid catheterization whenever possible
	Use condom catheters or intermittent catheterization whenever possible
At time of catheter insertion	Adhere to hand hygiene practices by health care workers
	Use proper aseptic techniques when inserting the catheter
	Use smaller catheters to decrease urethral trauma
After catheter insertion	Promote early catheter removal whenever possible
	Secure the catheter
	Maintain a closed drainage system
	Avoid unnecessary system disconnections
	Use aseptic technique when handling the catheter, including for sample collection
	Maintain unobstructed urine flow
	Empty the collecting bag regularly, using a separate collecting container for each patient
	Keep the collecting bag below the level of the bladder

of asymptomatic bacteriuria but do not significantly reduce the risk for symptomatic UTI. Antiseptic-coated catheters cost more than standard urinary catheters. In the absence of new evidence demonstrating their efficacy, they should not be used as a primary modality for preventing CAUTI. **H**

KEY POINTS

- Catheter-acquired urinary tract infection is the most common type of hospital-acquired infection.
- Pyuria is not a reliable indicator of a urinary tract infection in a catheterized patient.
- Antiseptic-coated catheters should not be used as a primary modality for preventing catheter-acquired urinary tract infection.

Surgical Site Infections

Surgical site infections (SSIs) are diagnosed when the following two criteria are met: (1) infection occurs within 30 days after an operative procedure and (2) infection involves either the skin or soft tissue (incisional SSI) or an organ/space that was operated on or manipulated during the surgical procedure (organ/space SSI). Incisional SSIs are further classified as superficial (involving only the skin and/or subcutaneous tissue) and deep (involving the soft tissue). Primary incisional infections are those that develop in the primary surgical incision; secondary incisional infections are those that develop in the secondary incision in patients who have had surgery with more than one incision (for example, the donor site [leg] in coronary artery bypass surgery). In organ/space SSI, any part of the body can be involved, excluding the skin incision, fascia, or muscle layers. If an implant is placed during surgery, SSI can occur up to 1 year postoperatively. Implant infections are not associated with a superficial incisional SSI and should always be considered to be deep incisional or organ/space infections.

SSIs occur in 2% to 5% of patients undergoing surgery in the United States each year and account for 300,000 to 500,000 infections annually. *Staphylococcus aureus* is the most common cause, accounting for approximately 20% to 37% of SSIs. Methicillin-resistant *S. aureus* (MRSA) is a leading cause of SSIs in some tertiary care and community hospitals. SSIs lead to increased duration of hospitalization (>1 week of additional postoperative hospital days), a 2- to 11-fold increased risk of death for infected patients, and increased health care costs ($3000 to $29,000 per patient and approximately 10 billion dollars annually for the U.S. health care system). Risk factors for SSI are shown in **Table 44**.

Diagnosis

SSI typically manifests during the second or third postoperative week, although it can occur much later if an implant was placed during surgery. Diagnosis of superficial incisional SSI is typically based on signs and symptoms, including purulent drainage, pain, tenderness, redness, or heat. Patients with

TABLE 44. Risk Factors for Surgical Site Infection

Period	Risk Factors
Preoperative	Modifiable factors: obesity, tobacco use, use of immunosuppressants, length of preoperative hospitalization
	Unmodifiable factors: age, diabetes mellitus
Perioperative	Wound class, length of surgery, shaving of hair, hypoxia, hypothermia
Postoperative	Hyperglycemia, substandard wound care, blood transfusion

deep incisional SSI or organ/space SSI are typically more symptomatic than patients with superficial SSI owing to inflammation or abscess involving an organ or soft tissues. Frequently, cultures obtained during incision and drainage or debridement are positive.

Cultures should be obtained whenever deep incisional or organ/space SSI is suspected. Optimal cultures are taken from the deepest layer involved and should be obtained under controlled conditions such as in the operating room or by needle aspiration. Superficial swab cultures are potentially misleading and have a specificity of less than 30%. If necessary for evaluation of possible SSI, advanced imaging (CT or MRI) is more reliable than plain radiographs for diagnosing SSI.

The diagnosis of SSI in a patient with an implant or prosthetic joint can be challenging. Radiographic findings are usually nonspecific, and clinical signs and symptoms may be subtle. Multiple cultures should be obtained from deep infected tissues surrounding the prosthetic joint. Sonication, the use of ultrasound to agitate and dislodge bacteria from a removed and infected implant, is another method used to increase the yield of cultures to establish an accurate microbiologic diagnosis; however, because of the complexities associated with this technique, it is not practiced routinely in many laboratories (see MKSAP 16 Rheumatology for further discussion of Prosthetic Joint Infections).

Treatment

Surgical opening of the incision with debridement and removal of necrotic tissue is the most important aspect of treatment of deep incisional and organ/space SSIs. Antimicrobial therapy is an important adjunct. The type of debridement and duration of postoperative antimicrobial therapy depend on the anatomic site of infection, the invasiveness of the SSI, and whether foreign material was implanted or fully removed.

Prevention

The major measures to prevent SSIs are listed in **Table 45**. Checklists have played an important role in decreasing SSI rates, because they help to ensure compliance with multiple infection control measures. The impact of preoperative nasal

TABLE 45. Prevention of Surgical Site Infection

Preoperative Preventive Measures	Comments
Control/eliminate modifiable risk factors	Including uncontrolled diabetes mellitus or hyperglycemia, obesity, tobacco use, use of immunosuppressive agents, and length of preoperative hospitalization
Provide antibiotic prophylaxis	Administer 30 to 60 min before incision (60-120 min before incision for vancomycin and the fluoroquinolones)
	Maintain therapeutic antibiotic levels until wound closure, even if additional doses are needed intraoperatively
	Do not give prophylactic antibiotics for longer than 24 h after surgery

Perioperative Preventive Measures	Comments
Avoid shaving of hair	If necessary, clipping is preferred
Use chlorhexidine-based surgical preparation	May be superior to povidone iodine–based antiseptics
Minimize traffic in and out of operating room	None
Administer supplemental oxygen	Still controversial (most experience in procedures involving colorectal surgery)
Use checklists to improve compliance with preventive processes	None

Postoperative Preventive Measures	Comments
Optimize glucose control	Maintaining plasma glucose levels below 200 mg/dL (11.1 mmol/L) for 48 h postoperatively is recommended
Monitor and report risk-adjusted SSI rates to surgeons	None

SSI = surgical site infection.

decolonization of *S. aureus* on risk for SSI is controversial. The results of controlled clinical trials have been mixed, with the most convincing evidence in cardiothoracic surgery in the setting of preoperative nasal decolonization combined with chlorhexidine bathing. Based on current evidence, if nasal decolonization of *S. aureus* is performed, it should be conducted in conjunction with chlorhexidine bathing.

KEY POINTS

- Surgical site infections are diagnosed when infection occurs within 30 days after an operative procedure and involves the skin/soft tissue or an organ/space that underwent surgery or was manipulated during the procedure.
- *Staphylococcus aureus* is the most common cause of surgical site infections.
- Radiographic findings in patients with surgical site infections who have an implant or prosthetic joint are usually nonspecific, and clinical signs and symptoms may be subtle.

Central Line–Associated Bloodstream Infections

Central line–associated bloodstream infection (CLABSI) is a bloodstream infection originating from a central line without another recognizable focus of infection. Catheter-related bloodstream infection (CRBSI) is a type of CLABSI in which cultures of the catheter tip grow the same organism found in blood culture specimens. In the United States, 80,000 episodes of CLABSI occur in intensive care units (ICUs) each year and are attributed with causing 28,000 deaths annually. The epidemiology of CLABSI outside the intensive care unit is less well studied, but rates are lower. Independent risk factors for CLABSI are shown in **Table 46**.

Diagnosis

CLABSI should be highly suspected in patients who do not have an obvious source of infection from a site other than the central line and in whom the same pathogen is isolated from a peripheral blood culture specimen and from either a blood culture specimen obtained by aspirating blood through the central line or a culture of the catheter tip. It is important to recognize that central venous catheter tips are often colonized with bacteria in the absence of clinical infection. Thus, a positive culture of a central venous catheter performed as part of a routine screening protocol in the absence of positive blood cultures or signs of infection does not require treatment. Blood cultures (at least two sets) should be obtained from different anatomic sites (at least one peripheral site). A threefold greater colony count from the culture drawn through a catheter compared with a peripheral blood culture is a strong predictor for CLABSI. "Time to positivity" is the time between blood culture incubation and growth detection. When blood cultures are drawn from a central line and from

TABLE 46. Independent Risk Factors for Central Line–Associated Bloodstream Infection

Period	Risk Factors
Before central line insertion	Premature birth
	Neutropenia
	Prolonged hospitalization
During central line insertion	Catheterization in a site other than the subclavian vein[a]
	Substandard catheter care
	Heavy microbial colonization of the skin at the insertion site
After central line insertion	Prolonged duration of catheterization
	Total parenteral nutrition delivered through the catheter
	Heavy microbial colonization of the catheter hub

[a]Femoral vein placement is associated with greatest infection risk, and internal jugular vein placement with the second greatest infection risk.

Note: Female sex and subclavian vein insertion site were independently associated with decreased risk for infection.

a peripheral site within 30 minutes of one another, if the central line culture turns positive at least 2 hours before growth is reported on the peripheral culture, a central line infection is strongly supported. The semiquantitative roll-plate method for culturing the distal tip of a central venous catheter is a validated method for detecting catheter colonization and contributes diagnostic information when the same pathogen is recovered from both the catheter tip and the blood culture specimen. Typically, blood cultures should become negative once an infected central line is removed and appropriate therapy is administered. If bacteremia persists, a diagnostic workup for a deeper source of infection is appropriate.

Treatment

Removal of the central line is the most important intervention in treating CLABSI and is especially important when the pathogen is *S. aureus*, *Pseudomonas aeruginosa*, or *Candida* species. If salvage of a central line is attempted, use of an antibiotic lock is an optional adjunct to administration of systemic antibiotics.

Prevention

Early CLABSI occurs in the first 5 to 7 days following central line insertion and is typically caused by pathogens introduced during insertion. Late CLABSI occurs 5 to 7 days or more after insertion and is generally caused by pathogens introduced during catheter use or care. Methods to prevent early CLABSI mostly relate to improving catheter insertion techniques. Hand hygiene, basic aseptic techniques, and full

barrier precautions are mandatory. In adults, the femoral vein should be avoided for venous access whenever possible, and use of chlorhexidine-based antiseptics (in preference to iodines or alcohol) for skin preparation is advocated. Once a catheter is inserted, it should be removed as soon as the indication for placement has resolved. Appropriate disinfection before and after accessing any part of the catheter helps prevent late CLABSI. Antiseptic sponge products are effective in preventing CLABSI and should be changed every 5 to 7 days or sooner if they become soiled. If a gauze dressing is used, the insertion site should be inspected, prepped again, and dressed every 48 hours using sterile technique, and dressings should be replaced when they become damp, loosened, or soiled. If a transparent dressing is used, the dressing should be changed every 7 days or sooner if it becomes non-intact. Whenever central line dressings are changed, the insertion site and catheter hub should be disinfected with a chlorhexidine-based antiseptic. In patients with central lines in place, especially patients in the ICU, daily bathing with chlorhexidine body wash has been shown to reduce the risk for CLABSI. Intravenous administration sets should be replaced every 96 hours. Hemodialysis catheter insertion sites may be treated with povidone-iodine ointment or polymyxin ointment whenever the dialysis catheter is accessed as long as these antiseptics do not interfere with the catheter material (based on the manufacturer's recommendations).

Use of antiseptic- or antimicrobial-coated or impregnated central venous catheters for adult patients has been shown to reduce rates of CLABSI, although there is a lack of consensus about the cost-benefit ratio of their use. However, their use is recommended if the CLABSI rate is not decreasing in centers after successful implementation of a comprehensive strategy to reduce CLABSI rates. Use of antibiotic or alcohol locks as prophylaxis, systemic antimicrobial prophylaxis, and routine replacement of central lines are not recommended, although the use of an antibiotic lock solution can be considered in patients with long-term catheters who have a history of multiple CRBSIs despite maximal adherence to aseptic technique.

The Institute for Healthcare Improvement launched a campaign in 2004 introducing a bundle of evidence-based interventions for reducing CLABSI. The bundle includes a checklist that lists the following processes associated with reduced risk for CLABSI: (1) hand hygiene prior to line insertion, (2) use of maximal barrier precautions, (3) use of chlorhexidine skin antiseptic, and (4) optimal catheter site selection (preferring the subclavian site and avoiding the femoral site). Subsequent additions to this bundle include use of daily chlorhexidine-based body washes, use of prepackaged central line insertion kits, and daily review of central line necessity. Increased education of staff regarding use of central line bundles, checklists, and central line kits or carts has been shown to significantly reduce rates of CLABSI. For example, rates in the United States decreased in 2008-2009 compared with those in 2001. ◨

TABLE 47. Risk Factors for Hospital-Acquired Pneumonia and Ventilator-Associated Pneumonia

Risk Factors	Variables
Comorbid conditions, exposures, and events	Advanced age
	Altered mental status
	Underlying chronic lung disease
	Rapidly or ultimately fatal disease
	Neurologic disease
	Trauma
	Previous antibiotic use
	Abdominal or thoracic surgery
	Mechanical ventilation
	Recent large-volume aspiration
	Nasogastric intubation
Medications	H_2 blockers
	Corticosteroids

Hospital-Acquired Pneumonia and Ventilator-Associated Pneumonia

Hospital-acquired pneumonia (HAP) is defined as a pneumonia that occurs 48 hours or more after hospital admission and was not incubating at the time of admission. Ventilator-associated pneumonia (VAP) is a subset of HAP and refers to pneumonia that develops more than 48 to 72 hours after mechanical ventilation was begun.

HAP is the second leading cause of hospital-acquired infection after catheter-associated urinary tract infection and is a common cause of infection in the ICU. Most cases of HAP in the ICU are due to VAP. The frequency of HAP is reportedly higher in certain patient populations, such as the elderly, newborns, and adult ICU patients. In one multinational study, HAP was the single most common type of infection. More than 50% of the antibiotics prescribed in the ICU are for the treatment of HAP, and HAP increases hospital stays by an average of 7 to 9 days per patient and increases health care costs by more than $40,000 per patient. The crude mortality rate may be as high as 70%. Multiple risk factors for HAP and VAP have been identified (**Table 47**). Mechanical ventilation is the single strongest independent risk factor for HAP; the incidence of pneumonia is 6- to 20-fold greater in ventilated than nonventilated patients. Re-intubation is an additional risk factor for VAP.

Diagnosis

Diagnosis of HAP and VAP is challenging. The two primary approaches to diagnosing these infections are through clinical and radiographic findings and bacteriologic test results. HAP should be suspected in patients with a new or progressive pulmonary infiltrate on chest radiograph with clinical findings suggesting infection (new onset of fever, purulent sputum, leukocytosis, and decreased oxygenation). When fever, leukocytosis, purulent sputum, and a positive lower respiratory tract culture are present without a new lung infiltrate, the diagnosis of nosocomial tracheobronchitis should be considered. Tracheobronchitis may mimic many of the clinical signs and symptoms of HAP and may respond to antibiotics. Bacterial colonization of the lower respiratory tract is common in intubated patients, and a positive culture does not necessarily indicate clinical infection. Additional components of diagnosing VAP include (1) obtaining blood cultures, (2) performing a diagnostic thoracentesis if a significant pleural effusion is present (or if a patient has a pleural effusion and appears toxic) to rule out empyema or a complicated parapneumonic effusion, and (3) obtaining lower respiratory tract samples for culture, ideally before antibiotics are initiated or changed.

Samples of lower respiratory tract secretions should be obtained from all patients with suspected HAP and should be ideally collected before antibiotic therapy is initiated or changed. Samples can include an endotracheal aspirate, bronchoalveolar lavage sample, or protected specimen brush sample.

Treatment

Delay in initiating appropriate antimicrobial therapy for HAP is associated with adverse outcomes. That some patients are at risk for HAP caused by multidrug-resistant organisms (see following discussion) should be considered when empiric therapy is selected. Risk factors for multidrug-resistant organisms include recent use of antibiotics, current hospitalization of 5 days or more, immunosuppression, and recent health care–associated exposures. If the presence of multidrug-resistant organisms is suspected, broad-spectrum antibiotic coverage for both gram-positive and gram-negative organisms (including MRSA and *P. aeruginosa*) should be prescribed as guided by the local hospital antibiogram. Antifungal and antiviral agents are not routinely prescribed.

"De-escalation," or narrowing of empiric antimicrobial coverage once culture results are available and the patient has stabilized (typically on hospital day 3 or 4), is another important component of treating HAP. Treatment for 8 days is sufficient for patients with VAP, as long as empiric therapy was effective and patients do not have pneumonia due to *Pseudomonas* species or *Acinetobacter* species. The four important components of treating HAP and VAP are to (1) treat early, (2) administer empiric broad-spectrum antimicrobial agents, (3) de-escalate antimicrobial coverage when appropriate, and (4) consider short-duration therapy (8 days) whenever feasible.

Prevention

The most effective way to prevent VAP is to avoid unnecessary mechanical ventilation. Use of noninvasive ventilation techniques whenever possible and aggressive weaning efforts for patients who do require mechanical ventilation are advocated. Adherence to an evidence-based VAP-prevention "bundle" of interventions is recommended, which includes (1) keeping the head of the bed elevated at greater than 30 degrees, (2) daily assessments of readiness to wean, and (3) use of chlorhexidine mouth care. Respiratory equipment has been associated with outbreaks of VAP, and equipment should be disinfected or sterilized according to published guidelines. Continuous intermittent subglottic suctioning has been demonstrated to reduce the risk for VAP. The data regarding use of endotracheal tubes coated with antiseptics in preventing VAP are promising, but coated tubes are not currently recommended by guidelines. Selective use of oral and digestive decontamination has been demonstrated to be an effective preventive intervention in Europe but not in the United States, where the prevalence of antibiotic-resistant pathogens is higher. **H**

KEY POINTS

- Hospital-acquired pneumonia is defined as a pneumonia that occurs 48 hours or more after hospital admission that was not incubating at the time of admission.
- Ventilator-associated pneumonia is defined as pneumonia that develops more than 48 to 72 hours after beginning mechanical ventilation.
- Mechanical ventilation is the single strongest independent risk factor for development of hospital-acquired pneumonia and ventilator-associated pneumonia.
- The four important components for treating hospital-acquired pneumonia and ventilator-associated pneumonia are to (1) treat early, (2) administer empiric broad-spectrum antimicrobial agents, (3) de-escalate antimicrobial coverage when appropriate, and (4) consider short-duration therapy (8 days) whenever feasible.

Hospital-Acquired Infections Caused by Multidrug-Resistant Organisms

Hospital-acquired infections (HAIs) are commonly caused by multidrug-resistant organisms. Examples of gram-positive multidrug-resistant organisms include MRSA and vancomycin-resistant enterococci. The vast majority of HAIs caused by MRSA are due to hospital-acquired MRSA, although community-associated MRSA has also been implicated. Frequently encountered gram-negative multidrug-resistant organisms include extended-spectrum β-lactamase (ESBL)–producing Enterobacteriaceae, carbapenem-resistant Enterobacteriaceae, *Acinetobacter baumannii*, and multidrug-resistant strains of *P. aeruginosa*.

The prevalence of multidrug-resistant organisms as causative pathogens for HAIs is continually increasing. Infections caused by multidrug-resistant organisms are associated with worse outcomes compared with infections caused by drug-susceptible strains of the same species. Multidrug-resistant infections were historically acquired only in nosocomial settings but are now being encountered in long-term care facilities (for example, nursing homes) and in patients without any contact with health care environments. Although the development of multidrug resistance is complex, its rapid expansion and increasing clinical significance highlight the need for diligent stewardship in using antibiotics in all settings.

Treatment of HAIs caused by multidrug-resistant organisms is frequently complicated by delays in beginning effective antimicrobial therapy. Treatment principles include the following:

1. MRSA infection is often treated with vancomycin. However, if the minimal inhibitory concentration to vancomycin is elevated (≥2 micrograms/mL) and the patient is not clinically responding to therapy, other agents may be considered, such as linezolid or clindamycin for pneumonia and daptomycin for bloodstream infections.

2. Linezolid and daptomycin are generally used to treat invasive infections due to vancomycin-resistant enterococci. However, if ampicillin is active against the causative organism, it should be used as the preferred therapeutic agent.

3. Carbapenems are the antibiotics of choice for invasive infections such as bacteremia caused by ESBL-producing pathogens. Group 1 carbapenems (for example, ertapenem) can be used to treat these infections as long as they are not caused by *Pseudomonas* or *Acinetobacter* species. Fluoroquinolones are also a therapeutic option if the pathogen is susceptible. Cephalosporins and penicillins, including cefepime and β-lactam/β-lactamase combinations, should not be used.

4. Therapeutic options for infections caused by carbapenem-resistant Enterobacteriaceae are limited. Polymyxins, tigecycline, and sometimes, aminoglycosides are often the only

CONT.

available active antimicrobial agents. Tigecycline monotherapy should not be used when bacteremia is suspected.

5. Some strains of non-fermenter, multidrug-resistant gram-negative organisms, such as *A. baumannii* and *P. aeruginosa*, may only be susceptible to polymyxins. *A. baumannii* sometimes retains susceptibility to tigecycline and/or minocycline. Minocycline, if active against the *A. baumannii* strain being treated, is preferred over tigecycline for treatment of urinary tract infection because it achieves higher urinary concentrations.

6. The role of polymyxin-based combination therapy (vs. monotherapy) for multidrug-resistant organisms such as *Acinetobacter* species, *P. aeruginosa*, and carbapenem-resistant Enterobacteriaceae remains uncertain as does the role of aerosolized colistin for treatment of ventilator-associated pneumonia.

Although contact precautions are effective measures to prevent nosocomial spread of multidrug-resistant organisms, their success depends on the compliance of health care workers. Cohort units with dedicated staff are an additional measure to control spread of these organisms. Communication between hospitals and surrounding long-term care facilities can help to identify suspected and known carriers of multidrug-resistant organisms at the time of hospital admission. A surveillance system to monitor rates of multidrug-resistant infections is an important component of hospital infection control. **H**

KEY POINTS

- The prevalence of multidrug-resistant organisms as causative pathogens for hospital-acquired infections is continually increasing.

- Treatment of hospital-acquired infections caused by multidrug-resistant organisms is frequently complicated by delays in beginning effective antimicrobial therapy.

- Although contact precautions are effective measures to prevent nosocomial spread of multidrug-resistant organisms, their success depends on the compliance of health care workers.

Infective Endocarditis Prevention

Background

Infective endocarditis is the net result of the several separate events. Damage to the heart valve or other surface can serve as a nidus for a thrombus composed of platelets, fibrin, and microbes. Turbulent blood flow contributes to this process as does foreign material, including prosthetic valves and pacemakers.

The intensity of bacteremia in the setting of infective endocarditis is variable. Spontaneous bacteremia can occur, but even minor trauma such as that associated with toothbrushing or interventions that manipulate the teeth and periodontal tissues, oropharynx, or gastrointestinal, urologic, and gynecologic tracts can elicit brief periods of bacteremia. Even though numerous bacteria may transiently enter the bloodstream, the risk for infective endocarditis is higher with bacteria such as streptococci, staphylococci, and enterococci, in which specific mediators of bacterial adherence are present (see MKSAP 16 Cardiovascular Medicine for discussion of Infective Endocarditis diagnosis and treatment).

KEY POINT

- Even though numerous bacteria may transiently enter the bloodstream, the risk for infective endocarditis is higher with bacteria such as streptococci, staphylococci, and enterococci, in which specific mediators of bacterial adherence are present.

Rationale

Interventions to prevent infective endocarditis have included correction of predisposing conditions, reduction of skin and oropharyngeal bacterial colonization, and elimination of the point of entry for potential pathogens. Administration of systemic antimicrobial agents, given before invasive procedures associated with transient bacteremia containing organisms causing infective endocarditis, has received the greatest attention as a preventive strategy. The American Heart Association (AHA) infective endocarditis prophylaxis recommendations, which were revised in 2007, acknowledge that this infection is much more likely to result from regular exposure to random bacteremia associated with daily activities than from bacteremia caused by a dental, gastrointestinal, genitourinary, or gynecologic tract procedure. It is likely that the risk of antibiotic-associated adverse events exceeds the benefit, if any, from prophylactic antibiotic therapy in these settings; therefore, the recommended indications for prophylaxis have been narrowed significantly relative to prior guidelines. These changes and their rationale will need to be discussed with patients, particularly low-risk patients who had previously received prophylaxis for dental procedures and are accustomed to this practice.

The AHA currently recommends prophylaxis for patients with cardiac conditions with the highest risk for adverse outcome from infective endocarditis rather than prophylaxis for those with an increased lifetime risk for this infection. Infective endocarditis prophylaxis is recommended for patients with (1) a prosthetic cardiac valve; (2) a previous episode of infective endocarditis; (3) congenital heart disease characterized by unrepaired cyanotic congenital heart disease, including palliative shunts and conduits; a completely repaired congenital heart defect with prosthetic material or device during the first 6 months after the procedure; and repaired congenital heart disease with residual defects; or (4) for cardiac transplantation recipients in whom cardiac valvulopathy develops. **H**

- Infective endocarditis is now thought to be much more likely to result from regular exposure to random bacteremia associated with daily activities than from bacteremia caused by a dental, gastrointestinal, genitourinary, or gynecologic tract procedure.

- The risk for antibiotic-associated adverse events exceeds the benefit, if any, from infective endocarditis prophylaxis.

- The American Heart Association currently recommends infective endocarditis prophylaxis for patients with a prosthetic cardiac valve, a history of infective endocarditis, certain types of congenital heart disease, or those who are cardiac transplantation recipients in whom cardiac valvulopathy develops.

Recommended Prophylactic Regimens

In patients who meet current AHA infective endocarditis criteria, a single dose of a prophylactic antimicrobial agent should be given 30 to 60 minutes before all dental procedures involving manipulation of gingival tissue, the periapical region of teeth, or perforation of the oral mucosa in those patients with cardiac conditions discussed previously. If the antimicrobial agent is inadvertently not administered before the procedure, the medication may be given up to 2 hours after the procedure. **Table 48** lists the preferred antimicrobial regimens for use before a dental procedure.

Although a link between invasive respiratory tract procedures and infective endocarditis has never been demonstrated, antimicrobial prophylaxis (see Table 48) may be considered for patients with the cardiac conditions discussed previously who undergo an invasive respiratory tract procedure. Infective endocarditis prophylaxis is not recommended for patients who undergo genitourinary or gastrointestinal procedures, including upper endoscopy or colonoscopy with or without biopsy.

Appropriate treatment for patients with bacteriuria is recommended to prevent wound infection or infection from genitourinary tract procedures. In patients at risk for infective endocarditis who are about to undergo a surgical procedure that involves infected skin and/or related tissues, it is recommended that the treatment regimen for the infection have adequate activity against staphylococci and β-hemolytic streptococci, because these organisms have a greater propensity to cause infective endocarditis. **H**

- In patients who meet current American Heart Association infective endocarditis criteria, a single dose of a prophylactic antimicrobial agent should be given 30 to 60 minutes before all dental procedures involving manipulation of gingival tissue, the periapical region of teeth, or perforation of the oral mucosa.

- In patients who meet current American Heart Association infective endocarditis criteria, if the antibiotic dose is inadvertently not administered before the procedure, the medication may be given up to 2 hours after the procedure.

TABLE 48. Prophylactic Regimens for Infective Endocarditis Before a Dental Procedure

Situation	Agent[a]	Adults	Children
Oral	Amoxicillin	2 g	50 mg/kg
Unable to take oral medication	Ampicillin	2 g IM or IV	50 mg/kg IM or IV
	or		
	Cefazolin or ceftriaxone	1 g IM or IV	50 mg/kg IM or IV
Allergic to penicillin or ampicillin – oral	Cephalexin	2 g	50 mg/kg
	or		
	Clindamycin	600 mg	20 mg/kg
	or		
	Azithromycin or clarithromycin	500 mg	15 mg/kg
Allergic to penicillin or ampicillin and unable to take oral medication	Cefazolin or ceftriaxone	1 g IM or IV	50 mg/kg IM or IV
	or		
	Clindamycin	600 mg IM or IV	20 mg/kg IM or IV

IM = intramuscular; IV = intravenous.

[a]Regimen consists of a single dose 30 to 60 minutes before the dental procedure, or, if inadvertently not administered, drug may be given up to 2 hours after the procedure.

Adapted from Wilson W, Taubert KA, Gewitz M, et al; American Heart Association. Prevention of infective endocarditis: guidelines from the American Heart Association: a guideline from the American Heart Association Rheumatic Fever, Endocarditis and Kawasaki Disease Committee, Council on Cardiovascular Disease in the Young, and the Council on Clinical Cardiology, Council on Cardiovascular Surgery and Anesthesia, and the Quality of Care and Outcomes Research Interdisciplinary Working Group. J Am Dent Assoc. 2008;139 Suppl:3S-24S. [PMID: 18167394]. Copyright 2008 American Dental Association.

HIV/AIDS

Epidemiology and Prevention

In the United States in 2009, one million persons were estimated to be infected with HIV, with about one third unaware of their diagnosis. The infrastructure for testing and early treatment is established in most developed countries and in many developing countries, but failure to seek testing and financial and other barriers to treatment still exist. Untested and untreated persons may be responsible for ongoing viral spread.

HIV is spread through sexual contact, contaminated blood such as from injection drug use or occupational exposure, or perinatally; barrier precautions, including condoms, can decrease the risk for sexually transmitted infection. In addition, in 2012, the FDA approved the drug emtricitabine/tenofovir disoproxil fumarate for pre-exposure prophylaxis against HIV infection in uninfected individuals who are at high risk of HIV infection and who may engage in sexual activity with HIV-infected partners. The drug is contraindicated for pre-exposure prophylaxis in persons with unknown or positive HIV status.

Postexposure prophylaxis, which can significantly lower the risk of infection if initiated early enough, is standard after occupational exposure and is becoming more accepted following sexual or other exposures. Pre-exposure prophylaxis has been found to be effective in reducing the risk of acquiring HIV infection; however, the merits of taking indefinite antiretroviral therapy are controversial (see Management of the Pregnant Patient with HIV Infection for discussion of perinatal HIV prevention).

KEY POINTS

- HIV is spread through sexual contact, contaminated blood, or perinatally; barrier precautions, including condoms, can decrease the risk for infection.
- Postexposure HIV prophylaxis can significantly lower the risk of infection if initiated early enough and is standard procedure after occupational exposure.

Pathophysiology and Natural History

HIV is a retrovirus that primarily infects CD4 cells, including T-helper lymphocytes, which replicate and integrate into the host cell genome. Infection leads to destruction of these cells and, eventually, to immune system compromise, predisposing to opportunistic infections and AIDS.

Acute Retroviral Syndrome

Up to 90% of persons who become infected with HIV experience an acute symptomatic illness within 2 to 4 weeks of infection, although an accurate diagnosis is not established in most patients during this time. Symptoms typically last 2 to 3 weeks and may range from a simple febrile illness to a full-blown, mononucleosis-like syndrome (**Table 49**). Because of the lack of immune response in early infection, virus levels tend to be very high, resulting in high levels of infectivity during this period. Patients presenting with the acute retroviral syndrome are usually in the "window period," during which time seroconversion of the disease has not yet occurred and results of HIV antibody testing are negative. However, viral-specific tests, such as those for nucleic acid, are usually positive at quite high levels during this time frame and can be used to establish the diagnosis. Symptoms of acute HIV infection resolve with or without treatment, and most acute infections are undiagnosed. The benefit of beginning antiretroviral therapy during acute infection has not been proved but is suggested by theoretical considerations and retrospective data.

Chronic HIV infection

After acute retroviral syndrome, a period of years of asymptomatic, but still active, infection occurs, during which depletion of CD4 T-lymphocytes progresses. Patients may develop symptoms of chronic HIV infection during this period (**Table 50**). Before progression to AIDS (see Opportunistic Infections), patients may experience common infections that do not qualify as opportunistic infections but are more prolonged or severe in the context of HIV infection. Examples include recurrent or refractory vaginal candidiasis, severe oral or genital herpes simplex virus infection, pneumococcal pneumonia, and herpes zoster virus infection.

AIDS

A diagnosis of AIDS is established with development of certain AIDS-indicator opportunistic infections or malignancies (see Opportunistic Infections) or when the CD4 cell count decreases to less than 200/microliter.

TABLE 49. Signs and Symptoms of the Acute Retroviral Syndrome (Primary HIV Infection)

Sign/Symptom	Frequency (%)
Fever	96
Lymphadenopathy	74
Pharyngitis	70
Rash	70
Myalgia/arthralgia	54
Diarrhea	32
Headache	32
Nausea/vomiting	27
Hepatosplenomegaly	14
Weight loss	13
Thrush	12
Neurologic symptoms	12

TABLE 50.	Signs and Symptoms of Chronic HIV Infection
Lymphadenopathy	
Fevers, night sweats	
Fatigue	
Weight loss	
Chronic diarrhea	
Seborrheic dermatitis, psoriasis, tinea, onychomycosis	
Oral aphthous ulcers, oral hairy leukoplakia, gingivitis/periodontitis	
Peripheral neuropathy	
Leukopenia, anemia, thrombocytopenia	
Nephropathy	

KEY POINTS

- Up to 90% of persons who become infected with HIV experience an acute symptomatic illness within 2 to 4 weeks of infection, although an accurate diagnosis is not established in most patients during this time.

- Symptoms of acute retroviral syndrome typically last 2 to 3 weeks and may range from a simple febrile illness to a full-blown, mononucleosis-like syndrome.

- An AIDS diagnosis is established when certain AIDS-indicator opportunistic infections or malignancies develop or when the CD4 cell count falls below 200/microliter.

Screening and Diagnosis

Because previous testing guidelines excluded many undiagnosed persons with HIV infection, the Centers for Disease Control and Prevention (CDC) released new HIV testing recommendations in 2006, significantly widening the scope of testing and encouraging reduction of barriers to widespread testing. Most, but not all, states have since revised or repealed laws requiring written consent for HIV testing, consistent with the CDC's recommendations for adoption of "opt-out" screening (the patient is informed and testing proceeds unless the patient declines). All adolescents and adults aged 13 to 64 years are recommended to undergo testing at least once unless the prevalence in the specific population is less than 0.1%. In addition, the American College of Physicians has issued a guidance statement recommending that this age range be expanded to include persons through age 75 years because of increased rates of infection in this population. Persons at high risk for HIV infection (injection drug users and their sex partners, persons who exchange sex for money or drugs, sex partners of those with HIV infection, men who have sex with men, and persons and their sex partners who have had more than one sex partner since their last HIV test) should undergo repeat testing at least annually. The guidelines reinforce the importance of HIV screening in all pregnant women as early as possible in

pregnancy to implement measures to minimize perinatal transmission. In addition, in 2012, the FDA approved an at-home, rapid HIV screening test. The self-administered test uses swabs of oral fluids from the upper and lower gums to identify HIV antibodies, and results are available within 20 to 40 minutes. Physicians should advise patients that a positive test result requires confirmatory testing in the office. Moreover, because HIV antibodies may not appear during the window period (see Acute Retroviral System, discussed previously) patients with negative home test results should undergo repeat testing within 3 months.

The diagnosis of HIV infection is established by a two-stage serologic testing process. The initial test is an enzyme immunoassay (EIA). A negative EIA is generally considered adequate to exclude infection except during the acute phase following primary infection (the window period) before seroconversion occurs and when serologic testing, including Western blot assay, may be falsely negative. In these patients, EIA testing should be repeated 6 to 12 weeks later when seroconversion is established. If an acute diagnosis is necessary during the window period, a specific viral test such as the quantitative RNA polymerase chain reaction assay may be useful; in acute infection, the viral load is usually very high (often >100,000 copies/mL). However, use of a viral load study for routine diagnosis or in situations other than during the acute phase of infection is discouraged because of decreased sensitivity and specificity of the test at lower viral loads and the significant cost relative to EIA. In a patient with a positive EIA, the test should be repeated. Repeatedly positive EIA results are confirmed by Western blot assay. Combination testing with EIA followed by Western blot assay has a sensitivity of 99.5% and specificity of 99.99%. Rapid HIV tests are now available in kits that can be used in the clinical setting. These are EIA tests, and positive results require standard follow-up confirmatory testing. Because the EIA requires confirmatory testing, it is never appropriate to tell patients they have HIV infection based on results of any EIA alone before the Western blot results are known.

A negative Western blot assay indicates a false-positive EIA result. An indeterminate Western blot assay indicates the presence of antibody bands to certain viral antigens, but results are insufficient to establish the diagnosis of HIV infection. This may occur during the "window period" of acute infection when patients are just beginning to develop antibodies to HIV. Repeatedly indeterminate Western blot results usually indicate a cross-reacting antibody caused by infections or immunologic diseases other than HIV infection. Indications for HIV testing are shown in **Table 51**.

KEY POINTS

- All persons aged 13 to 64 years are recommended to undergo HIV testing at least once unless the prevalence in the specific population is less than 0.1%.
- Persons likely to be at high risk for HIV infection should undergo repeat HIV testing at least annually.

- The diagnosis of HIV infection is established by a two-stage serologic testing process consisting of enzyme immunoassay (EIA) followed by Western blot assay confirmatory testing of positive EIA results.
- Standard HIV testing may be unreliable in early infection, and repeat testing or other tests such as quantitative RNA polymerase chain reaction assay can help to establish the diagnosis.

Initiation of Care

Initial Evaluation and Laboratory Testing

Initial evaluation of the newly diagnosed patient with HIV infection includes a complete history, including social and sexual history, and physical examination with attention to signs and symptoms of opportunistic infections and other complications. Counseling on HIV transmission and prevention is also appropriate.

Laboratory tests indicated for patients with newly diagnosed HIV infection are shown in **Table 52**. Baseline testing assesses the patient's hematologic and metabolic status and assesses for coinfections that would need to be addressed.

Baseline viral resistance testing is now recommended for all newly diagnosed patients with HIV infection to guide the choice of antiretroviral therapy (See Drug Resistance Testing). The CD4 T-lymphocyte cell count (CD4 cell count) and quantitative measurement of HIV RNA (viral

TABLE 52. Laboratory Testing as Part of the Evaluation of HIV Infection

Repeat HIV antibody testing if no documentation

Viral resistance testing at baseline and for treatment failure

Quantitative HIV RNA assay (viral load)

T-cell subsets (CD4 cell count)

Complete blood count with differential

Chemistries, including kidney function and fasting plasma glucose

Liver chemistry studies/liver enzymes

Fasting serum lipid profile

Tuberculin skin test or interferon-γ release assay for tuberculosis exposure

Serologic testing for hepatitis A, B, and C virus infection

Serologic testing for syphilis; testing for other sexually transmitted infections

Pap test

Toxoplasma serology

Varicella and cytomegalovirus serologies in high-risk individuals

load) are the most important tests for monitoring disease stage and effectiveness of treatment. The baseline CD4 cell count may be important in deciding when to initiate antiretroviral therapy. Follow-up monitoring of the viral load is critical in assessing the adequacy of the therapeutic regimen. Repeat testing of CD4 cell count, viral load, complete blood count, and kidney and liver function should be performed whenever HIV regimens are begun or modified, 2 to 8 weeks after therapy is changed, and every 3 to 6 months in patients whose regimens remain stable.

Immunizations and Prophylaxis for Opportunistic Infections

Because of their increased risk for pneumococcal pneumonia and other invasive pneumococcal diseases, all patients with HIV infection should receive pneumococcal polysaccharide vaccine immunization. Three doses of the hepatitis B virus (HBV) vaccine are indicated in patients who are not already immune to or infected with HBV. Annual influenza vaccination is appropriate, and recommendations for tetanus, diphtheria, and acellular pertussis; hepatitis A virus; human papillomavirus; and meningococcal vaccines are the same as those for the general population. Live virus vaccines, such as the measles-mumps-rubella and varicella-zoster vaccines, are not appropriate in patients with HIV infection, although studies evaluating the safety and effectiveness of the zoster vaccine in individuals with HIV infection with high CD4 cell counts are ongoing.

Indications and preferred agents for primary prophylaxis of opportunistic HIV/AIDS infections are shown in

TABLE 51. Indications for HIV Testing

Symptoms/signs of acute retroviral syndrome

Symptoms/signs of chronic HIV infection

Opportunistic infection

Severe, recurrent, or persistent infection that does not qualify as opportunistic

Presence of tuberculosis, HBV infection, HCV infection, other sexually transmitted infections, hemophilia

History of at-risk behavior (multiple sex partners, men who have sex with men, injection drug use) or sexual partner of someone who engages in at-risk behavior

Persons aged 13-64 years, unless in population areas with low (<0.1%) prevalence

Known or suspected HIV exposure

Victim of sexual assault

Patient request

All pregnant women

Child born to mother infected with HIV

Occupational exposure to blood/body fluid (both source patient and exposed worker)

Blood/semen/organ donor

HBV = hepatitis B virus; HCV = hepatitis C virus.

Table 53. It is important to exclude active infection with *Mycobacterium avium* complex clinically and with negative blood cultures, because the single agent selected as prophylaxis would not be effective treatment for the active infection, and resistance could emerge, making the active infection even more difficult to treat. Similarly, it is important to exclude active tuberculosis with tuberculin skin testing or the interferon-γ release assay to determine whether prophylactic treatment or treatment for active disease is necessary.

KEY POINTS

- A thorough history, including social and sexual history, and physical examination with attention to signs and symptoms of opportunistic infections and other complications, as well as counseling on HIV transmission and prevention, are appropriate in patients with newly diagnosed HIV.

- Baseline viral resistance testing is now recommended for all newly diagnosed patients with HIV infection to guide the choice of antiretroviral therapy.

- The CD4 T-lymphocyte cell count and quantitative measurement of HIV RNA viral load are the most important tests for monitoring disease stage and effectiveness of treatment.

- All patients with HIV infection should receive pneumococcal polysaccharide vaccine immunization; hepatitis B virus vaccine (if not already immune to or infected by); annual influenza vaccination; and vaccines for tetanus, diphtheria, and acellular/pertussis; hepatitis A; human papillomavirus; and meningococcal vaccines as indicated in the general population.

- In patients with HIV infection, it is important to exclude active infection with *Mycobacterium avium* complex clinically and with negative blood cultures and active tuberculosis with tuberculin skin testing or the interferon-γ release assay to determine whether prophylactic treatment or treatment for active disease is necessary.

Complications of HIV Infection in the Antiretroviral Therapy Era

The development of medication regimens that effectively lower HIV viral loads to undetectable levels has transformed HIV infection from a uniformly fatal illness into a manageable chronic disease. However, as opportunistic infections and AIDS-related malignancies occur less frequently, other complications of HIV have increased in importance. These medication regimens have been referred to as highly active antiretroviral therapy (HAART), a term that initially was used to differentiate more aggressive, usually multiple-drug therapy, from single- or double-drug therapy that was once the standard approach. Currently, combination therapy is used routinely, and the distinction between antiretroviral therapy (ART) and HAART is less meaningful. Consequently, the term ART will be used in the discussion of HIV therapy in this section.

Metabolic Disorders

Metabolic changes in patients with HIV infection can be caused by antiretroviral medications or the infection itself. HIV infection is associated with decreased total, HDL, and LDL serum cholesterol levels and increased serum triglyceride levels. ART tends to reverse some of these changes: total and LDL cholesterol increase, but HDL cholesterol remains decreased and triglycerides remain elevated. Some antiretroviral agents, including many protease inhibitors, are particularly associated with hyperlipidemia. Atorvastatin has been shown to be effective in treating hyperlipidemia in patients with HIV infection; however, because of interactions with the protease inhibitor ritonavir, atorvastatin should be started at a lower dose in these patients.

Insulin resistance may also develop or worsen with treatment of HIV infection. Measurement of fasting lipids and fasting glucose or hemoglobin A_{1c} levels is appropriate after initiation of or a change in antiretroviral regimens and requires periodic follow-up during therapy.

Changes in lipids may be accompanied by lipodystrophy as well as changes in body fat distribution, including truncal and visceral fat accumulation and loss of subcutaneous fat in the face and extremities. This peripheral

TABLE 53. Prophylaxis for Opportunistic Infections in HIV/AIDS		
Opportunistic Infection	**Indication**	**Preferred Drug**
Pneumocystis jirovecii	CD4 cell count <200/μL	TMP/SMX, double-strength tablet once daily or three times weekly
Toxoplasmosis	CD4 cell count <100/μL and positive serology	TMP/SMX, double-strength tablet once daily
Mycobacterium avium complex	CD4 cell count <50/μL	Azithromycin, 1200 mg/week
Tuberculosis	TST >5 mm or positive IGRA	INH, 300 mg/d for 9 months

IGRA = interferon-γ release assay; INH = isoniazid; TMP/SMX = trimethoprim-sulfamethoxazole; TST = tuberculin skin test; μL = microliter.

lipoatrophy may be reduced with avoidance of the thymidine analogue reverse transcriptase inhibitors (RTIs) (stavudine and zidovudine).

Mitochondrial toxicity leading to lactic acidosis, which can be fatal if not recognized early, has decreased with replacement of stavudine, didanosine, and zidovudine with lamivudine or emtricitabine and tenofovir in most regimens.

Osteopenia and osteoporosis may also be increased in patients with HIV infection; bone densitometry screening is not recommended for all patients but should be considered for those older than 50 years or with other risk factors.

HIV can also lead to chronic kidney disease through development of HIV-associated nephropathy. HIV-associated nephropathy, when diagnosed early, can be reversed with treatment of HIV. Patients in whom HIV-associated nephropathy progresses may require kidney dialysis or transplantation.

Liver disease is also increasing in patients with HIV infection, partly because of the high prevalence of coinfection with HBV or hepatitis C virus (HCV). Patients with HIV infection with chronic HBV infection requiring treatment should be given a multidrug regimen with agents active against both HBV and HIV infection. Patients co-infected with HIV and HCV have an increased risk for progression to chronic liver disease and cirrhosis.

KEY POINT

- Metabolic disorders, including hyperlipidemia, insulin resistance, body fat distribution changes, chronic kidney or liver disease and cirrhosis, and osteopenia and osteoporosis, are associated with HIV infection and HIV treatment.

Cardiovascular Disease

An increased risk for cardiovascular disease is associated not only with the use of some antiretroviral agents but also with HIV infection itself. The SMART study, which randomized subjects with CD4 cell counts greater than 350/microliter to continuous ART versus CD4 cell count–guided treatment interruptions, found that patients in the treatment-interruptions arm not only had more infectious complications (as expected), but they also experienced more cardiovascular disease end points and death, which led to early termination of the study. These results suggest that any increased cardiovascular risk caused by the metabolic side effects of treatment is more than offset by the risk from uncontrolled HIV infection, at least in those patients with CD4 cell counts less than 350/microliter. This increased risk is thought to be related to ongoing chronic inflammation, contributing to increased atherosclerosis. Chronic care of patients with HIV infection requires attention to modifiable cardiovascular risk factors, such as smoking, hyperlipidemia, hypertension, and diabetes.

KEY POINTS

- Any increased cardiovascular risk caused by the metabolic side effects of HIV treatment is more than offset by the risk from uncontrolled HIV infection.

- Chronic care of patients with HIV infection requires attention to modifiable cardiovascular risk factors, such as smoking, hyperlipidemia, hypertension, and diabetes mellitus.

Immune Reconstitution Inflammatory Syndrome

With the initiation of ART, viral load levels fall sharply, CD4 cell counts increase, and immune responses improve. In the presence of an opportunistic infection, which may not have been clinically recognized previously, this reconstitution of the immune response can lead to dramatic inflammatory responses as the newly revived immune system reacts to high burdens of antigens. This inflammatory presentation of infections is called immune reconstitution inflammatory syndrome (IRIS) and usually occurs a few weeks to a few months after initiation of ART. IRIS occurs with various opportunistic infections but most commonly in patients with mycobacterial infections, such as tuberculosis or *M. avium* complex, or disseminated fungal infections. Continuation of treatment is appropriate in patients with IRIS, but concomitant corticosteroids may be required to moderate excessive inflammation. ◨

KEY POINTS

- Immune reconstitution inflammatory syndrome can occur after initiation of antiretroviral therapy as a dramatic inflammatory response to a previously clinically unrecognized opportunistic infection when the newly revived immune system reacts to high burdens of antigens.

- Continuation of treatment is appropriate in patients with immune reconstitution inflammatory syndrome, but concomitant corticosteroids may be required to moderate excessive inflammation.

Opportunistic Infections

Most opportunistic infections are unlikely to occur in patients with a CD4 cell count higher than 200/microliter, which is why this is the threshold value used to define AIDS.

Oral candidiasis (thrush) may occur in patients with CD4 cell counts greater than 200/microliter, especially in those with other risk factors, such as history of use of inhaled corticosteroids or broad-spectrum antibiotics, but extension to esophageal candidiasis occurs more often in patients with AIDS. Diagnosis is usually based on findings of visual inspection showing characteristic whitish plaques on the oral mucosa. Treatment of oral candidiasis includes topical agents such as clotrimazole troches. Dysphagia or other swallowing symptoms in patients with visible thrush suggest esophageal candidiasis, which requires treatment with a systemic agent such as fluconazole.

Cryptococcal infection starts in the lung but rarely presents until it is disseminated, most commonly to the meninges or skin. Cryptococcal meningitis may occur in patients with higher CD4 cell counts but occurs more typically in those with counts less than 100/microliter. It has a subacute or chronic presentation, characterized by headaches and changes in mental status, and systemic symptoms such as fever, sweats, and weight loss. Focal neurologic deficits usually involve cranial nerves. Diagnosis is established by culture or cryptococcal antigen testing on cerebrospinal fluid or serum. Treatment consists of induction therapy with amphotericin B deoxycholate or the lipid formulation of amphotericin B, combined with flucytosine, followed by consolidation therapy with fluconazole. Attention to increased intracranial pressure is crucial to reduce the risk for mortality and neurologic sequelae such as blindness. Even with effective treatment, there is significantly increased risk of early mortality in patients with disseminated cryptococcal disease.

Pneumocystis jirovecii pneumonia occurs in patients with CD4 cell counts less than 200/microliter and usually presents subacutely with dyspnea, dry cough, and fever. The chest radiograph typically shows diffuse bilateral interstitial or alveolar infiltrates, and diagnosis can be confirmed by identification of stains of the organism in sputum or bronchoalveolar lavage fluid. The preferred treatment is high-dose trimethoprim-sulfamethoxazole. The patient may worsen clinically following initiation of appropriate treatment, and corticosteroids should be used as adjunctive therapy in those with an arterial Po_2 of less than 70 mm Hg (9.3 kPa) while breathing ambient air or an alveolar-arterial oxygen gradient of greater than 35 mm Hg.

Toxoplasma gondii is a protozoan transmitted through the ingestion of undercooked meat or contact with cat feces. Toxoplasmosis primarily causes encephalitis in patients with CD4 cell counts less than 100/microliter. The illness is characterized by fever, headache, focal neurologic deficits, and, possibly, seizures. Contrast-enhanced CT of the head or MRI of the brain usually shows multiple ring-enhancing lesions. MRI is the imaging modality of choice because it has higher sensitivity and can better differentiate toxoplasmosis from other infections and central nervous system lymphoma. Treatment is typically empiric (pyrimethamine plus sulfadiazine or pyrimethamine plus clindamycin, or alternatively, trimethoprim-sulfamethoxazole), with clinical and radiologic responses occurring within 1 to 2 weeks.

The most common mycobacterial diseases in AIDS are tuberculosis and disseminated *M. avium* complex infection. Unlike in HIV-negative individuals, the presentation of tuberculosis in patients with AIDS is more likely to be extrapulmonary or associated with atypical chest radiographic findings without upper lobe cavitary lesions. Treatment of tuberculosis in patients with AIDS is complicated by drug interactions with antiretroviral agents and usually requires the use of reduced doses of rifabutin instead of rifampin. Disseminated *M. avium* complex infection usually is characterized by CD4 cell counts less than 50/microliter and fever, sweats, weight loss, lymphadenopathy, hepatosplenomegaly, and cytopenia. Specific mycobacterial blood cultures are usually positive. Treatment consists of a macrolide-based (clarithromycin or azithromycin) multidrug regimen.

Patients with cytomegalovirus (CMV) infection usually have CD4 cell counts less than 50/microliter. Gastrointestinal involvement is most commonly characterized by ulcers in the esophagus or colon, although CMV infection may occur anywhere in the gastrointestinal tract. CMV may infect the central nervous system, causing encephalitis or polyradiculitis. Prior to ART, the most common and significant presentation of CMV was CMV retinitis. The incidence of this illness has decreased significantly and is currently limited to patients with advanced immunosuppression who have not responded to ART. Patients with CMV retinitis may initially present with only floaters, but their condition will progress to blindness. Urgent ophthalmologic evaluation and initiation of ganciclovir, valganciclovir, or foscarnet therapy are necessary in patients with suspected CMV retinitis.

Molluscum contagiosum, caused by a poxvirus, is characterized by dome-shaped papules with central umbilication, most commonly occurring on the face and neck; these papules usually resolve with initiation of ART (**Figure 12**).

Bacillary angiomatosis is the most common manifestation of *Bartonella* infection in patients with AIDS and is characterized by skin lesions that may be confused with Kaposi sarcoma. Kaposi sarcoma presents with red, purple, or brown macules,

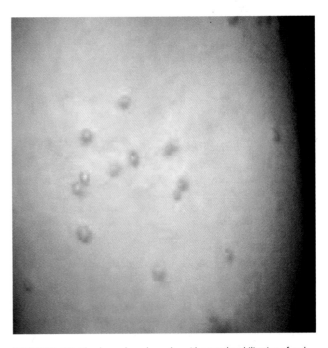

FIGURE 12. The dome-shaped papules with central umbilication of molluscum contagiosum.

CONT.

papules, plaques, or nodules on the skin or mucous membranes and is now known to be caused by a human herpesvirus (HHV-8). It occurs primarily in men who have sex with men and is rare in other HIV risk groups (**Figure 13**). 🄷

KEY POINTS

- Dysphagia or other swallowing symptoms in patients with HIV infection and visible oral thrush are suggestive of esophageal candidiasis, which requires treatment with a systemic agent such as fluconazole.

- Disseminated cryptococcal infection is characterized by headaches and neurologic deficits with changes in mental status, cranial nerve involvement, and systemic symptoms such as fever, sweats, and weight loss.

- Increased intracranial pressure in patients with disseminated cryptococcus can cause death and neurologic sequelae such as blindness.

- *Pneumocystis jirovecii* pneumonia occurs in patients with CD4 cell counts less than 200/microliter.

- Toxoplasmosis primarily causes encephalitis in patients with CD4 cell counts less than 100/microliter and is characterized by fever, headache, focal neurologic deficits, and possibly, seizures.

- The presentation of tuberculosis in patients with AIDS, unlike in HIV-negative individuals, is more likely to be extrapulmonary or associated with atypical chest radiographic findings without upper lobe cavitary lesions.

- Patients with cytomegalovirus disease usually have CD4 cell counts less than 50/microliter and retinitis or gastrointestinal involvement.

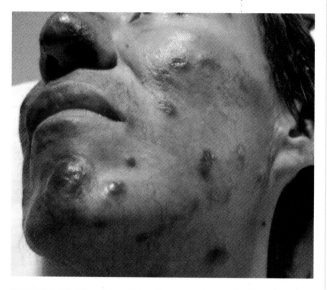

FIGURE 13. The lesions of Kaposi sarcoma, characterized by red, purple, or brown macules, papules, plaques, or nodules on the skin or mucous membranes.

Management of HIV Infection

The management of HIV infection continues to evolve rapidly. The U.S. Department of Health and Human Services (DHHS) and the National Institutes of Health regularly update guidelines on management of HIV infection, including the use of antiretroviral agents, prevention and treatment of opportunistic infections, and HIV testing and prophylaxis. The most recent guidelines are available at the AIDS info Web site (www.aidsinfo.nih.gov).

When to Initiate Treatment

Because the benefits of treating HIV earlier have been demonstrated, and the treatment regimens have become less complex and better tolerated, indications for when to begin ART have expanded. Current indications for initiation of ART, according to the DHHS guidelines, are listed in **Table 54**. In addition, the International AIDS Society U.S.A. Panel recommends treatment of those with active HCV coinfection and those who are at high risk for or have active cardiovascular disease, regardless of CD4 cell count. Whether to initiate treatment in all patients with HIV infection, even those with a CD4 cell count greater than 500/microliter, is an area of considerable controversy. A large NIH-sponsored prospective randomized controlled trial with clinical end points (the START study) is ongoing to address this question.

KEY POINT

- Antiretroviral therapy is recommended for patients with active hepatitis B or C virus coinfection, high risk for or active cardiovascular disease, a history of AIDS-defining opportunistic infection or malignancy, symptomatic HIV infection, a CD4 cell count <500 cells/microliter, HIV-associated nephropathy, or pregnancy.

TABLE 54. Indications for Initiation of Antiretroviral Therapy in HIV Infection

History of AIDS-defining opportunistic infection or malignancy[a]
Symptomatic HIV infection
CD4 cell count <500/μL
Presence of HIV-associated nephropathy
Active coinfection with hepatitis B or C virus
Pregnancy, to prevent perinatal transmission

μL = microliter.

[a]AIDS-defining illnesses include esophageal or pulmonary candidiasis; invasive cervical cancer; extrapulmonary coccidioidomycosis, cryptococcosis, or histoplasmosis; chronic intestinal cryptosporidiosis or isosporiasis; cytomegalovirus retinitis or infection other than liver, spleen, or lymph nodes; herpes simplex virus infection (chronic ulcers, bronchitis, pneumonitis, esophagitis); HIV encephalopathy; Kaposi sarcoma; lymphoma (Burkitt, immunoblastic, primary brain); lymphoid interstitial pneumonia; *Mycobacterium tuberculosis* at any site; extrapulmonary *Mycobacterium avium* complex or *Mycobacterium kansasii*; *Pneumocystis jirovecii* infection; progressive multifocal leukoencephalopathy; recurrent *Salmonella* bacteremia; toxoplasmosis of brain; HIV wasting syndrome; or recurrent bacterial pneumonia.

Antiretroviral Regimens

The objective of HIV treatment is to fully suppress viral replication to prevent the development of viral drug resistance, resulting in a rapid and progressive decrease of viral load levels within the first few weeks of treatment, and, within a few months of treatment, undetectable viral load levels that remain undetectable during therapy. Adhering to such a regimen requires a level of commitment often difficult for patients to maintain. Consequently, clinicians must discuss adherence with patients before initiation of therapy and at every follow-up visit. Maximal suppression of the virus generally requires the use of at least three drugs from at least two different classes. See **Table 55** for a list of agents currently in use in the United States.

The current preferred initial regimen in patients without viral drug resistance combines two nucleoside analogue RTIs (tenofovir and emtricitabine) with a nonnucleoside RTI (efavirenz), available as a once-daily, combination single pill. The use of a combination pill improves adherence and effectiveness. However, efavirenz should not be used in women who are or may become pregnant because of its association with neural tube defects (see Management of Pregnant Patients with HIV Infection). Other preferred regimens for patients who cannot take efavirenz use the same nucleoside "backbone," consisting of tenofovir and emtricitabine, with an integrase inhibitor (raltegravir) or a protease inhibitor (atazanavir or darunavir) as the third drug rather than efavirenz. Protease inhibitors are almost always given with a small dose of ritonavir, which is used to boost the drug levels of protease inhibitors, rather than as an antiretroviral agent itself. Ritonavir, even at small doses, has potent actions on multiple pathways of drug metabolism, including inhibition of the cytochrome P-450 enzyme system responsible for metabolism of many drugs. The use of ritonavir allows smaller and less frequent dosing of the regimen's other protease inhibitor, yet results in more steady and reliable drug levels, improving tolerability and effectiveness. Other drug interactions in patients with HIV infection are also common. For example, atazanavir should not be given with proton pump inhibitors, and protease inhibitors should not be given with lovastatin or simvastatin.

TABLE 55. Antiretroviral Agents Available in the United States to Treat HIV Infection	
Class	**Agents[a]**
Nucleoside analogue RTIs	Abacavir
	Didanosine
	Emtricitabine
	Lamivudine
	Stavudine
	Tenofovir
	Zidovudine
Nonnucleoside RTIs	Efavirenz
	Etravirine
	Nevirapine
	Rilpivirine
Protease inhibitors	Atazanavir
	Darunavir
	Fosamprenavir
	Indinavir
	Lopinavir
	Nelfinavir
	Ritonavir
	Saquinavir
	Tipranavir
Entry inhibitors	Enfuvirtide
	Maraviroc
Integrase inhibitor	Raltegravir

[a]Some agents are also available as components of combination medications.

RTIs = reverse transcriptase inhibitors.

KEY POINTS

- Clinicians must discuss the importance of adherence with their patients with HIV infection before initiation of antiretroviral drug therapy and at every follow-up visit.

- Maximal suppression of HIV generally requires the use of at least three drugs from at least two different classes.

- The current preferred initial HIV antiretroviral regimen in patients without viral drug resistance combines two nucleoside analogue reverse transcriptase inhibitors with a nonnucleoside reverse transcriptase inhibitor in a once-daily, combination single pill.

- Protease inhibitors are almost always given with a small dose of ritonavir, which is used to boost the drug levels of protease inhibitors rather than as an antiretroviral agent itself.

Resistance Testing

Baseline testing of a patient's HIV isolate for antiretroviral resistance should be performed to guide the choice of agents, because previous infection with a resistant virus may have occurred. Resistance testing is also appropriate in the setting of treatment failure as evidenced by suboptimally controlled viral loads (lack of decreased or suppressed viral load, or previously undetectable viral loads that have become detectable on repeated testing). Generally, about 500 copies of virus/mL of blood are required for resistance testing to be adequately performed. Testing for treatment failure should be done while the patient is still receiving therapy, because false-negative results may occur with removal of the selective pressure provided by the drugs.

- Resistance testing of a patient's HIV isolate should be performed to guide the choice of agents at baseline and in treatment failure as evidenced by suboptimally controlled viral loads.

- Testing for treatment failure should be done while the patient is still receiving therapy.

Management of Pregnant Patients with HIV Infection

HIV testing for all pregnant women is appropriate. About one in four neonates born to women with HIV infection will acquire HIV infection perinatally if antiretroviral therapy is not given. Appropriate antiretroviral therapy can reduce the risk of HIV transmission to the newborn to less than 2%. Because HIV infection can be transmitted through breast milk, mothers with HIV infection should not breastfeed their infants if an alternative method is available. The preferred antiretroviral regimen in pregnancy is zidovudine, lamivudine, and lopinavir/ritonavir; efavirenz is teratogenic and should not be given in pregnancy. Indications for antiretroviral therapy in women after delivery are the same as those for the nonpregnant adult.

- HIV testing for all pregnant women is appropriate.

- In pregnant women with HIV infection, appropriate antiretroviral therapy can reduce the risk of HIV transmission to the newborn to less than 2%.

- The preferred antiretroviral regimen in pregnancy is zidovudine, lamivudine, and lopinavir/ritonavir; efavirenz is teratogenic and should not be given in pregnancy.

Viral Infections

Influenza Viruses

Overview

Influenza virus infection is a highly contagious, acute, febrile respiratory illness that causes outbreaks annually and is responsible for approximately 36,000 deaths annually. Influenza A, B, and C viruses are human pathogens, although influenza C infection is rare. Influenza A viruses infect a wide range of hosts and are classified into subtypes based on their surface proteins, hemagglutinin and neuraminidase. Influenza virus variants result from frequent minor antigenic changes (drifts) caused by point mutations and recombination events that occur during viral replication. Major changes in the surface glycoproteins are referred to as antigenic shifts. Antigenic shifts are associated with epidemics and pandemics of influenza A virus infection, whereas antigenic drifts are associated with more localized outbreaks. Antigenic shifts only occur among influenza A viruses. New influenza A virus subtypes can cause a pandemic when they bring about illness in humans, are transmitted efficiently from human to human, and when little or no preexisting immunity is present among humans. In the spring of 2009, infection of humans with a novel influenza A virus (H1N1) was identified, and this virus caused a worldwide pandemic. Outbreaks caused by influenza B viruses are generally less severe than those caused by influenza A viruses; however, it is impossible to clinically differentiate between influenza A and B virus infection.

Outbreaks of influenza have a seasonal distribution and occur almost exclusively during the winter months in the Northern and Southern Hemispheres. In tropical regions, influenza occurs throughout the year. Although influenza viruses can cause disease among persons in any age group, rates of infection are highest among children. Serious illness and death are highest among children younger than 2 years and adults older than 65 years and those who have medical conditions that confer risk for complications. Seasonal influenza is estimated to cause approximately 36,000 deaths annually.

- New influenza A virus subtypes can cause a pandemic when they cause illness in humans, are transmitted efficiently from human to human, and when there is little or no preexisting immunity present among humans.

- Outbreaks caused by influenza B viruses are generally less severe than those caused by influenza A virus; however, it is impossible to clinically differentiate between influenza A and B virus infection.

Clinical Features and Evaluation

Typical symptoms of influenza in adults are fever, headache, myalgia, nonproductive cough, sore throat, and nasal discharge. Gastrointestinal symptoms may occur in children. The incubation period is 1 to 4 days.

The most common complication of influenza is pneumonia, occurring in patients with underlying chronic illnesses. Primary viral pneumonia, secondary bacterial pneumonia, or both may occur. The most common bacterial pathogens are *Streptococcus pneumoniae, Staphylococcus aureus,* and *Haemophilus influenzae.* Other less common influenza complications include myocarditis, pericarditis, myositis, rhabdomyolysis, encephalitis, aseptic meningitis, transverse myelitis, and Guillain-Barré syndrome. ■

When influenza has been documented in the community, a clinical diagnosis can be made based on signs and symptoms. The standard laboratory study used to confirm influenza virus infection is reverse transcriptase polymerase chain reaction or viral culture. Rapid influenza diagnostic tests are immunoassays that can identify the presence of influenza A and B viral nucleoprotein antigens in respiratory secretions and display results qualitatively as positive or negative. Several rapid influenza diagnostic tests are commercially available, and results are generally available within 15 minutes or less. Rapid influenza diagnostic tests are helpful in confirming disease if positive. However, because they have limited sensitivity, negative results do not exclude the diagnosis, and other studies are indicated if confirmation is necessary. However, these tests are useful for public health purposes in detecting influenza virus outbreaks and guiding decisions about implementation of prevention and control measures.

KEY POINTS

- Typical symptoms of influenza in adults are fever, headache, myalgia, nonproductive cough, sore throat, and nasal discharge; the incubation period is 1 to 4 days.

- The most common complication of influenza is pneumonia, occurring in patients with underlying chronic illnesses.

- When influenza has been documented in the community, a clinical diagnosis can be made based on signs and symptoms.

Management

Influenza vaccination is the most effective method for preventing influenza infection and its complications. Two types of influenza vaccine are available: trivalent inactivated influenza vaccine and live intranasal influenza vaccine. The trivalent inactivated influenza vaccine can be used in persons older than 6 months, including healthy persons, those with chronic medical conditions, and pregnant women. Live intranasal influenza vaccine is administered as a nasal spray. It can be used for healthy persons aged 2 to 49 years who are not pregnant or immunocompromised. In 2010, the Centers for Disease Control and Prevention's (CDC's) Advisory Committee on Immunization Practices (ACIP) began recommending annual influenza vaccination for all persons older than 6 months.

Antiviral medications with activity against influenza viruses are an important adjunct to influenza vaccination in preventing and treating influenza. Two FDA-approved influenza antiviral medications, oseltamivir and zanamivir, were recommended for use as influenza treatment and chemoprophylaxis in the United States during the 2011-2012 influenza season. These agents are neuraminidase inhibitors and are active against influenza A and B viruses. Because of high rates of adamantane resistance in the United States, the CDC-ACIP advised against the use of amantadine and rimantadine for the treatment or chemoprophylaxis of influenza A virus infection. Because resistance patterns may change rapidly, treatment recommendations should be reviewed each year.

Treatment is indicated for hospitalized patients; those with severe, complicated, or progressive illness; and those at high risk for influenza complications. However, prophylactic or therapeutic treatment in individuals at low risk or those with equivocal clinical findings of influenza infection should be avoided. When indicated, treatment should be started within the first 2 days of symptom onset and may reduce the duration of illness and decrease the risk for serious complications. Prompt initiation of treatment without awaiting confirmation of laboratory studies is recommended. For pregnant women and patients with severe or progressive illness, antiviral treatment started within 3 to 4 days of symptom onset may still be beneficial. **H**

KEY POINTS

- All persons older than 6 months are now recommended to receive annual influenza vaccination.

- Antiviral treatment of influenza is indicated for hospitalized patients; those with severe, complicated, or progressive illness; or those at high risk for influenza complications.

- When indicated, antiviral treatment of influenza should be started within the first 2 days of symptom onset and may reduce the duration of illness and decrease the risk for serious complications.

Herpes Simplex Viruses

Overview

Herpes simplex virus (HSV) infection can occur at any skin location. Lesions on abraded skin or the fingers (herpetic whitlow) were once common among health care workers before improvements in hand hygiene and the use of gloves emerged. Recurrent HSV-1 keratitis is a primary cause of corneal blindness in industrialized nations and is characterized by dendritic ulcers, which are detected by fluorescein staining.

HSV is the most common cause of sporadic encephalitis **H** in the United States. HSV encephalitis begins unilaterally in the temporal lobe and then spreads contralaterally, causing hemorrhagic necrosis. Manifestations include personality and behavioral changes, headache, fever, decreased consciousness, and abnormal speech. Focal seizures may also occur. Focal lesions are usually disclosed on imaging studies. Examination of the cerebrospinal fluid reveals pleocytosis and sometimes the presence of erythrocytes; the glucose level is usually normal. Cerebrospinal fluid testing for HSV DNA by polymerase chain reaction is appropriate. Prompt treatment is required as soon as the diagnosis is suspected. In patients who are immunocompromised, HSV may cause pneumonia, aseptic meningitis, esophagitis, colitis, hepatitis, or disseminated cutaneous disease. Oral and genital lesions may be particularly extensive. **H**

The clinical manifestations, evaluation, and diagnosis of herpes simplex virus infection and herpes zoster virus infection are discussed in MKSAP 16 Dermatology and the Sexually Transmitted Infection section.

- Clinical manifestations of herpes simplex encephalitis include personality and behavioral changes, headache, fever, decreased consciousness, and abnormal speech.

Management

Acyclovir, valacyclovir, and famciclovir are efficacious for treating mucocutaneous and visceral HSV infection, preventing HSV reactivation in immunocompromised hosts, and preventing symptomatic reactivation of recurrent genital herpes. Consideration of suppressive therapy is warranted for patients with a history of frequent (more than six per year) recurrences or severe recurrences of genital HSV or who are immunocompromised.

 For patients with HSV encephalitis and other serious life-threatening infections or for those who cannot tolerate oral therapy, intravenous acyclovir is the treatment of choice. Topical agents, such as trifluorothymidine, vidarabine, and cidofovir, are available for treating HSV ocular infections. Topical corticosteroids are contraindicated in patients in whom HSV is known or suspected to be the cause of an ocular infection.

Patients with resistance to acyclovir, which is more common in those who are severely immunocompromised, are treated with foscarnet or cidofovir. Valacyclovir, in high doses, has been associated (rarely) with thrombotic thrombocytopenic purpura after extended use in patients with AIDS.

- Acyclovir, valacyclovir, and famciclovir are efficacious for treating mucocutaneous and visceral herpes simplex virus (HSV) infection, preventing HSV reactivation in immunocompromised hosts, and preventing symptomatic reactivation of recurrent genital herpes.

- For herpes simplex virus encephalitis and other serious life-threatening infections or in the setting of intolerance to oral therapy, intravenous acyclovir is the treatment of choice.

- Topical corticosteroids are contraindicated in patients in whom herpes simplex virus is known or suspected to be the cause of an ocular infection.

Varicella-Zoster Virus

Overview

Varicella-zoster virus, a herpesvirus, causes two distinct forms of clinical disease: varicella (chickenpox) infection and herpes zoster (shingles).

Varicella represents the primary infection with varicella-zoster virus and is a highly contagious disease characterized by a generalized vesicular rash (**Figure 14**). It is characterized by a vesicular eruption that spreads from the face and extremities toward the trunk (centripetally). Several stages of lesions, including macules, papules, vesicles, pustules, and scabbed

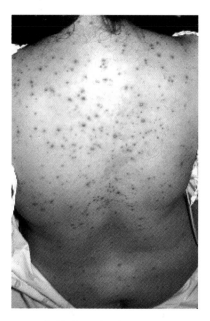

FIGURE 14. Varicella (chickenpox) rash is a vesicular eruption in which several stages of lesions (macules, papules, vesicles, pustules, and scabbed lesions) may be present simultaneously.

lesions, may be present simultaneously. Systemic symptoms are more pronounced in adults. Varicella can be more severe and disseminate in patients who are immunocompromised and in pregnant women. Complications may include secondary bacterial infections of the skin, including invasive streptococcal superinfection; pneumonia; encephalitis; optic neuritis; transverse myelitis; and Guillain-Barré syndrome.

Varicella is usually diagnosed clinically based on its characteristic appearance and history of exposure, although viral culture and immunohistochemical tests can be done.

Herpes zoster virus infection represents reactivation of prior infection with varicella-zoster virus and generally manifests as a vesicular rash in a dermatomal distribution. It should be considered in patients with pain along an affected dermatome, followed in 2 to 3 days by the typical diagnostic vesicular eruption (**Figure 15**).

- Varicella represents primary infection with varicella-zoster virus and is characterized by a vesicular eruption that spreads centripetally and encompasses several stages of lesions, including macules, papules, vesicles, pustules, and scabbed lesions, simultaneously.

- Herpes zoster is a reactivation of prior varicella-zoster virus infection and typically results in a vesicular rash in a dermatomal distribution.

Management

Varicella vaccine is highly effective and is recommended for routine vaccination in children between 12 to 15 months of

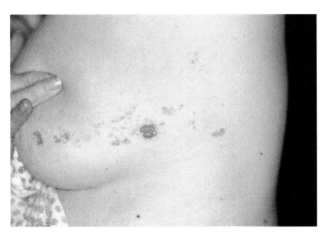

FIGURE 15. Pink to red papules and vesicles in a unilateral dermatomal distribution characteristic of herpes zoster virus infection.

KEY POINTS

- Varicella vaccine is recommended for routine vaccination in children between 12 and 15 months of age, with a second dose recommended at 4 to 6 years of age.
- Herpes zoster vaccine is indicated for the prevention of herpes zoster in persons aged 60 years or older.
- In patients with varicella-zoster virus infection, acyclovir shortens the duration of lesion formation, reduces the number of new lesions, and diminishes systemic symptoms and is recommended for adolescents, adults, and those at high risk for complications.

age, with a second dose given at 4 to 6 years of age. In patients 13 years or older who have not been immunized or have no evidence of immunity, two doses of vaccine should be given 4 to 8 weeks apart; a second ("catch-up") dose should also be given to patients older than 13 who previously received only one dose of vaccine as a child.

Varicella-zoster immune globulin, if it can be procured, or varicella-zoster immune globulin product (VariZIG), is useful in preventing and lessening symptomatic varicella after a significant exposure in high-risk patients, such as those who are immunocompromised, have a negative or unknown history of chickenpox, and have not been vaccinated against varicella-zoster virus infection. It is also recommended for pregnant women who are seronegative for varicella-zoster virus infection and who have had significant exposure to the virus as well as for newborn infants of mothers who had varicella less than 5 days before delivery or 48 hours postpartum. 🅗

Herpes zoster vaccine is indicated for the prevention of herpes zoster infection in persons aged 60 years or older. It has been found to reduce the incidence of herpes zoster infection and decrease the incidence and severity of postherpetic neuralgia.

Acyclovir is approved for the treatment of varicella and herpes zoster virus infection. This agent reduces the duration of lesion formation and number of new lesions and decreases systemic symptoms in normal hosts. Treatment is recommended for adolescents, adults, and those at high risk for complications. Treatment should be initiated within 24 hours of onset of lesions.

Acyclovir, valacyclovir, and famciclovir are approved oral agents for the treatment of herpes zoster. Valacyclovir and famciclovir have better oral bioavailability than acyclovir and are better for hastening healing of skin lesions and reducing the risk for postherpetic neuralgia. Concomitant administration of corticosteroids with antiviral therapy for herpes zoster virus infection remains controversial.

New Topics in Anti-infective Therapy 🅗

Introduction

Several newer antimicrobial agents have been licensed over the past decade that have improved the options for treatment of various infections caused by gram-positive and gram-negative bacteria. Their introduction is particularly important because antimicrobial resistance to many currently used antibiotics is becoming increasingly widespread. However, these new antibiotics are extremely expensive, and the risk of inappropriate use or overuse of these drugs could lead to low-value care and further resistance, potentially making treatment of many common infections problematic. Consequently, these medications should be used only when clearly indicated and when other appropriate treatment options are not available.

Emergence of resistant microorganisms has also led to a reexamination of older, well-known, and economical antibiotics that have retained activity against certain resistant pathogens. Indications are increasingly being recognized for these familiar agents in the treatment of infections involving organisms that are resistant to many currently used antibiotics. 🅗

KEY POINTS

- Several newer antimicrobial agents have improved the options for treatment of various gram-positive and gram-negative infections, but these agents should be used only when clearly indicated and when other appropriate treatment options are unavailable.
- Indications are increasingly being recognized for older, well-known agents in the treatment of infections with organisms that are resistant to many currently used antibiotics.

Newer Antibacterial Drugs 🅗
Lipopeptides and Glycolipopeptides

Daptomycin is a lipopeptide with bactericidal activity against gram-positive aerobic organisms, including methicillin-resistant

CONT.

Staphylococcus aureus (MRSA) and vancomycin-resistant enterococci (VRE) (**Table 56**). Daptomycin retains activity against many strains of *S. aureus* that have elevated minimal inhibitory concentrations (MICs) to vancomycin (≥2 micrograms/mL). Daptomycin is indicated for the treatment of complicated skin and soft tissue infections involving staphylococci, streptococci, and *Enterococcus faecalis*. Daptomycin is also an important agent in the treatment of bloodstream infections, including right-sided endocarditis caused by sensitive staphylococci (including MRSA) that are nonresponsive to vancomycin, particularly when the MIC to vancomycin is 2 micrograms/mL or higher. Daptomycin is not effective in

the treatment of pneumonia because it is inactivated by pulmonary surfactant. An important side effect of daptomycin is rhabdomyolysis; serum creatine kinase levels should be monitored weekly in patients receiving daptomycin, with discontinuation of treatment in patients whose creatine kinase level is elevated more than five times the upper limit of normal. Serious eosinophilic pneumonia developing during daptomycin treatment that has regressed on discontinuation of daptomycin has also been noted.

Telavancin is a glycolipopeptide with activity against grampositive aerobic bacteria, including MRSA (see Table 56). Telavancin has lower MICs to *S. aureus* than vancomycin as

TABLE 56.	**Newer Antimicrobial Agents**					
Agent	**Route**	**Dose for Patients with Normal Kidney and/or Liver Function**	**Relative Cost**	**Adverse Events**	**Issues/ Limitations**	**FDA Indications**
Ceftaroline	IV	600 mg every 12 h	$$	Similar to other cephalosporins; generally well tolerated	No clinical experience for MRSA outside of skin infections; limited activity against gram-negative bacilli	Community-acquired bacterial pneumonia except that caused by MRSA; acute bacterial skin and skin structure infections
Daptomycin	IV	6 mg/kg/d	$$$	Well tolerated; creatine kinase elevations	Inactivated by pulmonary surfactant; optimal dose still unknown	Complicated skin and skin structure infections; *S. aureus* bloodstream infections (bacteremia), including those with right-sided infective endocarditis, caused by methicillin-susceptible and methicillin-resistant isolates
Doripenem	IV	500 mg every 8 h	$$	Similar to other carbapenems, but lower risk for seizures	CNS penetration not well defined	Complicated intraabdominal infections; complicated urinary tract infections, including pyelonephritis
Linezolid	IV, PO	600 mg every 12 h	$$$	Thrombocytopenia; neuropathies	Toxicities may limit duration of therapy; selective serotonin reuptake inhibitor (SSRI) interaction	Vancomycin-resistant *Enterococcus faecium* infections, including cases with concurrent bacteremia; nosocomial pneumonia; complicated skin and skin structure infections, including diabetic foot infections without concomitant osteomyelitis; uncomplicated skin and skin structure infections; community-acquired pneumonia
Telavancin	IV	10 mg/kg/d	$$$	Nephrotoxicity	Significant interaction with coagulation tests; optimal doses unknown in patients with kidney dysfunction	Complicated skin and skin structure infections
Tigecycline	IV	100 mg x 1; 50 mg every 12 h	$$$	Nausea/vomiting; pancreatitis	Low serum concentrations	Complicated skin and soft tissue infection; complicated intraabdominal infection; community-acquired bacterial pneumonia

IV = intravenous; MRSA = methicillin-resistant *Staphylococcus aureus*; CNS = central nervous system; PO = orally.

well as a longer half-life than that of vancomycin, which allows for a simpler dosing regimen. Telavancin can cause nephrotoxicity; patients receiving this agent require monitoring of kidney function. Telavancin is FDA approved for the treatment of skin and soft tissue infections.

Oxazolidinones

Linezolid is an oxazolidinone agent with bacteriostatic activity against gram-positive aerobic bacteria, including MRSA and VRE (see Table 56). Major uses for linezolid are oral therapy for indicated MRSA infections (see Table 56) and intravenous or oral therapy for pneumonia. The high penetration of linezolid into respiratory secretions contributes to its efficacy in the treatment of pneumonia. Urinary concentrations are also high, facilitating bactericidal concentrations against enterococci. An important side effect of linezolid is myelosuppression, notably thrombocytopenia, with an incidence as high as 10% with long-term use. Patients treated with linezolid should receive weekly complete blood counts. Long courses of linezolid therapy are associated with mitochondrial toxicity, including potentially irreversible peripheral or optic neuropathy.

β-Lactam Antibiotics

Ceftaroline is an advanced-generation cephalosporin with activity against gram-positive aerobic bacteria, including MRSA, and some gram-negative aerobic bacteria, including nonextended-spectrum β-lactamase–producing Enterobacteriaceae. Ceftaroline is not considered effective against strains of *Pseudomonas aeruginosa* and *Acinetobacter baumannii*. This drug is approved for the treatment of skin and soft tissue infections, including those caused by MRSA, and community-acquired pneumonia, except for pneumonia caused by MRSA because ceftaroline's efficacy against MRSA pneumonia has not been studied in clinical trials.

Doripenem is a group 2 carbapenem with in vitro activity similar to that of imipenem and meropenem except that doripenem is more active against *P. aeruginosa* than imipenem and meropenem. Although doripenem may still retain activity against strains of *P. aeruginosa* that are resistant to other carbapenems, the true clinical efficacy of this finding is unclear. This agent is approved for the treatment of complicated intraabdominal and urinary tract infections and also is used to treat health care–associated infections such as hospital-acquired and ventilator-associated pneumonia. No seizure events directly attributable to doripenem have been reported.

Glycylcyclines

Tigecycline is a glycylcycline agent with bacteriostatic activity against aerobic gram-positive bacteria (including MRSA and VRE), gram-negative bacteria (including carbapenem-resistant Enterobacteriaceae [CRE] and *A. baumannii*, but not *P. aeruginosa*), and some anaerobes. It is approved for the treatment of complicated skin and skin structure infections, complicated intraabdominal infections, and community-acquired pneumonia. Tigecycline does not attain high serum concentrations and should not be used for treating bacteremia. Nor does it achieve adequate urine concentrations; consequently, it is not indicated for treating urinary tract infections. An important treatment niche for this agent is possible management of patients with highly resistant gram-negative organisms. Resistance to tigecycline may occur in patients receiving this agent, and treatment failures have been reported. Nausea and vomiting are the most common side effects; cases of pancreatitis have also been reported. ◧

KEY POINTS

- Daptomycin is indicated for complicated skin and soft tissue infections involving staphylococci, streptococci, and *Enterococcus faecalis*.
- Telavancin is active against gram-positive aerobic bacteria, including methicillin-resistant *Staphylococcus aureus*.
- Telavancin has a lower minimal inhibitory concentration to *Staphylococcus aureus* than vancomycin and a longer half-life than that of vancomycin, allowing for a simpler dosing regimen.
- Major uses for linezolid are oral therapy for methicillin-resistant *Staphylococcus aureus* infections and intravenous or oral therapy for pneumonia.
- Linezolid causes myelosuppression, notably thrombocytopenia, with an incidence as high as 10% with long-term use; patients receiving linezolid require weekly complete blood counts.
- Ceftaroline is approved for treating skin and soft tissue infections, including those caused by methicillin-resistant *Staphylococcus aureus* (MRSA), and community-acquired pneumonia, except for pneumonia caused by MRSA.
- Doripenem is approved for complicated intraabdominal and urinary tract infections and also is used to treat health care–associated infections.

New Uses for Older Antimicrobial Agents ◧
Trimethoprim-sulfamethoxazole

Trimethoprim-sulfamethoxazole (TMP-SMX) is a combination antimicrobial agent that is bactericidal against many pathogens (**Table 57**). TMP-SMX is used as a primary therapeutic agent against *Stenotrophomonas maltophilia* and *Pneumocystic (carinii) jirovecii*. TMP-SMX has retained excellent activity against MRSA, is orally bioavailable, and is an important agent in the treatment of skin and soft tissue infections caused by community-associated MRSA. The role of TMP-SMX in treating bacteremia or pneumonia remains unclear. Limitations of this drug include allergy (including Stevens-Johnson syndrome), hyperkalemia, and possible kidney toxicity.

TABLE 57. Older Antimicrobial Agents for New Indications

Drug	Route	Dosage[a]	Daily cost	Adverse Events	Issues/Limitations	Emerging Uses
Colistin	IV	5 mg/kg/d	$$	Nephrotoxicity; neurotoxicity	Pharmacologic properties poorly defined; significant unknowns on dosing	Treatment of multidrug-resistant gram-negative bacilli
Fosfomycin	PO, IV	3 g x 1 PO; 1-16 g/d IV	PO: $$; IV: unavailable	Gastrointestinal	Only available orally in United States; systemic experience limited to combination therapy	Urinary tract infection due to VRE or multidrug- resistant gram-negative (e.g., ESBL-producing organism or CRE)
Trimethoprim-sulfamethoxazole	IV, PO	5 mg/kg every 12 h (dose based on TMP component)	IV: $$; PO: $	Hypersensitivity; hyperkalemia	Limited data in ESKAPE pathogens; shortage of IV formulation	Skin and soft tissue infection from MRSA

IV = intravenous; PO = oral; ESBL – extended-spectrum β-lactamase; CRE – carbapenem-resistant Enterobacteriaceae; MRSA = methicillin-resistant *Staphylococcus aureus*; VRE = vancomycin-resistant enterococci; TMP = trimethoprim-sulfamethoxazole; ESKAPE = *Enterococcus faecium, Staphylococcus aureus, Klebsiella pneumoniae, Acinetobacter baumannii, Pseudomonas aeruginosa,* and *Enterobacter* species.

[a]Refers to the dosage for patients with normal kidney and/or liver function.

Polymyxins

CONT.

Colistin (polymyxin E) and polymyxin B are the two commercially available polymyxin antimicrobial agents (see Table 57) with bactericidal activity against many strains of gram-negative bacilli, including *P. aeruginosa, A. baumannii,* and the Enterobacteriaceae. Polymyxins are important in the treatment of gram-negative bacilli that are resistant to all other antimicrobials, including CRE, *P. aeruginosa,* and *A. baumannii.* Colistin, which is administered in the form of its prodrug, colistimethate sodium, has become the most commonly used form of polymyxin for parenteral administration and has also been used as nebulization therapy for pneumonia in patients with cystic fibrosis and pneumonia caused by multidrug-resistant gram-negative organisms as well as for intrathecal or intraventricular therapy in patients with meningitis caused by resistant strains of *A. baumannii.* Given concerns of risk for prescribing errors in the United States, colistin dosing is based on milligrams of colistin base activity (CBA). Limitations of colistin include nephrotoxicity and neurotoxicity.

Fosfomycin

Fosfomycin is a phosphonic acid derivative with bactericidal activity against many gram-positive and gram-negative organisms, including MRSA, VRE, and multidrug-resistant gram-negative organisms (see Table 57). Only the oral formulation is available in the United States, although it is not widely available, and attainable serum concentrations are low. An important use of this agent is in the treatment of lower urinary tract infection (cystitis). Fosfomycin can be especially useful in patients with allergies to multiple antibiotics because it is not cross-allergenic with any other agent.

Aminoglycosides

Aminoglycosides are bactericidal antimicrobials that are primarily used as companion drugs to broaden activity or provide synergy against treatment of gram-negative bacilli or to provide synergistic activity against gram-positive bacteria. However, these agents have retained activity against some multidrug-resistant strains of gram-negative bacilli, including *A. baumannii, P. aeruginosa,* and CRE, and have become important agents of last resort in the treatment of infections caused by these bacteria. Once-daily dosing of these agents is becoming the preferred mode of administration for treatment of infection caused by gram-negative bacilli. The major limitations of the aminoglycosides are nephrotoxicity and ototoxicity (vestibular and cochlear).

Rifamycins

Rifampin is a rifamycin that has retained activity against many strains of MRSA and is often used in combination with other agents for the treatment of infections caused by MRSA and coagulase-negative staphylococci, especially in patients who also have infection associated with indwelling foreign bodies. A major limitation of rifampin is its potential to induce hepatic microsomal enzymes, causing multiple drug-drug interactions. Rifampin should not be used as monotherapy for the treatment of bacterial infection because of the rapid emergence of resistance. Rifaximin is a nonabsorbable rifamycin derivative that has been useful in the treatment and prophylaxis of travelers' diarrhea. It has also shown benefit in the management of hepatic encephalopathy.

- Trimethoprim-sulfamethoxazole is used as a primary agent against *Stenotrophomonas maltophilia* and *Pneumocystis jirovecii*, and it has retained excellent activity against methicillin-resistant *Staphylococcus aureus* (MRSA), is orally bioavailable, and is important in treating skin and soft tissue infections caused by community-associated MRSA.

- Polymyxins are important in the treatment of gram-negative bacilli that are resistant to all other antimicrobials, including carbapenem-resistant Enterobacteriaceae, *Pseudomonas aeruginosa*, and *Acinetobacter baumannii*.

- Fosfomycin is active against many gram-positive and gram-negative organisms, including methicillin-resistant *Staphylococcus aureus*, vancomycin-resistant enterococci, and multidrug resistant gram-negative organisms.

- Aminoglycosides have retained activity against some multidrug-resistant strains of gram-negative bacilli, including *Acinetobacter baumannii*, *Pseudomonas aeruginosa*, and carbapenem-resistant Enterobacteriaceae.

- Once-daily dosing of aminoglycosides is becoming the preferred mode of administration for treatment of infection caused by gram-negative bacilli.

- Rifampin has retained activity against many strains of methicillin-resistant *Staphylococcus aureus* (MRSA) and is often used in conjunction with other agents to treat infections caused by MRSA and coagulase-negative staphylococci, especially in patients who also have infection associated with indwelling foreign bodies.

- Rifampin should not be used as monotherapy for the treatment of bacterial infection because of the rapid emergence of resistance.

Antimicrobial Stewardship

Antimicrobial stewardship focuses on optimizing antimicrobial therapy through appropriate empiric therapy, narrowing the spectrum of coverage once clinical data become available, and shortening the duration of therapy whenever possible. Once a specific organism is isolated and its sensitivities to available antibiotics known, it is beneficial to focus or "de-escalate" therapy to avoid the selection of organisms resistant to currently effective broad-spectrum antibiotics. Important goals of stewardship are to limit the emergence of antimicrobial resistance and reduce inappropriate antimicrobial usage.

Core members of the stewardship team include an infectious diseases physician, an infectious diseases pharmacist (or professionals with interest and experience in antimicrobial therapeutics), a health care epidemiologist, a clinical microbiologist, and an information systems specialist. Support from hospital administration to provide the necessary infrastructure and involvement of quality assurance and patient safety programs are important to the success of antimicrobial stewardship programs. **H**

- Important goals of antimicrobial stewardship are to limit the emergence of antimicrobial resistance and reduce inappropriate antimicrobial usage.

Outpatient Antimicrobial Therapy

Outpatient antimicrobial therapy (OPAT) encompasses intravenous, intramuscular, and subcutaneous antimicrobial therapy administered without hospitalization. OPAT can be delivered at home or in other nonhospital settings. Patients receiving OPAT should be clinically stable. OPAT requires teamwork among a physician, nurse, pharmacist, and case manager. Creation of a schedule of visits and periodic laboratory monitoring are also required. The home situation should include family/caregiver support, transportation, availability of emergency services (if needed), telephone, running water, and refrigeration. Conditions commonly treated with OPAT include skin and soft tissue infections, osteomyelitis, and bacteremia. It is preferable to use agents for OPAT that are dosed infrequently, such as ceftriaxone or vancomycin, and the first dose of therapy should be administered in a supervised setting. OPAT can be delivered through peripheral short catheters, peripherally inserted central catheters, and tunneled or nontunneled central catheters.

- Outpatient antimicrobial therapy encompasses intravenous, intramuscular, and subcutaneous antimicrobial therapy administered without hospitalization, and it can be delivered at home or in other nonhospital settings.

- Patients for whom outpatient antimicrobial therapy is being considered require a home situation with family/caregiver support, transportation, availability of emergency services, telephone, running water, and refrigeration.

- It is preferable to use agents for outpatient antimicrobial therapy that are dosed infrequently, such as ceftriaxone or vancomycin, and the first dose should be administered in a supervised setting.

Hyperbaric Oxygen **H**

Hyperbaric oxygen is sometimes used to promote wound healing. Data are limited regarding use of this modality for treatment of acute, life-threatening soft tissue infections, although the recognized infectious diseases for which

CONT.

hyperbaric oxygen is used include clostridial gangrene, necrotizing fasciitis, and refractory osteomyelitis.

Hyperbaric oxygen is also sometimes used to treat chronic nonhealing ulcers. Some studies have reported decreased amputation rates associated with use of hyperbaric oxygen. Hyperbaric oxygen might be used as adjunctive therapy for severe diabetic foot infections or nonhealing infections despite appropriate antimicrobial and surgical therapy.

Absolute contraindications to hyperbaric oxygen therapy include untreated pneumothorax and recent chemotherapy with doxorubicin or cisplatin. The most common adverse effect is barotrauma to the middle ear, cranial sinuses, or the teeth; oxygen toxicity is a rare complication. **H**

KEY POINTS

- In patients with chronic, nonhealing ulcers, decreased amputation rates have been reported with use of hyperbaric oxygen.

- Absolute contraindications to hyperbaric oxygen therapy include untreated pneumothorax and recent chemotherapy with doxorubicin or cisplatin.

Bibliography

Central Nervous System Infections

Bloch KC, Glaser C. Diagnostic approaches for patients with suspected encephalitis. Curr Infect Dis Rep. 2007;9(4):315-322. [PMID: 17618552]

Boström A, Oertel M, Ryang Y, et al. Treatment strategies and outcome in patients with non-tuberculous spinal epidural abscess—a review of 46 cases. Minim Invasive Neurosurg. 2008;51(1):36-42. [PMID: 18306130]

Brouwer MC, McIntyre P, de Gans J, Prasad K, van de Beek D. Corticosteroids for acute bacterial meningitis. Cochrane Database Syst Rev. 2010;9:CD004405. [PMID: 20824838]

Brouwer MC, Tunkel AR, van de Beek D. Epidemiology, diagnosis, and antimicrobial treatment of acute bacterial meningitis. Clin Microbiol Rev. 2010;23:467-492. [PMID: 20610819]

Carpenter J, Stapleton S, Holliman R. Retrospective analysis of 49 cases of brain abscess and review of the literature. Eur J Clin Microbiol Infect Dis. 2007;26(1):1-11. [PMID: 17180609]

Centers for Disease Control and Prevention (CDC). Licensure of a 13-valent pneumococcal conjugate vaccine (PCV13) and recommendations for use among children – Advisory Committee on Immunization Practices (ACIP), 2010. MMWR Morb Mortal Wkly Rep. 2010;59(9):258-261. [PMID: 20224542]

Darouiche RO. Spinal epidural abscess. N Engl J Med. 2006;355(19):2012-2020. [PMID: 17093252]

Glaser CA, Honarmand S, Anderson LJ, et al. Beyond viruses: clinical profiles and etiologies associated with encephalitis. Clin Infect Dis. 2006;43(12):1565-1577. [PMID: 17109290]

Hsu HE, Shutt KA, Moore MR, et al. Effect of pneumococcal conjugate vaccine on pneumococcal meningitis. N Engl J Med. 2009;360(3):244-256. [PMID: 19144940]

Ihekwaba UK, Kudesia G, Mckendrick MW. Clinical features of viral meningitis in adults: significant differences in cerebrospinal fluid findings among herpes simplex virus, varicella zoster virus, and enterovirus infections. Clin Infect Dis. 2008;47(6):783-789. [PMID: 18680414]

Lee TH, Chang WN, Su TM, et al. Clinical features and predictive factors of intraventricular rupture in patients who have bacterial brain abscess. J Neurol Neurosurg Psychiatry. 2007;78(3):303-309. [PMID: 17012340]

Lu CH, Chang WN, Lui CC. Strategies for the management of bacterial brain abscess. J Clin Neurosci. 2006;13(10):979-985. [PMID: 17056261]

Mailles A, Stahl JP; Steering Committee and Investigators Group. Infectious encephalitis in france in 2007: a national prospective study. Clin Infect Dis 2009;49(12):1838-1847. [PMID: 19929384]

Murray KO, Walker C, Gould E. The virology, epidemiology, and clinical impact of West Nile virus: a decade of advancements in research since its introduction into the Western Hemisphere. Epidemiol Infect. 2011;139(6):1-11. [PMID: 21342610]

Nathoo N, Nadvi SS, Gouws E, van Dellen JR. Craniotomy improves outcome for cranial subdural empyema: computed tomography–era experience with 699 patients. Neurosurgery. 2001;49(4):872-878. [PMID: 11564248]

Osborn MK, Steinberg JP. Subdural empyema and other suppurative complications of paranasal sinusitis. Lancet Infect Dis. 2007:7(1):62-67. [PMID: 17182345]

Sendi P, Bregenzer T, Zimmerli W. Spinal epidural abscess in clinical practice. QJM. 2008;101(1):1-12. [PMID: 17982180]

Tebruegge M, Curtis N. Epidemiology, etiology, pathogenesis, and diagnosis or recurrent bacterial meningitis. Clin Microbiol Rev. 2008;21(3):519-537. [PMID: 18625686]

Thigpen MC, Whitney CG, Messonnier N, et al; Emerging Infections Program Network. Bacterial meningitis in the United States, 1998-2007. N Engl J Med. 2011;364(21):2016-2025. [PMID: 21612470]

Tunkel AR, Glaser CA, Bloch KC, et al; Infectious Diseases Society of America. The management of encephalitis: clinical practice guidelines by the Infectious Diseases Society of America. Clin Infect Dis. 2008;47(3):303-327. [PMID: 18582201]

Tunkel AR, Hartman BJ, Kaplan SL, et al. Practice guidelines for the management of bacterial meningitis. Clin Infect Dis. 2004;39(9):1267-1284. [PMID: 15494903]

van de Beek D, Drake JM, Tunkel AR. Nosocomial bacterial meningitis. N Engl J Med. 2010;362(2):146-154. [PMID: 20071704]

Werno AM, Murdoch DR. Medical microbiology: laboratory diagnosis of invasive pneumococcal disease. Clin Infect Dis. 2008;46(6):926-932. [PMID: 18260752]

Prion Diseases of the Central Nervous System

Holman RC, Belay ED, Christensen KY, et al. Human prion diseases in the United States. PLoS One. 2010;5(1):e8521. [PMID: 20049325]

Rosenbloom MH, Atri A. The evaluation of rapidly progressive dementia. Neurologist. 2011;17(2):67-74. [PMID: 21364356]

Ryou C. Prions and prion diseases: fundamentals and mechanistic details. J Microbiol Biotechnol. 2007;17(7):1059-1070. [PMID: 18051314]

Skin and Soft Tissue Infections

Anaya DA, Pellinger EP. Necrotizing soft tissue infection: diagnosis and management. Clin Infect Dis. 2007;44(5):705-710. [PMID: 17278065]

Björnsdóttir S, Gottfredsson M, Thórisdóttir AS, et al. Risk factors for acute cellulitis of the lower limb: a prospective case-control study. Clin Infect Dis. 2005;41(10):1416-1422. [PMID: 16231251]

Lipsky BA, Berendt AR, Cornia PB, et al. 2012 Infectious Diseases Society of America clinical practice guideline for the diagnosis and treatment of diabetic foot infections. Clin Infect Dis. 2012;54(12):132-173. [PMID: 22619242]

Liu C, Bayer A, Cosgrove SE, et al; Infectious Diseases Society of America. Clinical practice guidelines by the Infectious Diseases Society of America for the treatment of methicillin-resistant Staphylococcus aureus infections in adults and children. Clin Infect Dis. 2011;52(3):e18-55. Epub 2011 Jan 4. [PMID: 21208910]

Semel JD, Goldin H. Association of athlete's foot with cellulitis of the lower extremities: diagnostic value of bacterial cultures of ipsilateral interdigital space samples. Clin Infect Dis. 1996;23(5):1162–1164. [PMID: 8922818]

Stevens DL, Bisno AL, Chambers HF, et al; Infectious Diseases Society of America. Practice guidelines for the diagnosis and management of skin and soft tissue infections. Clin Infect Dis. 2005;41(10):1373-1406. [PMID: 16231249]

Stevens DL, Eron LL. Cellulitis and soft-tissue infections. Ann Intern Med. 2009;150(1):ITC11. [PMID: 19124814]

Wong CH, Khin LW, Heng KS, Tan KC, Low CO. The LRINEC (Laboratory Risk Indicator for Necrotizing Fasciitis) score: a tool for distinguishing necrotizing fasciitis from other soft tissue infections. Crit Care Med. 2004;32(7):1535-1541. [PMID: 15241098]

Community-Acquired Pneumonia

Chalmers JD, Singanayagam A, Akram AR, et al. Severity assessment tools for predicting mortality in hospitalized patients with community-acquired pneumonia. Systematic review and meta-analysis. Thorax. 2010;65(10):878-883. [PMID: 20729231]

Christ-Crane, Opal SM. Clinical review: the role of biomarkers in the diagnosis and management of community-acquired pneumonia. Crit Care. 2010;14(1):203. [PMID: 20236471]

Jackson ML, Nelson JC, Jackson LA. Risk factors for community-acquired pneumonia in immunocompetent seniors. J Am Geriatr Soc. 2009;57(5):822-828. [PMID: 19453307]

Lewis PF, Schmidt MA, Lu X, et al. A community-based outbreak of severe respiratory illness caused by human adenovirus serotype 14. J Infect Dis. 2009;199(10):1427-1434. [PMID: 19351259]

Mandell LA, Wunderink RG, Anzueto A, et al; Infectious Diseases Society of America; American Thoracic Society. Infectious Diseases Society of America/American Thoracic Society consensus guidelines on the management of community-acquired pneumonia in adults. Clin Infect Dis. 2007;(44)(suppl 2):S27-72. [PMID: 17278083]

Mortensen EM, Copeland LA, Pugh MJ, et al. Diagnosis of pulmonary malignancy after hospitalization for pneumonia. Am J Med. 2010;123(1):66-71. [PMID: 20102994]

Niederman N. In the clinic. Community-acquired pneumonia. Ann Intern Med. 2009;151(7):ITC4-2-ITC4-14; quiz ITC4-16. [PMID: 19805767]

Restrepo MI, Mortensen EM, Rello J, Brody J, Anzueto A. late admission to the ICU in patients with severe community-acquired pneumonia is associated with higher mortality. Chest. 2010;137(3):552-557. [PMID: 19880910]

Ruhnke GW, Coca-Perraillon M, Kitch BT, Cutler DM. Marked reduction in 30-day mortality among elderly patients with community-acquired pneumonia. Am J Med. 2011;124(2):171-178.e1. [PMID: 21295197]

Waterer GW, Rello J, Wunderink RG. Management of community-acquired pneumonia in adults. Am J Respir Crit Care Med. 2011;183(2):157-164. [PMID: 20693379]

Tick-Borne Diseases

Chapman AS, Bakken JS, Folk SM, et al; Tickborne Rickettsial Diseases Working Group; CDC. Diagnosis and management of tickborne rickettsial diseases: Rocky Mountain spotted fever, ehrlichiosis, and anaplasmosi—United States: a practical guide for physicians and other health-care and public health professionals. MMWR Recomm Rep. 2006;55(RR-4):1-27. [PMID: 16572105]

Halperin JJ, Shapiro ED, Logigian E, et al; Quality Standards Subcommittee of the American Academy of Neurology. Practice parameter: treatment of nervous system Lyme disease (an evidence-based review): report of the Quality Standards Subcommittee of the American Academy of Neurology. Neurology. 2007;69(1):91-102. [PMID: 17522387]

Ismail N, Bloch KC, McBride JW. Human ehrlichiosis and anaplasmosis. Clin Lab Med. 2010;30(1):261-292. [PMID: 20513551]

Murray TS, Shapiro ED. Lyme disease. Clin Lab Med. 2010;30(1):311-328. [PMID: 20513553]

O'Connell S. Lyme borreliosis: current issues in diagnosis and management. Curr Opin Infect Dis. 2010;23(3):231-235. [PMID: 20407371]

Stanek G, Wormser GP, Gray J, Strle F. Lyme borreliosis. Lancet. 2012;379(9814):461-473. [PMID: 21903253]

Wormser GP, Dattwyler RJ, Shapiro ED, et al. The clinical assessment, treatment, and prevention of lyme disease, human granulocytic anaplasmosis, and babesiosis: clinical practice guidelines by the Infectious Diseases Society of America. Clin Infect Dis. 2006;43(9):1089-1134. [PMID: 17029130]

Urinary Tract Infections

Dielubanza EJ, Schaeffer AJ. Urinary tract infections in women. Med Clin North Am. 2011;95(1):27-41. [PMID: 21095409]

Foxman B. The epidemiology of urinary tract infection. Nat Rev Urol. 2010;7(12):653-660. [PMID: 21139641]

Gupta K, Hooton TM, Naber KG, et al; Infectious Diseases Society of America; European Society for Microbiology and Infectious Diseases. International clinical practice guidelines for the treatment of acute uncomplicated cystitis and pyelonephritis in women: A 2010 update by the Infectious Diseases Society of America and the European Society for Microbiology and Infectious Diseases. Clin Infect Dis. 2011;52(5):e103-120. [PMID: 21292654]

Nicolle LE, Bradley S, Colgan R, Rice JC, Schaeffer A, Hooton TM; Infectious Diseases Society of America; American Society of Nephrology; American Geriatric Society. Infectious Diseases Society of America guidelines for the diagnosis and treatment of asymptomatic bacteriuria in adults. Clin Infect Dis. 2005;40(5):643-654. [PMID: 15714408]

Mycobacterium tuberculosis **Infection**

American Thoracic Society; CDC; Infectious Diseases Society of America. Treatment of tuberculosis. MMWR Recomm Rep. 2003;52(RR-11):1-77. [PMID: 12836625]

Blanc F-X, Sok T, Laureillard D, et al; CAMELIA (ANRS 1295–CIPRA KH001) Study Team. Earlier versus later start of antiretroviral therapy in HIV-infected adults with tuberculosis. N Engl J Med. 2011;365(16):1471-1481. [PMID: 22010913]

Caminero JA, Sotgiu G, Zumla A, Migliori GB. Best drug treatment for multidrug-resistant and extensively drug-resistant tuberculosis. Lancet Infect Dis. 2010;10(9):621-629. [PMID: 20797644]

Centers for Disease Control and Prevention (CDC). Recommendations for use of an isoniazid-rifapentine regimen with direct observation to treat latent Mycobacterium tuberculosis infection. MMWR Morb Mortal Wkly Rep. 2011;60(48):1650-1653. [PMID: 22157884]

Centers for Disease Control and Prevention (CDC). Reported tuberculosis in the United States, 2010. Atlanta, GA: U.S. Department of Health and Human Services, CDC, October 2011.

Centers for Disease Control and Prevention (CDC). Updated guidelines for the use of nucleic acid amplification tests in the diagnosis of tuberculosis. MMWR Morb Mortal Wkly Rep. 2009;58(01):7-10. [PMID: 19145221]

Diagnostic Standards and Classification of Tuberculosis in Adults and Children. This official statement of the American Thoracic Society and the Centers for Disease Control and Prevention was adopted by the ATS Board of Directors, July 1999. This statement was endorsed by the Council of the Infectious Disease Society of America, September 1999. Am J Respir Crit Care Med. 2000;161(4 pt 1):1376-1395. [PMID: 10764337]

Mazurek GH, Jereb J, Vernon A, LoBue P, Goldberg S, Castro K; IGRA Expert Committee; Centers for Disease Control and Prevention (CDC). Updated guidelines for using Interferon Gamma Release Assays to detect Mycobacterium tuberculosis infection - United States, 2010. MMWR Recomm Rep. 2010;59(RR-5):1-25. [PMID: 20577159]

Nontuberculous Mycobacterial Infections

Griffith DE, Aksamit T, Brown-Elliot BA, et al; ATS Mycobacterial Diseases Subcommittee; American Thoracic Society; Infectious Disease Society of America. An official ATS/IDSA statement: diagnosis, treatment, and prevention of nontuberculous mycobacterial diseases. Am J Respir Crit Care Med. 2007;175(4):367-416. [PMID: 17277290]

Jarzembowski JA, Young MB. Nontuberculous mycobacterial infections. Arch Pathol Lab Med. 2008;132(8):1333-1341. [PMID: 18684037]

Piersimoni C, Scarparo C. Pulmonary infections associated with nontuberculous mycobacteria in immunocompetent patients. Lancet Infect Dis. 2008;8(5):323-334. [PMID: 18471777]

Tortoli E. Clinical manifestations of nontuberculous mycobacteria infections. Clin Microbiol Infect. 2009;15(10):906-910. [PMID: 19845702]

Fungal Infections

Billie J. New non-culture-based methods for the diagnosis of invasive candidiasis. Curr Opin Crit Care. 2010;16(5):460-464. [PMID: 20736833]

Chen SC, Playford EG, Sorrell TC. Antifungal therapy in invasive fungal infections. Curr Opin Pharmacol. 2010;10(5):522-530. Epub 2010 Jul 2. [PMID: 20598943]

Kauffman CA. Histoplasmosis. Clin Chest Med. 2009;30(2):217-225. [PMID: 19375629]

Pappas PG, Kauffman CA, Andes D, et al; Infectious Diseases Society of America. Clinical practice guidelines for the management of candidiasis: 2009 update by the Infectious Diseases Society of America. Clin Infect Dis. 2009;48(5):503-535. [PMID: 19191635]

Perfect JR, Dismukes WE, Dromer F, et al. Clinical practice guidelines for the management of cryptococcal disease: 2010 update by the Infectious Diseases Society of America. Clin Infect Dis. 2010;50(3):291-322. [PMID: 20047480]

Smith JA, Kauffman CA. Blastomycosis. Proc Am Thorac Soc. 2010;7(3):173-180. [PMID: 20463245]

Spellberg B, Ibrahim AS. Recent advances in the treatment of mucormycosis. Curr Infect Dis Rep. 2010;12(6):423-429. [PMID: 21308550]

Thursky KA, Playford EG, Seymour JF, et al. Recommendations for the treatment of established fungal infections. Intern Med J. 2008;38(6b):496-520. [PMID: 18588522]

Vyas KS, Bariola JR, Bradsher RW Jr. Treatment of endemic mycoses. Expert Rev Respir Med. 2010;4(1):85-95. [PMID: 20387295]

Walsh TJ, Anaissie EJ, Denning DW, et al; Infectious Diseases Society of America. Clin Infect Dis. 2008;46(3):327-360. [PMID: 18177225]

Sexually Transmitted Infections

Martin-Iguacel R, Llibre JM, Nielsen H, et al. Lymphogranuloma venereum proctocolitis: a silent endemic disease in men who have sex with men in industrialized countries. Eur J Clin Microbiol Infect Dis. 2010;29(8):917-925. [PMID: 20509036]

U.S. Preventive Services Task Force. Screening for chlamydial infection: U.S. Preventive Services Task Force recommendation statement. Ann Intern Med. 2007;147(2):128-134. [PMID: 17576996]

Wilson JF. In the clinic. Vaginitis and cervicitis. Ann Intern Med. 2009;151(5):ITC3-1-ITC3-15 [PMID: 19721016]

Workowski KA, Berman S; Centers for Disease Control and Prevention (CDC). Sexually transmitted diseases treatment guidelines, 2010. MMWR Recomm Rep. 2010;59(RR 1-12):1-110. [Erratum in MMWR Recomm Rep. 2011;60(1):18]. [PMID: 21160459]

Osteomyelitis

Conterno LO, da Silva Filho CR. Antibiotics for treating chronic osteomyelitis in adults. Cochrane Database Syst Rev. 2009;(3):CDO4439. [PMID: 19588358]

Lew DP, Waldvogel FA. Osteomyelitis. N Engl J Med. 1997;336(14):999-1007. [PMID: 9077380]

Pineda C, Vargas A, Rodriguez AV. Imaging of osteomyelitis: current concepts. Infec Dis Clin North Am. 2006;20(4):789-825. [PMID: 17118291]

Powlson AS, Coll AP. The treatment of diabetic foot infections. J Antimicrob Chemother. 2010;65(suppl 3):iii3-9. [PMID: 20876626]

Rao N, Lipsky BA. Optimizing antimicrobial therapy in diabetic foot infections. Drugs. 2007;67(2):195-214. [PMID: 17284084]

Zimmerli W. Clinical practice. Vertebral osteomyelitis. N Engl J Med. 2010;362(11):1022-1029. [PMID: 20237348]

Fever of Unknown Origin

Bleeker-Rovers CP, Vos FJ, de Kleijn EM, et al. A prospective multicenter study on fever of unknown origin: the yield of a structured diagnostic protocol. Medicine (Baltimore). 2007;86(1):26-38. [PMID: 17220753]

Hot A, Jaisson I, Girard C, et al. Yield of bone marrow examination in diagnosing the source of fever of unknown origin. Arch Intern Med. 2009;169(21):2018-2023. [PMID: 19933965]

Mourad O, Palda V, Detsky AS. A comprehensive evidence-based approach to fever of unknown origin. Arch Intern Med. 2003;163(5):545-551. [PMID: 12622601]

Vanderschueren S, Knockaert D, Adriaenssens T, et al. From prolonged febrile illness to fever of unknown origin: the challenge continues. Arch Intern Med. 2003;163(9):1033-1041. [PMID: 12742800]

Primary Immunodeficiencies

Maarschalk-Ellerbroek LJ, Hoepelman IM, Ellerbroek PM. Immunoglobulin treatment in primary antibody deficiency. Int J Antimicrob Agents. 2011;37(5):396-404. [PMID: 21276714]

Morimoto Y, Routes JM. Immunodeficiency overview. Prim Care. 2008;35(1):159-173. [PMID: 18206723]

Nelson KS, Lewis DB. Adult-onset presentations of genetic immunodeficiencies: genes can throw slow curves. Curr Opin Infect Dis. 2010;23(4):359-364. [PMID: 20581672]

Notarangelo LD. Primary immunodeficiencies. J Allergy Clin Immunol. 2010;125(2)(suppl 2):S182-194. Epub 2009 Dec 29. [PMID: 20042228]

Oliveira JB, Fleisher TA. Laboratory evaluation of primary immunodeficiencies. J Allergy Clin Immunol. 2010;125(2)(suppl 2):S297-S305. Epub 2009 Dec 29. [PMID: 20042230]

Park MA, Li JT, Hagan JB, Maddox DE, Abraham RS. Common variable immunodeficiency: a new look at an old disease. Lancet. 2008;372(9637):489-502. [PMID: 18692715]

Ram S. Lewis LA, Rice PA. Infections of people with complement deficiencies and patients who have undergone splenectomy. Clin Microbiol Rev. 2010;23(4):740-780. [PMID: 20930072]

Wood P, UK Primary Immunodeficiency Network. Clin Med. 2009;9(6):595-599. [PMID: 20095309]

Yel L. Selective IgA deficiency. J Clin Immunol. 2010;30(1):10-16. Epub 2010 Jan 26. [PMID: 20101521]

Bioterrorism

Arnon S, Schecter R, Inglesby TV, et al; Working Group on Civilian Biodefense. Botulinum toxin as a biological weapon: medical and public health management. JAMA. 2001;285(8):1059-1070. [PMID: 11209178]

Bartlett JG, Inglesby TV, Boria L. Management of anthrax. Clin Infect Dis. 2002;35(7):851-858. [PMID: 12228822]

Borchardt SM, Ritger KA, Dworkin MS. Categorization, prioritization, and surveillance of potential bioterrorism agents. Infect Dis Clin North Am. 2006;20(2):213-225, vii-viii. [PMID: 16762736]

Boria L, Inglesby TV, Peters CJ, et al; Working Group on Civilian Biodefense. Hemorrhagic Fever Viruses as Biological Weapons: medical and public health management. JAMA. 2002;287(18):2391-2405. [PMID: 11988060]

Breman JG, Henderson DA. Diagnosis and management of smallpox. N Engl J Med. 2002;346(17):1300-1308. [PMID: 11923491]

Bush LM, Abrams BH, Beall A, Johnson CC. Index case of fatal inhalational anthrax due to bioterrorism in the United States. N Engl J Med. 2001;345(22):1607-1610. [PMID: 11704685]

Dennis DT, Inglesby TV, Henderson DA, et al; Working Group on Civilian Biodefense. Tularemia as a biological weapon: medical and public health management. JAMA. 2001;285(21):2763-2773. [PMID: 11386933]

Inglesby TV, Dennis DT, Henderson DA, et al; Working Group on Civilian Biodefense. Plague as a biological weapon: medical and public health management. JAMA. 2000;283(17):2281-2290. [PMID: 10807389]

Inglesby TV, O'Toole T, Henderson DA, et al; Working Group on Civilian Biodefense. Anthrax as a biological weapon, 2002: updated recommendations for management. JAMA. 2002;287(17):2236-2252. [PMID: 11980524]

Travel Medicine

Ariza J, Bosilkovski M, Cascio A, et al; International Society of Chemotherapy; Institute of Continuing Medical Education of Ioannina. Perspectives for the treatment of brucellosis in the 21st century: the Ioannina recommendations. PLoS Med. 2007;4(12):e317. [PMID: 18162038]

Cao C, Liang L, Wang W, et al. Common reservoirs for Penicillium marneffei infection in humans and rodents, China. Emerg Infect Dis. 2011;17(2):209-214. [PMID: 21291590]

Centers for Disease Control and Prevention (CDC). Acinetobacter baumannii infections among patients at military medical facilities treating injured U.S. service members, 2002-2004. MMWR Morb Mortal Wkly Rep. 2004;53(45);1063-1066. [PMID: 15549020]

Cetron MS, Marfin AA, Julian KG, et al. Yellow Fever vaccine. Recommendations of the Advisory Committee on Immunization Practices (ACIP), 2002. MMWR Recomm Rep. 2002;51(RR-17):1-11; quiz CE1-4. [PMID: 12437192]

Galgiani JN, Ampel NM, Blair JE, et al; Infectious Diseases Society of America. Coccidioidomycosis. Clin Infect Dis. 2005;41(9):1217-1223. [PMID: 16206093]

Hill DR, Baird JK, Parise ME, Lewis LS, Ryan ET, Magill AJ. Primaquine: report from CDC expert meeting on malaria chemoprophylaxis I. Am J Trop Med Hyg. 2006;75(3):402-415. [PMID: 16968913]

Hill DR, Ericsson CD, Pearson RD et al; Infectious Diseases Society of America. The Practice of Travel Medicine: Guidelines by the Infectious Diseases Society of America. Clin Infect Dis. 2006;43(12):1499-1539. [PMID: 17109284]

Parola P, Paddock CD, Raoult D. Tick-borne rickettsioses around the world: emerging diseases challenging old concepts. Clin Microbiol Rev. 2005;18(4):719-756. [PMID: 16223955]

Steinberg EB, Bishop R, Haber P, et al. Typhoid fever in travelers: who should be targeted for prevention? Clin Infect Dis. 2004;39(2):186-191. [PMID: 15307027]

Teixeira MG, Barreto ML. Diagnosis and management of dengue. BJM. 2009;339:b4338. [PMID: 19923152]

Infectious Gastrointestinal Syndromes

Buchholz U, Bernard H, Werber D, et al. German outbreak of Escherichia coli O104:H4 associated with sprouts. N Engl J Med. 2011;365(19)1763-1770. [PMID: 22029753]

Cabada MM, White AC Jr. Treatment of cryptosporidiosis: do we know what we think we know? Curr Opin Infect Dis. 2010;23(5):494-499. [PMID: 20689422]

Cohen SH, Gerding DN, Johnson S, et al; Society for Healthcare Epidemiology of America; Infectious Diseases Society of America. Clinical practice guidelines for Clostridium difficile infection in adults: 2010 update by the society for healthcare epidemiology of America

(SHEA) and the infectious diseases society of America (IDSA). Infect Control Hosp Epidemiol. 2010;31(5):431-455. [PMID: 20307191]

Division of Viral Diseases, National Center for Immunization and Respiratory Diseases, Centers for Disease Control and Prevention. Updated norovirus outbreak management and disease prevention guidelines. MMWR Recomm Rep. 2011;60(RR-3):1-18. [PMID: 21368741]

Guerrent RL, Van Gilder T, Steiner TS, et al; Infectious Diseases Society of America. Practice guidelines for the management of infectious diarrhea. Clin Infect Dis. 2001;32(3):331-351. [PMID: 11170940]

Kelly CP, LaMont JT. Clostridium difficile—more difficult than ever. N Engl J Med. 2008;359(18):1932-1940. [PMID: 18971494]

Kent AJ, Banks MR. Pharmacological management of diarrhea. Gastroenterol Clin North Am. 2010;39(3):495-507. [PMID: 20951914]

Loo VG, Poirier L, Miller MA, et al. A predominantly clonal multi-institutional outbreak of Clostridium difficile-associated diarrhea with high morbidity and mortality. N Engl J Med. 2005;353(23):2442-2449. [PMID: 16322602]

Louis TJ, Miller MA, Mullane KM, et al; OPT-80-003 Clinical Study Group. Fidaxomicin versus vancomycin for Clostridium difficile infection. N Engl J Med. 2011;364(5):422-431. [PMID: 21288078]

Orth D, Grif K, Zimmerhackl LB, Würzner R. Prevention and treatment of enterohemorrhagic Escherichia coli infections in humans. Expert Rev Anti Infect Ther. 2008;6(1):101-108. [PMID: 18251667]

Tan KS, Mirza H, Teo JD, Wu B, Macary PA. Current views on the clinical relevance of Blastocystis spp. Curr Infect Dis Rep. 2010;12(1):28-35. [PMID: 21308496]

Valdez Y, Ferreira RB, Finlay BB. Molecular mechanisms of Salmonella virulence and host resistance. Curr Top Microbiol Immunol. 2009;337:93-127. [PMID: 19812981]

Infections in Transplant Recipients

Avery RK. Infectious disease following kidney transplant: core curriculum 2010. Am J Kidney Dis. 2010;55(4):755-771. [PMID: 20338466]

Eid AJ, Razonable RR. New developments in the management of cytomegalovirus infection after solid organ transplantation. Drugs. 2010;70(8):965-981. [PMID: 20481654]

Nishi SPE, Valentine VG, Duncan S. Emerging bacterial, fungal, and viral respiratory infections in transplantation. Infect Dis Clin North Am. 2010;24(3):541-555. [PMID: 20674791]

Nucci M, Anaissie E. Fungal infections in hematopoietic stem cell transplantation and solid-organ transplantation—focus on aspergillosis. Clin Chest Med. 2009;30(2):295-306, vii. [PMID: 19375636]

AST Infectious Diseases Community of Practice. The American Society of Transplantation Infectious Diseases Guidelines, Second Edition. Am J Transplant. 2009;9(suppl 4):S1-S281.

Tomblyn M, Chiller T, Einsele H, et al; Center for International Blood and Marrow Research; National Marrow Donor program; European Blood and MarrowTransplant Group; American Society of Blood and Marrow Transplantation; Canadian Blood and Marrow Transplant Group; Infectious Diseases Society of America; Society for Healthcare Epidemiology of America; Association of Medical Microbiology and Infectious Disease Canada; Centers for Disease Control and Prevention. Guidelines for preventing infectious complications among hematopoietic cell transplantation recipients: a global perspective. Biol Blood Marrow Transplant. 2009;15(10):1143-1238. [PMID: 19747629]

Hospital-Acquired Infections

American Thoracic Society, Infectious Diseases Society of America. Guidelines for the management of adults with hospital-acquired, ventilator-associated, and healthcare-associated pneumonia. Am J Respir Crit Care Med. 2005;171(4):388–416. [PMID: 15699079]

Anderson DJ. Surgical site infections. Infect Dis Clin North Am. 2011;25(1):135-153. [PMID: 21315998]

Boucher HW, Talbot GH, Bradley JS, et al. Bad bugs, no drugs: no ESKAPE! An update from the Infectious Diseases Society of America. Clin Infect Dis. 2009;48(1):1-12. [PMID: 19035777]

Burke JP. Infection control - a problem for patient safety. N Engl J Med. 2003;348(7):651-656. [PMID: 12584377]

Chenoweth CE, Saint S. Urinary tract infections. Infect Dis Clin North Am. 2011;25(1):103-115. [PMID: 21315996]

Hidron AI, Edwards JR, Patel J, et al; National Healthcare Safety Network Team; Participating National Healthcare Safety Network Facilities. NHSN annual update: antimicrobial-resistant pathogens associated with healthcare-associated infections: annual summary of data reported to the National Healthcare Safety Network at the Centers for Disease Control and Prevention, 2006-2007. Infect Control Hosp Epidemiol. 2008;29(11):996-1011. [PMID: 18947320]

Hooton TM, Bradley SF, Cardenas DD, et al; Infectious Diseases Society of America. Diagnosis, prevention, and treatment of catheter-associated urinary tract infection in adults: 2009 International Clinical Practice Guidelines from the Infectious Diseases Society of America. Clin Infect Dis. 2010;50(5):625-663. [PMID: 20175247]

Horan TC, Andrus M, Dudeck MA. CDC/NHSN surveillance definition of health care-associated infection and criteria for specific types of infections in the acute care setting. Am J Infect Control. 2008;36(5):309-332. [PMID: 18538699]

Lin MY, Hota B, Khan YM, et al; CDC Prevention Epicenter Program. Quality of traditional surveillance for public reporting of nosocomial bloodstream infection rates. JAMA. 2010;304(18):2035-2041. [PMID: 21063013]

Mermel LA, Allon M, Bouza E, et al. Clinical practice guidelines for the diagnosis and management of intravascular catheter-related infection: 2009 Update by the Infectious Diseases Society of America. Clin Infect Dis. 2009;49(1):1-45. [PMID: 19489710]

O'Grady NP, Alexander M, Burns LA, et al; Healthcare Infection Control Practices Advisory Committee (HICPAC) (Appendix 1). Summary of recommendations: Guidelines for the Prevention of Intravascular Catheter-related Infections. Clin Infect Dis. 2011;52(9):1087-1099. [PMID: 21467014]

Weber DJ, Rutala WA. Central line-associated bloodstream infections: prevention and management. Infect Dis Clin North Am. 2011;25(1):77-102. [PMID: 21315995]

Yokoe DS, Mermel LA, Anderson DJ, et al. A compendium of strategies to prevent healthcare-associated infections in acute care hospitals. Infect Control Hosp Epidemiol. 2008;29(suppl 1):S12-S21. [PMID: 18840084]

Infective Endocarditis Prevention

Gould FK, Elliott TS, Foweraker J, et al; Working Party of the British Society for Antimicrobial Chemotherapy. Guidelines for the prevention of endocarditis: report of the Working Party of the British Society for Antimicrobial Chemotherapy. J Antimicrob Chemother. 2006;57(6):1035-1042. [PMID: 16624872]

Wilson W, Taubert KA, Gewitz M, et al; American Heart Association. Prevention of infective endocarditis: guidelines from the American Heart Association: a guideline from the American Heart Association Rheumatic Fever, Endocarditis, and Kawasaki Disease Committee, Council on Cardiovascular Disease in the Young, and the Council on Clinical Cardiology, Council on Cardiovascular Surgery and Anesthesia, and the Quality of Care and Outcomes Research Interdisciplinary Working Group. Circulation. 2007;116(15):1736-1754. [PMID: 17446442]

HIV/AIDS

Aberg JA, Kaplan JE, Libman H, et al; HIV Medicine Association of the Infectious Diseases Society of America. Primary care guidelines for the management of persons infected with human immunodeficiency virus: 2009 update by the HIV Medicine Association of the Infectious Diseases Society of America. Clin Infect Dis. 2009;49(5):651-681. [PMID: 19640227]

Branson BM, Handsfield HH, Lampe MA, et al; Centers for Disease Control and Prevention (CDC). Revised recommendations for HIV testing of adults, adolescents, and pregnant women in health-care settings. MMWR Recomm Rep. 2006;55(RR-14):1-17. [PMID: 16988643]

Cohen MS, Gay CL, Busch MP, Hecht FM. The detection of acute HIV infection. J Infect Dis. 2010;202(suppl 2):S270-S277. [PMID: 20846033]

Farrugia PM, Lucariello R, Coppola, JT. Human immunodeficiency virus and atherosclerosis. Cardiol Rev. 2009;17(5):211-215. [PMID: 19690471]

Feinberg, J. Management of newly diagnosed HIV infection. Ann Intern Med. 2011;155(7):ITC41. [PMID: 21969353]

Kaplan JE, Benson C, Holmes KH, Brooks JT, Pau A, Masur H; Centers for Disease Control and Prevention (CDC); National Institutes of Health; HIV Medicine Association of the Infectious Diseases Society of America. Guidelines for prevention and treatment of opportunistic infections in HIV-infected adults and adolescents: recommendations from the CDC, National Institutes of Health, and the HIV Medicine Association of the Infectious Diseases Society of America. MMWR Recomm Rep. 2009;58(RR-4):1-207. [PMID: 19357635]

Landovitz RJ, Currier JS. Postexposure prophylaxis for HIV infection. N Engl J Med. 2009;361(18):1768-1775. [PMID: 19864675]

Panel on Antiretroviral Guidelines for Adults and Adolescents. Guidelines for the use of antiretroviral agents in HIV-1-infected adults and adolescents. Department of Health and Human Services. January 10, 2011;1-166. Available at www.aidsinfo.nih.gov/ContentFiles/AdultandAdolescentGL.pdf. Accessed July 9, 2012.

Panel on Treatment of HIV-Infected Pregnant Women and Prevention of Perinatal Transmission. Recommendations for use of antiretroviral drugs in pregnant HIV-1-infected women for maternal health and interventions to reduce perinatal HIV transmission in the United States. May 24, 2010;1-117. Available at www.aidsinfo.nih.gov/ContentFiles/PerinatalGL.pdf. Accessed July 9, 2012.

Qaseem A, Snow V, Shekelle P et al. and the Clinical Efficacy Assessment Subcommittee, American College of Physicians. Screening for HIV in health care settings: a guidance statement from the American College of Physicians and HIV Medicine Association. Ann Intern Med. 2009 Jan 20;150(2):125-31. Epub 2008 Nov 30. PubMed [PMID: 19047022]

Taylor S, Jayasuriya A, Smit E. Using HIV resistance tests in clinical practice. J Antimicrob Chemother. 2009;64(2):218-222. [PMID: 19535382]

Thompson MA, Aberg JA, Cahn P, et al; International AIDS Society-USA. Antiretroviral treatment of adult HIV infection: 2010 recommendations of the International AIDS Society-USA Panel. JAMA. 2010;304(3):321-333. [PMID: 20639566]

Viral Infections

Bond D, Mooney J. A literature review regarding the management of varicella-zoster virus. Musculoskeletal Care. 2010;8(2):118-122. [PMID: 20301227]

Cernik C, Gallina K, Brodell RT. The treatment of herpes simplex infections: an evidence-based review. Arch Intern Med. 2008;168(11):1137-1144. [PMID: 18541820]

Fiore AE, Bridges CB, Cox NJ. Seasonal influenza vaccines. Curr Top Microbiol Immunol. 2009;333:43-82. [PMID: 19768400]

Fiore AE, Fry A, Shay D, Gubareva L, Bresee JS, Uyeki TM; Centers for Disease Control and Prevention (CDC). Antiviral agents for the treatment and chemoprophylaxis of influenz — recommendations of the Advisory Committee on Immunization Practices (ACIP). MMWR Recomm Rep. 2011;60(1):1-24. [PMID: 21248682]

Jefferson T, Jones M, Doshi P, Del Mar C, Dooley L, Foxlee R. Neuraminidase inhibitors for preventing and treating influenza in healthy adults. Cochrane Database Syst Rev. 2010;(2):CD001265. [PMID: 20166059]

Mubareka S, Leung V, Aoki FY, Vinh DC. Famciclovir: a focus on efficacy and safety. Expert Opin Drug Saf. 2010;9(4):643-658. [PMID: 20429777]

Oxman MN. Zoster vaccine: current status and future prospects. Clin Infect Dis. 2010;51(2):197-213. [PMID: 20550454]

Strasfeld L, Chou S. Antiviral drug resistance: mechanisms and clinical implications. Infect Dis Clin North Am. 2010;24(3):809-833. [PMID: 20674805]

Vigil KJ, Chemaly RF. Valacyclovir: approved and off-label uses for the treatment of herpes virus infections in immunocompetent and immunocompromised adults. Expert Opin Pharmacother. 2010;11(11):1901-1913. [PMID: 20536295]

Whitley RJ, Volpi A, McKendrick M, Wijck A, Oaklander AL. Management of herpes zoster and post-herpetic neuralgia now and in the future. J Clin Virol. 2010;48(suppl 1):S20-S28. [PMID: 20510264]

New Topics in Anti-infective Therapy

Chen LF, Kaye D. Current use for old antibacterial agents: polymyxins, rifamycins, and aminoglycosides. Infect Dis Clin North Am. 2009;23(4):1053-1075, x. [PMID: 19909897]

Dellit TH, Owens RC, McGowan JE Jr, et al; Infectious Diseases Society of America; Society for Healthcare Epidemiology of America. Infectious Diseases Society of America and the Society for Healthcare Epidemiology of America guidelines for developing an institutional program to enhance antimicrobial stewardship. Clin Infect Dis. 2007;44(2):159-177. [PMID: 17173212]

Eskes A, Ubbink DT, Lubbers M, Lucas C, Vermeulen H. Hyperbaric oxygen therapy for treating acute surgical and traumatic wounds. Cochrane Database Syst Rev. 2010;(10):CD008059. [PMID: 20927771]

Lipsky BA, Berendt AR, Deery HG, et al; Infectious Diseases Society of America. Diagnosis and treatment of diabetic foot infections. Plast Reconstr Surg. 2006;117(7 suppl):212S-238S. [PMID: 16799390]

Pogue JM, Marchaim D, Kaye D, Kaye KS. Re-visiting "older" antibiotics in the era of multi-drug resistance. Pharmacotherapy. 2011;31(9):912-921. [PMID: 21923592]

Tice AD, Rehm SJ, Dalovisio JR, et al; IDSA. Practice guidelines for outpatient parenteral antimicrobial therapy. IDSA guidelines. Clin Infect Dis. 2004;38(12):1651-1672. [PMID: 15227610]

Infectious Disease
Self-Assessment Test

This self-assessment test contains one-best-answer multiple-choice questions. Please read these directions carefully before answering the questions. Answers, critiques, and bibliographies immediately follow these multiple-choice questions. The American College of Physicians is accredited by the Accreditation Council for Continuing Medical Education (ACCME) to provide continuing medical education for physicians.

The American College of Physicians designates MKSAP 16 Infectious Disease for a maximum of 16 *AMA PRA Category 1 Credits*™. Physicians should claim only the credit commensurate with the extent of their participation in the activity.

Earn "Same-Day" CME Credits Online

For the first time, print subscribers can enter their answers online to earn CME credits in 24 hours or less. You can submit your answers using online answer sheets that are provided at mksap.acponline.org, where a record of your MKSAP 16 credits will be available. To earn CME credits, you need to answer all of the questions in a test and earn a score of at least 50% correct (number of correct answers divided by the total number of questions). Take any of the following approaches:

> ➤ Use the printed answer sheet at the back of this book to record your answers. Go to mksap.acponline.org, access the appropriate online answer sheet, transcribe your answers, and submit your test for same-day CME credits. There is no additional fee for this service.

> ➤ Go to mksap.acponline.org, access the appropriate online answer sheet, directly enter your answers, and submit your test for same-day CME credits. There is no additional fee for this service.

> ➤ Pay a $10 processing fee per answer sheet and submit the printed answer sheet at the back of this book by mail or fax, as instructed on the answer sheet. Make sure you calculate your score and fax the answer sheet to 215-351-2799 or mail the answer sheet to Member and Customer Service, American College of Physicians, 190 N. Independence Mall West, Philadelphia, PA 19106-1572, using the courtesy envelope provided in your MKSAP 16 slipcase. You will need your 10-digit order number and 8-digit ACP ID number, which are printed on your packing slip. Please allow 4 to 6 weeks for your score report to be emailed back to you. Be sure to include your email address for a response.

If you do not have a 10-digit order number and 8-digit ACP ID number or if you need help creating a username and password to access the MKSAP 16 online answer sheets, go to mksap.acponline.org or email custserv@acponline.org.

CME credit is available from the publication date of December 31, 2012, until December 31, 2015. You may submit your answer sheets at any time during this period.

Directions

*Each of the numbered items is followed by lettered answers. Select the **ONE** lettered answer that is **BEST** in each case.*

Self-Assessment Test

Item 1

An 18-year-old woman is evaluated 4 weeks following hospitalization for her second episode of pneumococcal pneumonia in 18 months. She received the pneumococcal vaccine 20 months ago. The patient was also diagnosed with giardiasis 2 years ago. She also has a history of asthma. Her mother has selective IgA deficiency, and her brother has lymphoma. Her review of systems is negative for findings associated with autoimmune disorders, including systemic lupus erythematosus.

On physical examination, vital signs are normal. Faint crackles are heard at the posterior left lung base.

Laboratory studies show a hemoglobin level of 8.6 g/dL (86 g/L), a mean corpuscular volume of 120 fL, and leukocyte count of 6800/µL (6.8 × 10⁹/L) with a normal differential. HIV serology results are negative.

Which of the following is most likely to establish the diagnosis?

(A) Check response to pneumococcal and tetanus vaccines
(B) Measure CD4 cell count
(C) Measure serum IgG, IgM, and IgA levels
(D) Measure total hemolytic complement level

Item 2

A 33-year-old man is evaluated after learning that a person living in his home was recently found to have active tuberculosis. The patient has no acute symptoms. He was recently diagnosed with HIV infection, and his CD4 cell count is 250/µL. He is a U.S. citizen and has no history of incarceration, homelessness, or travel to areas with an increased prevalence of tuberculosis. He takes no medications but had been planning to begin antiretroviral therapy at his next office visit.

On physical examination, vital signs are normal. The remainder of the examination, including cardiopulmonary findings, is normal.

A tuberculin skin test induces 0 mm of induration. A chest radiograph is normal.

Which of the following is the most appropriate next step in the management of this patient?

(A) Begin isoniazid and pyridoxine
(B) Begin isoniazid, rifampin, pyrazinamide, pyridoxine, and ethambutol
(C) Begin rifampin and pyrazinamide
(D) No additional evaluation or therapy is needed

Item 3

A 64-year-old woman is hospitalized for a 2-day history of fever and chills and a 1-day history of hypotension and dyspnea. Medical history is significant for adenocarcinoma of the colon diagnosed 3 weeks ago for which she had a partial colectomy. Her course was complicated by the

development of a polymicrobial intra-abdominal abscess. After drainage of the abscess, she received hyperalimentation through a central line catheter and ceftriaxone and metronidazole for 7 days.

On physical examination, temperature is 39.0 °C (102.2 °F), blood pressure is 90/60 mm Hg, pulse rate is 120/min, and respiration rate is 20/min. There are erythema and purulent drainage at the site of a right subclavian central venous catheter. The rest of the examination is normal.

Laboratory studies indicate a leukocyte count of 16,000/µL (16 × 10⁹/L). Serum creatinine level is 3.6 mg/dL (318.2 µmol/L) compared with a value of 1.2 mg/dL (106.1 µmol/L) at admission. Two sets of blood cultures obtained 2 days ago are growing yeast.

In addition to central venous catheter removal, which of the following is the most appropriate treatment option for this patient?

(A) Caspofungin
(B) Conventional amphotericin B
(C) Fluconazole
(D) Liposomal amphotericin B
(E) Voriconazole

Item 4

A 42-year-old man is evaluated for recurrent diarrhea. Four weeks ago, the patient was diagnosed with a mild *Clostridium difficile* infection and treated with a 14-day course of metronidazole, 500 mg orally every 8 hours, with resolution of his symptoms. He currently takes no medications.

One week after his last dose of metronidazole, he again develops recurrent watery stools without fever or other symptoms. There is no visible blood or mucus in the stools.

Physical examination findings are noncontributory.

Results of laboratory studies show a leukocyte count of 10,400/µL (10.4 × 10⁹/L) and a normal serum creatinine level. A stool sample tests positive for occult blood, and results of a repeat stool assay are again positive for *C. difficile* toxin.

Which of the following is the most appropriate treatment at this time?

(A) Oral metronidazole for 14 days
(B) Oral metronidazole taper over 42 days
(C) Oral vancomycin for 14 days
(D) Oral vancomycin plus parenteral metronidazole for 14 days
(E) Oral vancomycin taper over 42 days

Item 5

A 28-year-old woman is evaluated for a 2-day history of painful genital lesions accompanied by dysuria, generalized myalgia, malaise, and fever. She is sexually active.

On physical examination, temperature is 37.8 °C (100.0 °F), and the remaining vital signs are normal. Examination of the genital area discloses painful vesicular lesions on an erythematous base.

Which of the following is the most appropriate treatment?

(A) Acyclovir
(B) Benzathine penicillin G
(C) Ceftriaxone and azithromycin
(D) Fluconazole

Item 6

A 35-year-old man is evaluated in the emergency department for a 6-day history of fever, headache, malaise, myalgia, dry cough, shortness of breath, and vague chest pain. He recently returned from filming a documentary on hibernating Indiana bats in the caves of Ohio. Medical history is noncontributory.

On physical examination, temperature is 38.3 °C (100.9 °F). Pulmonary examination discloses a few bilateral wheezes. The remainder of the examination, including vital signs, is normal.

The hemoglobin level is 10.5 g/dL (105 g/L), and the leukocyte count is 8000/μL (8.0 × 10⁹/L) with 53% neutrophils, 35% lymphocytes, and 12% monocytes. HIV serologic testing is negative.

The chest radiograph shows hilar lymphadenopathy and interstitial infiltrates.

The preliminary blood and sputum cultures are negative for organisms.

Which of the following is the most likely diagnosis?

(A) Blastomycosis
(B) Coccidioidomycosis
(C) Cryptococcosis
(D) Histoplasmosis

Item 7

An 82-year-old woman is evaluated for a 3-week history of pain in the right knee. She underwent right knee arthroplasty 3 years ago. Ten months following her arthroplasty, she developed a methicillin-resistant *Staphylococcus aureus* (MRSA) infection that required removal of the prosthetic joint and a new total knee arthroplasty as well as 6 weeks of vancomycin and rifampin antimicrobial therapy.

On physical examination, vital signs are normal. Examination of the knee joint and surrounding tissues is unremarkable.

Leukocyte-tagged nuclear imaging studies demonstrate focal uptake at the proximal tibia, and radiographic findings are consistent with sequestrum formation at the same anatomic location.

Culture of the joint fluid reveals MRSA sensitive to vancomycin, daptomycin, linezolid, trimethoprim-sulfamethoxazole, tetracycline, and rifampin.

The patient refuses to undergo any further surgical procedures.

Which of the following is the most appropriate management of this patient?

(A) Lifelong oral rifampin
(B) Lifelong oral trimethoprim-sulfamethoxazole
(C) Six weeks of parenteral vancomycin and oral rifampin
(D) Symptomatic treatment

Item 8

A 47-year-old woman is evaluated in the emergency department for abdominal pain and diarrhea. The diarrhea began 3 days ago as semi-formed stools, but in the last 24 hours the patient has noted streaks of bright red blood in the stools. She has abdominal cramps that are unrelated to bowel movements but no fever. Five days before her symptoms developed, the patient attended a cookout where she ate potato salad, coleslaw, and a hamburger. Two other guests have also developed a diarrheal illness.

On physical examination, temperature and blood pressure are normal; the pulse rate is 115/min. Abdominal examination discloses hyperactive bowel sounds with diffuse tenderness to palpation. Remaining physical examination findings are noncontributory.

Results of laboratory studies show a leukocyte count 17,400/μL (17.4 × 10⁹/L) and a serum creatinine level 1.0 mg/dL (88.4 μmol/L). A stool sample shows gross blood.

Which of the following pathogens is most likely causing this patient's current illness?

(A) *Bacillus cereus*
(B) *Campylobacter jejuni*
(C) Shiga toxin–producing *Escherichia coli*
(D) *Staphylococcus aureus*
(E) *Yersinia enterocolitica*

Item 9

A 33-year-old woman is evaluated for a 2-day history of diarrhea. She describes the stools as mucoid but without visible blood. Bowel movements are associated with mild abdominal cramping. She has no nausea or vomiting. The patient works with infants in a day care center, and several children have recently had a diarrheal illness.

On physical examination, temperature is 37.8 °C (100.0 °F); other vital signs are normal. Abdominal examination discloses normal bowel sounds and diffuse mild tenderness to palpation.

A stool sample shows no gross blood, but results of guaiac testing and a test for fecal leukocytes are positive.

The patient is advised to increase fluid intake and take over-the-counter antipyretic agents for fever. No antibiotics are prescribed. Two days later, a stool culture is reported to be growing *Shigella sonnei*. The patient is contacted and reports that her diarrhea and fever have both resolved and that she wishes to return to work.

**hich of the following is the most appropriate treat-
ent at this time?**

(A) Azithromycin

(B) Ciprofloxacin

(C) Metronidazole

(D) No treatment is needed

em 10

52-year-old man is admitted to the hospital with fatigue
d fever of 3 days' duration. He is a health care worker and
s a bicuspid aortic valve. He takes no medications.

Blood cultures are obtained at the time of admission,
d he is started on empiric vancomycin for possible
docarditis.

On hospital day 2, his initial blood cultures become
sitive for gram-positive cocci in clusters, and on hospital
y 3, his blood cultures grow methicillin-resistant *Staphy-
coccus aureus*. Susceptibility to vancomycin is intermediate
IC = 4 µg/mL).

On hospital day 4, the patient continues to appear ill.
mperature is 38.6 °C (101.5 °F), blood pressure is
5/65 mm Hg, and pulse rate is 110/min. On car-
opulmonary examination, the lungs are clear, and a grade
/6 systolic ejection murmur is heard at the right upper
rnal border, but there is no evidence of heart failure or
ptic emboli.

**hich of the following is the most appropriate man-
ement?**

(A) Discontinue vancomycin and begin daptomycin

(B) Discontinue vancomycin and begin linezolid

(C) Discontinue vancomycin and begin trimethoprim-
sulfamethoxazole

(D) Increase vancomycin dose

em 11

1 18-year-old woman is evaluated for a 5-day history of a
ick yellow vaginal discharge that is occasionally tinged
th blood, especially after intercourse. She has no dys-
reunia or abdominal pain. She has been sexually active
th a single male partner for the past 3 months and uses
al contraceptives. Her partner has no symptoms.

On physical examination, temperature is 37.2 °C
8.9 °F), blood pressure is 105/65 mm Hg, pulse rate is
/min, and respiration rate is 10/min. A pelvic examina-
n reveals no abnormalities of the vulva or vaginal mucosa.
e cervix is inflamed, and copious mucopurulent secre-
ns are noted. No cervical motion tenderness, uterine ten-
rness, adnexal tenderness, or masses are identified on
manual examination.

A wet mount of vaginal secretions shows numerous
akocytes, with a pH of 5.5. The whiff test is negative.
ere are no trichomonads or clue cells. A urine pregnancy
st is negative.

**Which of the following is the most appropriate treat-
ment?**

(A) Oral cefixime

(B) Oral ciprofloxacin and oral azithromycin

(C) Parenteral ceftriaxone and oral azithromycin

(D) Parenteral cefoxitin and oral doxycycline

Item 12

A 63-year-old man undergoes annual screening for tuberculosis. The patient is a physician, and this screening is
required for maintaining his hospital appointment. His
medical history is significant for bladder cancer diagnosed 1
year ago that was treated with bacillus Calmette-Guérin.
There is no current evidence of active bladder cancer on follow-up cystoscopy, and he has no respiratory or systemic
symptoms.

On physical examination, vital signs are normal. The
remaining physical examination findings, including cardiopulmonary examination, are normal.

**Which of the following is the most appropriate next
step in management?**

(A) Chest radiograph

(B) Interferon-γ release assay

(C) Tuberculin skin test

(D) Two-step tuberculin skin testing

Item 13

A 28-year-old woman is evaluated in the emergency department for an injury to the hand sustained after punching
another woman in the mouth 5 hours ago. She is allergic to
penicillin, which causes hives, facial edema, and wheezing.
All immunizations are current, including tetanus toxoid,
diphtheria toxoid, and acellular pertussis vaccine administered 4 years ago.

On physical examination, temperature is normal, blood
pressure is 125/70 mm Hg, pulse rate is 75/min, and respiration rate is 14/min. The dorsum of the left hand has
several tiny punctures with minimal erythema and tenderness. There is no purulence or other evidence of infection,
and no underlying tissue is visible.

Results of a urine pregnancy test are negative. Radiographs of the left hand show no fracture, foreign body,
or gas.

**Which of the following is the most appropriate man-
agement?**

(A) Cephalexin

(B) Clindamycin and moxifloxacin

(C) Tetanus immunization

(D) Trimethoprim-sulfamethoxazole

(E) Observation

Item 14

A 20-year-old man is evaluated following exposure to a relative who was found to have an active varicella-zoster infection that developed about 2 days after their contact. The patient was recently diagnosed with acute myeloid leukemia and completed one cycle of induction therapy with standard-dose cytarabine and daunorubicin. He does not recall having had chickenpox as a child and has never received a varicella vaccine.

On physical examination, temperature is normal, blood pressure is 110/70 mm Hg, pulse rate is 70/min, and respiration rate is 12/min. There is no skin rash.

The leukocyte count is 600/µL (0.6 × 10⁹/L), and the absolute neutrophil count is 200/µL. Testing for varicella antibody is negative.

Which of the following is the most appropriate management of this patient?

(A) Acyclovir
(B) Varicella vaccine
(C) Varicella-zoster immune globulin product
(D) No treatment

Item 15

A 73-year-old woman is evaluated for a 2-day history of fatigue, fever, nausea, and vomiting but no localizing symptoms. She is otherwise healthy.

On physical examination, she appears ill. Temperature is 39.8 °C (103.6 °F), blood pressure is 125/75 mm Hg, pulse rate is 115/min, and respiration rate is 15/min. Cardiopulmonary and abdominal examinations are unremarkable.

Laboratory studies indicate a leukocyte count of 17,500/µL (17.5 × 10⁹/L) with 85% neutrophils. A urinalysis demonstrates more than 50 leukocytes/hpf and is positive for leukocyte esterase. Gram-negative rods are seen on microscopic examination. A chest radiograph is normal.

She is admitted to the hospital and treated with aggressive intravenous fluid therapy and empiric piperacillin-tazobactam. On hospital day 2, her urine and blood cultures become positive for *Escherichia coli* susceptible to piperacillin-tazobactam, imipenem, ciprofloxacin, ampicillin, and nitrofurantoin.

Which of the following is the most appropriate management?

(A) Continue piperacillin-tazobactam
(B) Discontinue piperacillin-tazobactam and begin ampicillin
(C) Discontinue piperacillin-tazobactam and begin ciprofloxacin
(D) Discontinue piperacillin-tazobactam and begin imipenem
(E) Discontinue piperacillin-tazobactam and begin nitrofurantoin

Item 16

A 55-year-old man is evaluated in the emergency department after experiencing fever and chills yesterday evening and bilateral arm pain and a rash on the upper extremit upon awakening this morning. The patient ate raw oyste from the Gulf Coast 3 nights ago. He was recently diag nosed with hemochromatosis.

On physical examination, the patient is ill appearin Temperature is 39.1 °C (102.4 °F), blood pressure 85/50 mm Hg, pulse rate is 130/min, and respiration ra is 28/min. Skin findings of the upper extremity are show

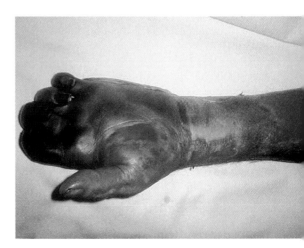

Cardiopulmonary examination findings are norm On abdominal examination, there is shifting dullness and guarding or rebound. No signs of meningeal irritation present.

Laboratory studies:

Leukocyte count	28,000/µL (28 × 10⁹/L) with 93% neutrophils, 6% lymphocytes, and 1% monocytes
Ferritin	1000 ng/mL (1000 µg/L
Albumin	2.3 g/dL (23 g/L)
Aspartate aminotransferase	145 units/L
Alanine aminotransferase	100 units/L

The peripheral blood smear is normal.

Which of the following pathogens is most likely cau ing this patient's current findings?

(A) *Babesia microti*
(B) *Capnocytophaga canimorsus*
(C) *Rickettsia rickettsii*
(D) *Vibrio vulnificus*

Item 17

A 23-year-old man was admitted to a hospital 2 days a with a 3-day history of fever, severe headache and backac vomiting, and sores in the back of his throat. The patien a soldier. Yesterday, he developed spots on his hands a face, and today, the spots have spread to his arms and tru d he has developed a papular rash on his face and hands; of the lesions are now at the same stage of development. he patient's nurse, a 28-year-old woman, did not use any rsonal protective equipment during her first 2 days of his re.

hich of the following interventions is most appro- iate for the nurse?

.) Acyclovir

) Cidofovir

C) Smallpox vaccine

D) Varicella vaccine

) No intervention is required

em 18

45-year-old woman is evaluated for nausea, anorexia, and igue. She had a kidney transplant 7 months ago and has en doing well since then, with normal blood pressure, a rmal serum creatinine level, and an at-goal tacrolimus vel on routine follow-up last month. Medications are crolimus, mycophenolate mofetil, and prednisone. She ports that 5 days ago, she also began taking some leftover rithromycin that she had at home because she thought e was getting a sinus infection.

On physical examination, temperature is 37.2 °C 9.0 °F), blood pressure is 142/90 mm Hg, pulse rate is 4/min, and respiration rate is 20/min. Cardiopulmonary amination is normal. The abdomen is soft and nontender. he surgical site of the transplanted kidney is well healed.

Laboratory studies indicate a blood urea nitrogen level 51 mg/dL (18.2 mmol/L) and a serum creatinine level 3.7 mg/dL (327.1 μmol/L).

Dipstick and microscopic urinalysis are normal.

hich of the following is the most likely cause of this tient's acute kidney injury?

) Clarithromycin-induced interstitial nephritis

) Mycophenolate mofetil toxicity

C) Organ rejection

D) Tacrolimus toxicity

em 19

32-year-old man is admitted to the hospital with a 5-day story of fever, chills, and myalgia. The patient works as a ldlife biologist. Most of his time is spent outdoors in rural eas. He removed an attached tick from his right leg 3 eks ago but recalls no rash.

On physical examination, temperature is 38.8 °C 01.8 °F), and pulse rate is 115/min. The patient is ori- ted and conversant. There is no nuchal rigidity. Neuro- gic examination is notable for right lower extremity weak- ss, with 2/5 strength with foot dorsiflexion and plantar xion, 2/5 strength with knee flexion and extension, and 5 strength with hip flexion. Right knee and ankle deep ndon reflexes are absent but are intact on the left side. nsation is preserved. Remaining physical examination dings are unremarkable.

Laboratory studies, including a complete blood count with differential and metabolic panel, are normal. A CT scan of the head without contrast is normal. Lumbar punc- ture is performed. The cerebrospinal fluid (CSF) leukocyte count is 227/μL (227×10^6/L), with 45% neutrophils. The CSF protein level is 75 mg/dL (750 mg/L). A Gram- stained CSF specimen is negative.

Which of the following CSF diagnostic studies should be performed next?

(A) Cytomegalovirus polymerase chain reaction (PCR)

(B) PCR for *Ehrlichia* species

(C) PCR for *Borrelia burgdorferi* species

(D) West Nile virus IgM antibody assay

Item 20

A 59-year-old woman is evaluated for a dry cough with moderate exertional dyspnea, which has remained stable in intensity over the past 7 months. The onset of her respira- tory symptoms does not correlate with any unusual expo- sures. She has intermittently been treated with oral antibi- otics for outpatient pneumonia without a change in her symptoms. She has no systemic signs or symptoms and oth- erwise feels well. Medical history is unremarkable. She does not smoke. She has lived most of her adult life in the south- eastern United States. She currently takes no medications.

On physical examination, vital signs are normal. Pul- monary auscultation reveals scattered rhonchi. The remain- der of the examination, including cardiac examination, is normal.

A CT scan of the lungs demonstrates scattered nodu- lar infiltrates, mostly confined to the right middle and bilat- eral upper lobes.

Normal respiratory flora grow from a sputum culture, and although the smear for acid-fast bacilli is negative, the culture eventually grows *Mycobacterium avium* complex by DNA gene-probe testing.

Which of the following is the most appropriate next step in management?

(A) Bronchoalveolar lavage

(B) Clarithromycin, ethambutol, and rifampin

(C) Repeat sputum acid-fast bacilli smear and culture

(D) Video-assisted thorascopic lung biopsy

(E) Observation

Item 21

A 40-year-old woman is admitted to the hospital for headaches, fever, and sweats of 3 weeks' duration as well as diplopia and increased somnolence that began yesterday. She was diagnosed with HIV infection 2 months ago with a CD4 cell count of 166/μL and an HIV RNA viral load of 66,923 copies/mL, and she immediately began taking antiretroviral therapy. She had been tolerating her medica- tions and felt well until her current symptoms started. Med- ications are tenofovir, emtricitabine, efavirenz, and trimethoprim-sulfamethoxazole.

CONT.

On physical examination, temperature is 38.2 °C (100.8 °F), blood pressure is 154/96 mm Hg, pulse rate is 64/min, and respiration rate is 18/min. She is awake but drowsy and is oriented to person and place but not time. The left eye cannot move laterally with leftward gaze. The rest of the neurologic examination is unremarkable.

CT scan of the head shows mildly increased ventricle size and mild cerebral atrophy, which is confirmed by MRI of the brain. Lumbar puncture is performed.

Cerebrospinal fluid analysis:

Leukocyte count	122/µL (122 × 10⁶/L) with 18% polymorphonuclear cells and 82% mononuclear cells
Glucose	62 mg/dL (3.4 mmol/L)
Protein	433 mg/dL (4330 mg/L)

The CD4 cell count is 251/µL, and the HIV RNA viral load is 675 copies/mL.

Infection with which of the following is the most likely cause of this patient's clinical presentation?

(A) *Cryptococcus neoformans*
(B) Cytomegalovirus
(C) *Histoplasma capsulatum*
(D) *Toxoplasma gondii*

 Item 22

An 18-year-old woman is evaluated in the emergency department for a 2-day history of fever, headache, vomiting, and photosensitivity. She noted painful ulcers on the vulva 10 days ago. Her boyfriend has had penile ulcers. Medical history is otherwise unremarkable.

On physical examination, temperature is 38.5 °C (101.3 °F), blood pressure is 100/60 mm Hg, pulse rate is 110/min, and respiration rate is 14/min. Nuchal rigidity is noted. The eyes appear normal. She has no oral or skin lesions. There are a few shallow ulcers on the vulva. There are no changes in sensorium. Neurologic examination is nonfocal.

Cerebrospinal fluid (CSF) analysis:

Leukocyte count	200/µL (200 × 10⁶/L) with 90% lymphocytes
Erythrocyte count	10/µL (10 × 10⁶/L)
Glucose	60 mg/dL (3.3 mmol/L)

Plasma glucose level is 100 mg/dL (5.6 mmol/L). A Gram stain of the CSF is negative.

Which of the following is the most likely diagnosis?

(A) Acute bacterial meningitis
(B) Acute retroviral syndrome
(C) Behçet disease
(D) Herpes simplex virus–induced aseptic meningitis

Item 23

A 22-year-old man is evaluated for a skin eruption on his leg. The patient lives in Virginia and is active outdoors. One week ago, he found a black tick on his lower leg, which his roommate removed with a tweezers. Yesterday he developed diffuse myalgia, neck stiffness, and fatigue. The symptoms have persisted, and today he notes erythema the site of the previously attached tick.

On physical examination, temperature is 38.1 (100.6 °F); other vital signs are normal. There is no nuch rigidity. Skin findings are shown.

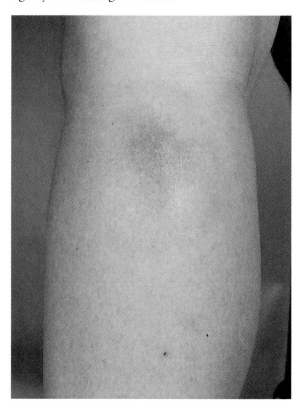

Which of the following is the most appropriate init management?

(A) *Borrelia burgdorferi* polymerase chain reaction on skin biopsy specimen
(B) Empiric intravenous ceftriaxone
(C) Empiric oral doxycycline
(D) Serologic testing for Lyme disease

Item 24

A 35-year-old woman is evaluated for a 1-day history fever, headache, myalgia, arthralgia, and neck stiffness. T patient is sexually active. She had a similar episode 2 ye ago, at which time results of cerebrospinal fluid (CS analysis showed lymphocytic meningitis. All culture resu were negative, and her symptoms resolved over the nex days.

On physical examination, temperature is 38.3 (101.0 °F), blood pressure is 110/70 mm Hg, pulse rate 90/min, and respiration rate is 12/min. There are no o or genital ulcers. There is mild neck stiffness. Remaini physical examination findings, including mental status ev uation and complete neurologic examination, are norm Funduscopic examination is normal.

Examination of the CSF shows a leukocyte count of 0/μL (90 × 10⁶/L) with 95% lymphocytes, a glucose level 68 mg/dL (3.8 mmol/L), and a protein level of 70 g/dL (700 mg/L). A Gram-stained CSF specimen is gative.

Which of the following diagnostic studies will most kely establish the cause of this patient's meningitis?

A) CSF cytology

B) CSF IgM assay for West Nile virus

C) CSF polymerase chain reaction for herpes simplex virus type 2

D) MRI of the brain

em 25

42-year-old man is admitted to the hospital for a 2-week story of headache and fever and a 1-week history of skin sions. He was diagnosed with AIDS 5 years ago. He has ot taken antiretroviral therapy for the past year. His only rrent medication is trimethoprim-sulfamethoxazole.

On physical examination, temperature is 38.0 °C 00.4 °F). Skin findings are shown.

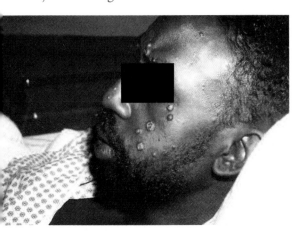

The remainder of the physical examination is normal.

Results of the serum cryptococcal antigen assay are sitive at a titer of 1:1024. Blood cultures from admission e growing budding yeast. Cerebrospinal fluid (CSF) ening pressure is 220 mm H₂0. CSF cryptococcal anti- n and culture results are pending. A Gram stain of the SF is negative.

erebrospinal fluid analysis:

eukocyte count	2/μL (2.0 × 10⁶/L)
rythrocyte count	10/μL (10 × 10⁶/L)
otein	70 mg/dL (700 mg/L)
lucose	70 mg/dL (3.9 mmol/L)

The plasma glucose level is 100 mg/dL (5.6 mol/L).

A CT scan of the head is normal.

hich of the following is the most appropriate initial eatment?

A) Conventional amphotericin B and flucytosine

B) Caspofungin

(C) Fluconazole

(D) Itraconazole

Item 26

A 23-year-old woman is evaluated for a 5-day history of yellow vaginal discharge accompanied by lower abdominal pain and dyspareunia. The remainder of the medical history is noncontributory.

On physical examination, temperature is 38.0 °C (100.4 °F), blood pressure is 110/60 mm Hg, pulse rate is 90/min, and respiration rate is 12/min. The cervix appears inflamed, with a small amount of mucopurulent discharge. There is no cervical motion tenderness, but there is tenderness to palpation of the uterus on bimanual examination. No adnexal tenderness or masses are noted.

A serum pregnancy test is negative.

Which of the following is the most appropriate treatment?

(A) Intravenous clindamycin and gentamicin for 7 days

(B) Oral ciprofloxacin and metronidazole for 14 days

(C) Single-dose intramuscular ceftriaxone and oral doxycycline for 14 days

(D) Single-dose intramuscular ceftriaxone and single-dose oral azithromycin

Item 27

A 31-year-old woman is evaluated for recurrent episodes of genital symptoms that consist of itching, irritation, and burning in the vulvar area without vaginal discharge. The patient has experienced two similar episodes over the past 3 years, but she has never noticed any lesions in the genital region. She has had six lifetime sexual partners.

On physical examination, vital signs are normal. An examination of the external genitalia reveals a linear fissure between the labia minora and the labia majora on the left. A pelvic examination is normal.

HIV and syphilis screening are performed.

Which of the following is the most appropriate next diagnostic test to perform?

(A) Herpes simplex virus polymerase chain reaction

(B) Serology for *Chlamydia trachomatis* serovars L1, L2, and L3

(C) Tzanck smear

(D) Wet mount with potassium hydroxide

Item 28

A 22-year-old man is evaluated for a painless penile lesion first noted 3 days ago. He has no fever or other symptoms. He has had three male sexual partners in the past 6 months and uses condoms inconsistently. He undergoes HIV testing every year, and his most recent results 7 months ago were negative.

On physical examination, vital signs are normal. Skin findings on the shaft of the penis are shown.

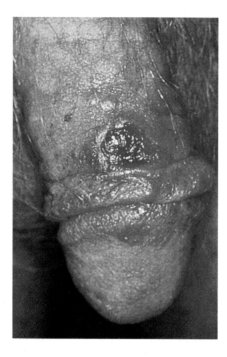

There is no evidence of penile discharge or other genital lesions. He has no other skin or oral lesions. Shotty, nontender inguinal lymphadenopathy is noted.

Which of the following is the most likely diagnosis?

(A) Chancroid
(B) Herpes simplex virus infection
(C) Human papillomavirus infection
(D) Syphilis

Item 29

A 24-year-old man is admitted to the hospital with a 4-day history of fever, malaise, and arthralgia of the elbows, wrists, and knees. Two days ago, he developed progressive pain and swelling of the right knee. He also has a rash on his right arm.

On physical examination, temperature is 38.2 °C (100.8 °F), blood pressure is 110/60 mm Hg, pulse rate is 95/min, and respiration rate is 12/min. There is evidence of tenosynovitis of the left wrist. The right knee is swollen and warm, with significant effusion. The rash on his arm is shown (see top of right-hand column).

Blood cultures are obtained, and an arthrocentesis of the right knee is performed. The synovial fluid leukocyte count is 60,000/µL (60 × 10⁹/L) with 90% polymorphonuclear neutrophils. The Gram stain is negative.

Which of the following is the most appropriate diagnostic test to perform next?

(A) Antinuclear antibody and rheumatoid factor assays
(B) Biopsy and culture of a skin lesion

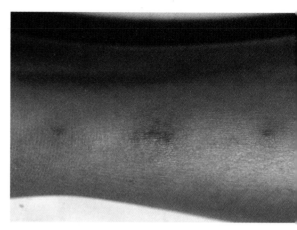

ITEM 29

(C) HLA B27 testing
(D) Nucleic acid amplification urine test for *Neisseria gonorrhoeae*

Item 30

A 35-year-old man is evaluated for a 2-week history of no productive cough and fever. He has a 20-year history asthma. Three weeks ago, he visited friends in Indiana. I has no dyspnea, hemoptysis, or worsening of his baseli asthma symptoms. His only medication is an albute inhaler as needed.

On physical examination, temperature is 38.0 (100.4 °F), blood pressure is 130/70 mm Hg, pulse rate 88/min, and respiration rate is 16/min. Crackles are hea in both lungs.

Laboratory studies show a normal leukocyte count a serum creatinine level.

Chest radiograph reveals patchy pulmonary infiltra with mild hilar lymphadenopathy.

Which of the following is the most appropriate ma agement?

(A) Lipid amphotericin B
(B) Fluconazole
(C) Itraconazole
(D) No treatment

Item 31

A 46-year-old man is admitted to the hospital with a ru tured gallbladder requiring emergent open cholecystecton

An indwelling urinary catheter is inserted prior to surge and a drain is left in his upper right abdominal quadrant.

The patient is stabilized and transferred to the surgi intensive care unit.

In addition to removing the urinary catheter at tl first possible moment, which of the following w decrease this patient's risk of catheter-associated u nary tract infection?

(A) Daily cleansing of the meatal area of the catheter with antiseptics

) Maintenance of urine-collecting bag below the level of the bladder

C) Routine catheter change every 5 days

D) Treatment of asymptomatic bacteriuria

E) Use of antiseptic-coated urinary catheters

em 32

46-year-old man with quadriplegia is evaluated for fever d increased muscle spasticity. He self-catheterizes inter-ittently four times daily because of chronic bladder dys-nction, although an indwelling urinary catheter was placed weeks ago because of difficulty with self-catheterization.

On physical examination, the temperature is 38.9 °C 02.0 °F). The remainder of the examination is consistent th the diagnosis of quadriplegia. An indwelling bladder theter is in place.

A urinalysis and culture are obtained.

hich of the following is required to establish the agnosis of catheter-associated urinary tract infection this patient?

A) Grossly cloudy urine

B) Positive urine dipstick for leukocyte esterase

C) Positive urine Gram stain

D) Urine culture with more than 10^3 colony-forming units/mL

em 33

29-year-old man is evaluated for newly diagnosed HIV fection. He has no symptoms and is willing to start com-ination antiretroviral therapy if necessary. He has no other edical problems and takes no medications.

Physical examination is normal.

The complete blood count, serum chemistries, and er enzymes are normal. CD4 cell count is 424/µL. HIV NA viral load is 21,317 copies/mL. HIV resistance test-g is negative for mutations. A hepatitis B virus surface tibody assay, serologic testing for syphilis, and a hepatitis virus antibody assay are negative.

addition to periodic follow-up monitoring, which the following is the most appropriate management this patient's HIV infection?

A) Begin combination antiretroviral therapy now

B) Withhold treatment until CD4 cell count falls below 350/µL

C) Withhold treatment until HIV RNA viral load exceeds 55,000 copies/mL

D) Withhold treatment until symptoms develop

em 34

26-year-old man is evaluated for a 3-day history of fever, yalgia, dry cough, and malaise. He has no known drug ergies, and the remainder of the medical history is non-ntributory.

On physical examination, temperature is 38.3 °C (100.9 °F), blood pressure is 125/75 mm Hg, pulse rate is 95/min, and respiration rate is 16/min. Oxygen saturation is 100% with the patient breathing ambient air. Crackles are heard in the left lung base.

Chest radiograph shows left lower lobe airspace disease.

Which of the following oral agents is the most appropriate treatment?

(A) Amoxicillin

(B) Azithromycin

(C) Cefuroxime

(D) Ciprofloxacin

Item 35

A 25-year-old woman is evaluated for a 1-week history of cough and fever, painful nodules on the extensor surfaces of the arms and the legs, and arthralgia of the knees and ankles. Her symptoms developed 3 weeks after she vacationed in the Arizona desert.

On physical examination, temperature is 39.0 °C (102.2 °F), blood pressure is 100/60 mm Hg, pulse rate is 110/min, and respiration rate is 18/min. Crackles and egophony are heard in the posterior left lower lung field. There is no evidence of joint effusions. Findings of the skin examination of the lower extremities are shown.

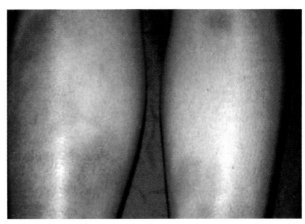

Laboratory studies indicate an erythrocyte sedimentation rate of 70 mm/h and a normal complete blood count.

A chest radiograph reveals a dense infiltrate of the left lower lobe and left hilar lymphadenopathy. Gram stains of sputum are negative.

Which of the following is the most likely diagnosis?

(A) Blastomycosis

(B) Coccidioidomycosis

(C) Histoplasmosis

(D) Sporotrichosis

Item 36

A 22-year-old woman is evaluated for a 1-day history of dysuria and urinary urgency and frequency. She had an episode of cystitis 2 years ago. The patient has a sulfa allergy.

On physical examination, temperature is normal, blood pressure is 110/60 mm Hg, pulse rate is 60/min, and respiration rate is 14/min. There is mild suprapubic tenderness, but no flank tenderness. The remainder of the examination is normal.

Urine dipstick analysis shows 3+ leukocyte esterase. A pregnancy test is negative.

Treatment with which of the following antibiotics is most appropriate?

(A) Amoxicillin
(B) Fosfomycin
(C) Levofloxacin
(D) Nitrofurantoin

Item 37

A 30-year-old man is admitted to the hospital with a 1-month history of fever, night sweats, cough, weight loss, and chest pain. The patient is homeless. A diagnosis of pericardial tamponade is established.

Pericardiocentesis is performed, following which there is no recurrence of a significant pericardial effusion. Microbiologic examination of pericardial fluid identifies *Mycobacterium tuberculosis*.

In addition to four-drug antituberculous therapy, which of the following is the most appropriate next treatment?

(A) Indomethacin and colchicine
(B) Pericardial window
(C) Prednisone
(D) Surgical pericardiectomy

Item 38

A 21-year-old man undergoes evaluation in the intensive care unit (ICU) before surgical intervention scheduled for tomorrow. He was admitted to the surgical ICU 17 days ago for multiple gunshot wounds. He is mechanically ventilated and had a central line catheter placed in the right femoral vein. *Acinetobacter baumannii* has been isolated from blood cultures drawn from the central line catheter, sputum, and one of the abdominal drains. The patient shares the room with one additional patient, who is also mechanically ventilated.

Which of the following is most likely to reduce spread of this patient's *Acinetobacter* infection to his roommate?

(A) Clean the patients' room with bleach
(B) Ensure strict staff adherence to hand hygiene practices
(C) Give prophylactic antimicrobial agents active against *Acinetobacter* species to the roommate
(D) Replace source patient's central line catheter, endotracheal tube, and abdominal drain with new devices

Item 39

A 59-year-old woman is evaluated for a 1-week history of increasing pain of the right foot. She recalls stepping on a nail about 1 month before her symptoms began. The patient has a 5-year history of heart failure secondary idiopathic dilated cardiomyopathy. She has an implantable cardioverter-defibrillator, and her current medications a carvedilol, lisinopril, furosemide, and spironolactone.

On physical examination, vital signs are normal. Examination of the foot reveals tenderness and warmth direct below the proximal fifth metatarsal bone.

A radiograph of the right foot is normal.

Which of the following is the most appropriate ne step to establish the diagnosis?

(A) CT scan
(B) Gallium scan
(C) MRI
(D) Three-phase bone scan

Item 40

A 54-year-old man is evaluated in the emergency depar ment for a 2-week history of fever and chills occurring eve 1 to 2 days. He also has a significant headache, muscle pai and intermittent diarrhea. The patient is an archeology pr fessor who returned 2 weeks ago from a 6-week "dig" Thailand in Southeast Asia. He received pre-travel proph lactic vaccinations, including combined hepatitis A and virus vaccines, as well as yellow fever, typhoid, and Japane encephalitis vaccines. In addition, he completed a regime of mefloquine for malaria chemoprophylaxis.

On physical examination, he appears ill but is awa and alert. Temperature is 39.4 °C (102.9 °F), blood pre sure is 100/62 mm Hg, pulse rate is 118/min, and resp ration rate is 20/min. Cardiopulmonary examination unremarkable. There is mild splenomegaly.

A complete blood count indicates a leukocyte count 8900/µL (8.9×10^9/L), a platelet count of 82,000/µL (8 $\times 10^9$/L), and a hemoglobin level of 10 g/dL (100 g/L He also has a mildly increased serum indirect bilirubin lev and elevated serum alanine and aspartate aminotransfera levels. A peripheral blood smear is shown.

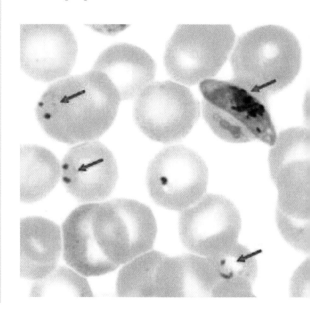

against which of the following malaria species should treatment be initiated in this patient?

) *Plasmodium falciparum*
) *Plasmodium malariae*
) *Plasmodium ovale*
) *Plasmodium vivax*

Item 41

25-year-old woman undergoes evaluation. Treatment active pulmonary tuberculosis was initiated 6 weeks o. The mycobacteria were susceptible to all first-line tituberculous agents, and a 2-month course of isoni- id, rifampin, ethambutol, and pyrazinamide was pre- ibed as initial therapy. However, the patient was lost to low-up for 3 weeks, during which time she discontin- d all medications.

On physical examination, temperature is 37.7 °C 9.9 °F), blood pressure is 110/70 mm Hg, pulse rate is /min, and respiration rate is 18/min. The remainder of r physical examination is normal.

hich of the following is the most appropriate man- ement?

) Continue the same treatment to complete the planned total number of doses, provided all doses are completed within 3 months
) Repeat sputum smear for acid-fast bacilli; if results are negative, treatment can be considered complete
) Restart different treatment with at least two new drugs to which the mycobacteria were originally sus- ceptible
) Restart the same treatment from the beginning

Item 42

70-year-old man is evaluated for a 6-month history of perkeratotic skin lesions. The patient lives in Michigan. e is otherwise healthy.

On physical examination, temperature is normal, blood essure is 150/78 mm Hg, pulse rate is 80/min, and res- ration rate is 14/min. The lungs are clear.

A representative skin lesion on the face is shown.

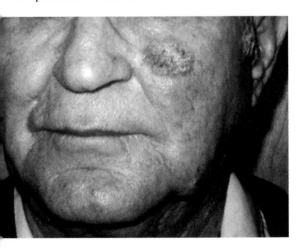

Skin biopsy shows a pyogranulomatous reaction and broad-based budding yeast. Chest radiograph is normal.

Which of the following is the most appropriate treat- ment of this patient?

(A) Amphotericin B
(B) Fluconazole
(C) Itraconazole
(D) Surgical excision

Item 43

A 42-year-old woman is evaluated for a 4-day history of mild fever, headache, myalgia, nonproductive cough, and sore throat. There is a confirmed influenza A (H1N1) outbreak in the local community. She has no other med- ical illnesses.

On physical examination, temperature is 38.2 °C (100.8 °F), blood pressure is 130/70 mm Hg, pulse rate is 88/min, and respiration rate is 14/min. She does not appear ill. There is diffuse muscle tenderness to palpation. The lungs are clear. The abdomen is soft and nontender.

Laboratory studies show a leukocyte count of 5600/µL (5.6×10^9/L) and a serum creatinine level of 1.0 mg/dL (88.4 µmol/L).

Which of the following is the most appropriate treat- ment?

(A) Amantadine
(B) Oseltamivir
(C) Rimantadine
(D) Zanamivir
(E) No treatment

Item 44

A 53-year-old man is evaluated for a 2-day history of swelling and pain of the right knee. Active tuberculosis was recently diagnosed, and the patient has been treated with isoniazid, rifampin, and pyrazinamide for the past 7 weeks. Ethambutol, which was also started 7 weeks ago, had to be discontinued 1 week ago after the patient experienced decreased visual acuity ascribed to optic neuritis. Mycobac- teria are fully susceptible to all first-line antituberculous agents. His medical history also includes hypertension for which he takes amlodipine.

On physical examination, vital signs are normal. The right knee is warm, erythematous, and swollen, and he has difficulty bearing weight on this leg because of intense pain. Range of motion of the knee is restricted and elicits pain.

A serum uric acid level obtained today is 10.5 mg/dL (0.62 mmol/L). A complete blood count reveals a leuko- cyte count of 14,700/µL (14.7×10^9/L) with 87% poly- morphonuclear cells and 13% lymphocytes. An arthrocen- tesis of the right knee is performed and reveals a synovial fluid leukocyte count of 30,000/µL (30×10^9/L) (90% polymorphonuclear cells, 10% lymphocytes). Gram stain is negative, but polarized light microscopy reveals intra- and extracellular monosodium urate crystals.

Which of the following is most likely responsible for this patient's clinical findings?

(A) Amlodipine
(B) Isoniazid
(C) Pyrazinamide
(D) Rifampin

Item 45

A 52-year-old man is admitted to the intensive care unit with fever and hypotension. He sustained a burn injury 1 year ago with involvement of approximately 20% of his skin surface area. Since his injury, he has been hospitalized frequently for skin grafting procedures, most recently 1 week ago involving the anterior left thigh. At the site of his latest skin graft, he has developed purulent drainage over the past 24 hours. The patient takes no medications, including antibiotics.

On physical examination, temperature is 38.8 °C (101.8 °F), blood pressure is 95/50 mm Hg, and the pulse rate is 115/min. Cardiopulmonary examination is unremarkable. He has multiple well-healed skin graft sites except for his recent graft site on the anterior left thigh, which shows an area of devitalized skin with eschar formation and peripheral erythema and drainage of a moderate amount of pus.

Empiric vancomycin is initiated.

Two sets of blood cultures obtained at the onset of fever on admission are positive for *Pseudomonas aeruginosa*. Empiric vancomycin and cefepime are initiated. Antibiotic sensitivity studies show that the organism is pan-resistant to all antimicrobial agents to which it was tested, including all β-lactam antimicrobial agents, carbapenems, fluoroquinolones, and aminoglycosides.

Which of the following is the most appropriate antibiotic treatment for this patient?

(A) Intravenous colistin
(B) Intravenous minocycline
(C) Intravenous rifampin
(D) Intravenous tigecycline

Item 46

A 47-year-old man is admitted to the hospital with community-acquired pneumonia. He has hypertension and a 25-pack-year smoking history. His only current medication is chlorthalidone.

On physical examination, the patient is in mild respiratory distress. Temperature is 40.1 °C (104.2 °F), blood pressure is 145/85 mm Hg, pulse rate is 130/min, and respiration rate is 16/min. Oxygen saturation is 89% with the patient breathing ambient air. Pulmonary examination demonstrates dullness to percussion with bronchial breath sounds localized to the right lung base.

A chest radiograph shows right lower lobe consolidation without significant pleural effusion. Intravenous ceftriaxone and azithromycin are initiated. On the second hospital day, blood cultures obtained on admission are positive

for gram-positive cocci in pairs and chains. The ceftriaxo is continued and the azithromycin is stopped.

On the morning of hospital day 3, the patient is fe ing better, has been afebrile for the past 12 hours, and is e ing and drinking well. The blood culture isolate is identifi as *Streptococcus pneumoniae* susceptible to penicillin. Te perature is 37.0 °C (98.6 °F), blood pressure is 140/ mm Hg, pulse rate is 88/min, and respiration rate 16/min. Oxygen saturation is 97% with the patient brea ing ambient air.

Which of the following is the most appropriate ma agement?

(A) Discharge on oral levofloxacin to complete 7 days therapy
(B) Discharge on oral amoxicillin to complete 14 days therapy
(C) Discharge on oral amoxicillin to complete 7 days of therapy
(D) Switch to oral amoxicillin and discharge tomorrow, stable

Item 47

A 56-year-old man is evaluated in the emergency depa ment for a 3-day history of fever, myalgia, dyspnea, a mid-anterior chest discomfort. He works at a local airp as an airplane mechanic where small aircraft are used crop-dusting nearby fields. The remainder of the medi history is unremarkable.

On physical examination, temperature is 38.7 (101.7 °F), blood pressure is 94/60 mm Hg, pulse rate 115/min, and respiration rate is 24/min. The patie appears confused. The skin is cool and mottled. No rash present. Pulmonary examination discloses diminish breath sounds bilaterally at the lung bases. Other than tant heart sounds and tachycardia, the cardiac examinati is normal. There are no focal neurologic findings.

A chest radiograph is shown.

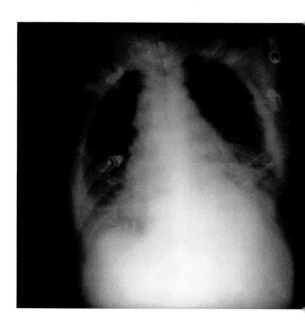

Which of the following is the most likely infectious agent?

(A) *Bacillus anthracis*
(B) *Erysipelothrix rhusiopathiae*
(C) *Listeria monocytogenes*
(D) *Nocardia* species

Item 48

A 55-year-old man undergoes follow-up evaluation for treatment of *Blastocystis* infection. Ten days ago, the patient went to a walk-in clinic because of diarrhea. Probable viral gastroenteritis was diagnosed, and loperamide was prescribed. Stool studies were performed at that time. Cultures for bacteria were negative, but a microscopic examination for ova and parasites showed *Blastocystis* species. He was contacted by the clinic and told to seek further medical attention because of his stool studies.

Diarrhea resolved within 24 hours of starting loperamide, and the patient is currently asymptomatic. He takes no medications.

On physical examination today, vital signs are normal. There is no abdominal tenderness.

Which of the following is the most appropriate intervention at this time?

(A) Begin ciprofloxacin
(B) Begin metronidazole
(C) Repeat stool examination for ova and parasites
(D) No additional evaluation or treatment is indicated

Item 49

A 62-year-old man is admitted to the hospital with confusion. His wife reports that he is a truck driver, but he has been unable to work for the past 3 weeks because he can no longer follow map directions. Yesterday, she found him putting his clothes in the dishwasher rather than the washing machine. The patient has insomnia and fatigue but no headache, photophobia, stiff neck, fever, or other localizing symptoms or signs. He has never traveled outside the United States.

On physical examination, vital signs are normal. He appears disheveled and is conversant but slow to respond to questions. Myoclonic movements of the upper extremities are noted at rest. Remaining physical examination findings are unremarkable.

Results of a complete blood count and metabolic panel are normal. Urine culture findings are negative. Lumbar puncture is performed. The cerebrospinal fluid (CSF) leukocyte count is 2/µL (2.0 × 10⁶/L). CSF protein and glucose levels are normal.

MRI of the brain shows atrophy appropriate for his age, but no focal lesions.

Which of the following is the most likely diagnosis?

(A) Cryptococcal meningitis
(B) Neurosyphilis
(C) Sporadic Creutzfeldt-Jakob disease
(D) Tuberculous meningitis

Item 50

A 48-year-old woman is admitted to the hospital with a 1-week history of nasal congestion, rhinorrhea, dry cough, fever, chills, and myalgia. She was beginning to feel better until 48 hours ago when she developed a recurrence of fever and chills, a cough productive of blood-streaked yellow sputum, and right-sided pleuritic chest pain. She has had no recent hospitalizations. Medical history is significant for type 2 diabetes mellitus. She has no history of tobacco, alcohol, or recreational drug use. Current medications are metformin and glipizide.

On physical examination, temperature is 39.0 °C (102.2 °F), blood pressure is 100/50 mm Hg, pulse rate is 110/min, and respiration rate is 24/min. Crackles are heard over the right lateral chest with egophony and increased fremitus.

Laboratory studies indicate a leukocyte count of 20,000/µL (20 × 10⁹/L), a blood urea nitrogen level of 28 mg/dL (10.0 mmol/L), and a serum creatinine level of 1.3 mg/dL (114.9 µmol/L). Chest radiograph shows right middle lobe airspace disease with a small area of cavitation and blunting of the right costophrenic angle.

Which of the following is the most appropriate empiric treatment of this patient?

(A) Aztreonam
(B) Ceftriaxone and azithromycin
(C) Ceftriaxone, azithromycin, and vancomycin
(D) Moxifloxacin

Item 51

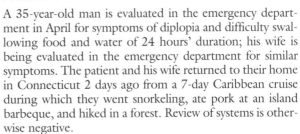

A 35-year-old man is evaluated in the emergency department in April for symptoms of diplopia and difficulty swallowing food and water of 24 hours' duration; his wife is being evaluated in the emergency department for similar symptoms. The patient and his wife returned to their home in Connecticut 2 days ago from a 7-day Caribbean cruise during which they went snorkeling, ate pork at an island barbeque, and hiked in a forest. Review of systems is otherwise negative.

On physical examination, vital signs are normal. The patient is alert and oriented. He has dysphonia and dysarthria, obvious bilateral ocular palsies, an absent gag reflex, and symmetric upper extremity motor weakness without any objective sensory abnormalities. The remainder of the examination is unremarkable.

Which of the following is the most likely diagnosis?

(A) Botulism
(B) Guillain-Barré syndrome
(C) Paralytic shellfish poisoning
(D) Tick paralysis

Item 52

A 33-year-old woman is evaluated for a 5-week history of whitish spots in the mouth and the back of the throat and discomfort with swallowing solid foods. This is her first episode of these symptoms. She has had no mouth pain, trouble ingesting liquids or pills, nausea, vomiting, diarrhea, fever, chills, sweats, or skin problems. She has a 3-year history of HIV infection and also has moderately severe asthma, which is now well controlled with inhaled medications that were recently prescribed. Her medications are tenofovir, emtricitabine, raltegravir, and inhaled fluticasone and salmeterol.

On physical examination, her vital signs are normal. Whitish plaques are seen on the palate and posterior pharynx. The remainder of the physical examination is normal.

Her last CD4 cell count was 458/μL. The HIV RNA viral load is undetectable.

Which of the following is the most appropriate management of this patient?

(A) Clotrimazole troches
(B) Fluticasone cessation
(C) Intravenous amphotericin B
(D) Nystatin swish-and-swallow
(E) Oral fluconazole

Item 53

A 74-year-old man is evaluated in the emergency department for a 3-day history of fever and chills as well as confusion. He has a 5-week history of a nonhealing ulcer on the plantar surface of his left foot. He has diabetes mellitus, hypertension, and peripheral vascular disease for which he takes metformin, glyburide, lisinopril, chlorthalidone, and aspirin. He has no known medication allergies.

On physical examination, temperature is 39.0 °C (102.2 °F), blood pressure is 92/60 mm Hg, pulse rate is 108/min, and respiration rate is 18/min. He appears ill and is slow to respond. Examination of the left foot discloses a 3.5 × 2.5-cm ulcer with surrounding erythema and warmth. A foul odor and edema and tenderness involving the entire foot are noted. Pedal pulses are absent. The underlying bone is detected with a metal probe.

Laboratory studies indicate a leukocyte count of 21,500/μL (21.5 × 10⁹/L) with 18% band forms. Serum electrolyte levels and kidney function tests are normal.

A radiograph of the left foot reveals soft tissue swelling with erosion of the cortex at the head of the metatarsal bone beneath the site of the ulceration.

Which of the following is the most appropriate empiric antimicrobial regimen?

(A) Aztreonam and metronidazole
(B) Cefazolin and metronidazole
(C) Clindamycin and gentamicin
(D) Vancomycin and meropenem

Item 54

A 25-year-old woman who is 12 weeks pregnant is found to be HIV positive during a routine pregnancy evaluation. She is asymptomatic. Her medical history is unremarkable, and her only medication is a prenatal vitamin.

On physical examination, vital signs are normal. No lymphadenopathy, thrush, or skin lesions are noted. The remainder of the examination is normal.

Hemoglobin is 11 g/dL (110 g/L). HIV antibody testing is positive by enzyme immunoassay and confirmed by Western blot analysis. CD4 cell count is 865/μL, and HIV RNA viral load is 510 copies/mL. Rapid plasma reagin and hepatitis B serologies are negative. HIV genotyping shows no resistance mutations. The remaining laboratory studies are unremarkable.

Which of the following is the most appropriate management?

(A) Begin antiretroviral therapy at the onset of labor
(B) Begin tenofovir, emtricitabine, and efavirenz now
(C) Begin zidovudine, lamivudine, and lopinavir-ritonavir now
(D) Repeat CD4 cell count and treat if 500/μL or lower

Item 55

A 19-year-old man is evaluated for a sore throat, daily fever, frontal headache, myalgia, and arthralgia of 5 days' duration. He also has severe discomfort in the lower spine and a rash on his trunk and extremities. He returned from a 2-day trip to the Caribbean 8 days ago. The remainder of the history is noncontributory.

On physical examination, temperature is 38.3 °C (100.9 °F), blood pressure is 104/72 mm Hg, pulse rate is 102/min, and respiration rate is 16/min. His posterior pharynx is notably injected but without exudate. He has a maculopapular rash on his chest, arms, and legs that spares the palms and soles. There is no palpable lymphadenopathy. The remainder of the examination, including cardiopulmonary and abdominal examinations, is normal.

Laboratory studies:

Leukocyte count	3100/μL (3.1 x 10⁹/L)
Platelet count	85,500/μL (85.5 x 10⁹/L)
Hemoglobin	13.9 g/dL (139 g/L)
Alanine aminotransferase	114 units/L
Aspartate aminotransferase	154 units/L
Total bilirubin	1.2 mg/dL (20.5 μmol/L)

Which of the following is the most likely diagnosis?

(A) Dengue fever
(B) Leptospirosis
(C) Malaria
(D) Syphilis
(E) Yellow fever

Item 56

A 24-year-old man is evaluated for an increasingly painful boil on his back that has been present for 3 days and has increased in size. The patient has had similar lesions on his back and chest previously, but these were smaller and spontaneously drained and resolved without requiring medical attention. The remainder of the medical history is noncontributory.

On physical examination, vital signs are normal, and ͻe patient is not ill appearing. Examination of the back dis- ͻses a 7-cm fluctuant, tender, oval-shaped lesion, with sur- ͻunding erythema extending 3 cm from the edge of the ͻsion. The remainder of the physical examination is normal.

An aspirate of the lesion reveals purulent material, a ͻram stain of which demonstrates many leukocytes and ͻany gram-positive cocci in clusters. A culture is sent for ͻrocessing. Incision and drainage of the lesion produces ͻpproximately 5 mL of pus.

**ʼhich of the following is the most appropriate antibi-
ͻic treatment for this patient?**

ͺ) Amoxicillin-clavulanate

ͻ) Azithromycin

ͻ) Moxifloxacin

ͻ) Rifampin

ͻ) Trimethoprim-sulfamethoxazole

ʼem 57

23-year-old man undergoes preliminary evaluation. He ͻs just been admitted to a detoxification center because of ͻjection drug use.

On physical examination, temperature is 36.8 °C ʼ8.2 °F), blood pressure is 125/75 mm Hg, pulse rate is ͻ)/min, and respiration rate is 18/min. Findings of physi- ͻl examination demonstrate evidence of injection drug use ͻ the bilateral upper extremities but are otherwise normal.

Tuberculin skin testing induces 6 mm of induration. ʼhe patient has not had previous tuberculin skin tests. ͻesults of a serologic test for HIV infection are negative.

**ʼhich of the following is the most appropriate next
ͻep in the management of this patient?**

ͺ) Chest radiograph

ͻ) Isoniazid

ͻ) Isoniazid, rifampin, pyrazinamide, and ethambutol

ͻ) No additional therapy or evaluation

ͼem 58

44-year-old woman is evaluated for a 1-week history of ͻw-grade fever, fatigue, and body aches. She had a kidney ͻansplant 5 months ago; at the time of transplantation, she ͻas seropositive for Epstein-Barr virus and seronegative for ͻtomegalovirus with a seropositive donor. Her recent ͻurse has been uncomplicated with no episodes of rejec- ͻon. She completed cytomegalovirus prophylaxis with val- ͻnciclovir last month. Medications are tacrolimus, ͻycophenolate mofetil, prednisone, and trimethoprim-sul- ͻmethoxazole.

On physical examination, temperature is 37.8 °C ʼ00.0 °F), blood pressure is 136/88 mm Hg, pulse rate is ʼ6/min, and respiration rate is 16/min. There is no lym- ͻhadenopathy. The transplant surgical wound site is with- ͻut erythema or drainage. Cardiopulmonary examination is ͻrmal. The abdomen is soft and nontender.

Laboratory studies:

Hematocrit	33%
Leukocyte count	3200/μL (3.2 × 10⁹/L)
Platelet count	112,000/μL (112 × 10⁹/L)
Alkaline phosphatase	155 units/L
Alanine aminotransferase	52 units/L
Aspartate aminotransferase	48 units/L
Bilirubin	0.6 mg/dL (10.3 μmol/L)
Blood urea nitrogen	18 mg/dL (6.4 mmol/L)
Creatinine	1.1 mg/dL (97.2 μmol/L)

Microscopic urinalysis is unremarkable. The chest radiograph is normal.

**Infection with which of the following is the most likely
diagnosis?**

(A) Cytomegalovirus

(B) Epstein-Barr virus

(C) *Listeria monocytogenes*

(D) Polyoma BK virus

Item 59

A 70-year-old man is evaluated in the emergency depart- ment for a 1-day history of fever and altered mental status. Medical history is significant for coronary artery disease and hypertension treated with hydrochlorothiazide, aspirin, lisinopril, and atenolol.

On physical examination, temperature is 38.3 °C (101.0 °F), blood pressure is 98/58 mm Hg, pulse rate is 100/min, and respiration rate is 20/min. The patient is confused and oriented only to person. He is unable to answer any questions. His neck is supple, and neurologic examination findings are nonfocal. He has no rash.

A CT scan of the head without contrast reveals evi- dence of mild cerebral edema.

Lumbar puncture is performed. Opening pressure is 300 mm H₂O. Cerebrospinal fluid (CSF) analysis demon- strates a leukocyte count of 1200/μL (1200 × 10⁶/L) with 60% neutrophils and 40% lymphocytes, a glucose level of 30 mg/dL (1.7 mmol/L), and a protein level of 350 mg/dL (3500 mg/L). A Gram-stained CSF specimen is negative.

Dexamethasone followed by vancomycin, ampicillin, and ceftriaxone are begun in the emergency department, and the patient is admitted to the hospital. The next day, his clinical condition is unchanged.

**Which of the following is the most appropriate man-
agement at this time?**

(A) Add rifampin

(B) Continue current management

(C) Place an external ventricular drain

(D) Repeat the CSF analysis

Item 60

A 68-year-old woman is admitted to the intensive care unit with severe community-acquired pneumonia complicated by hypercapnic respiratory failure. Medical history is signif- icant for COPD, with several exacerbations occurring in the past 6 months that were successfully managed with prednisone in the outpatient setting. She also has a 60-pack-year smoking history. Medications are prednisone, albuterol, fluticasone-salmeterol, and tiotropium.

The patient is intubated and placed on mechanical ventilation. On physical examination, temperature is 37.8 °C (100.0 °F), blood pressure is 160/100 mm Hg, pulse rate is 115/min, and respiration rate is 22/min. There are diminished breath sounds throughout the lung fields, with scattered rhonchi, wheezing, and marked prolongation of the expiratory phase.

A chest radiograph shows hyperinflation, with flattening of the diaphragms and right lower lobe consolidation with air bronchograms.

Results of a Gram stain and culture of the endotracheal aspirate show numerous polymorphonuclear cells, few epithelial cells, and moderate gram-negative rods.

Which of the following is the most appropriate initial treatment?

(A) Aztreonam and azithromycin

(B) Cefepime, tobramycin, and azithromycin

(C) Cefotaxime and azithromycin

(D) Cefotaxime, azithromycin, and levofloxacin

Item 61

A 57-year-old woman is admitted to the hospital with a 2-day history of fever and confusion. Medical history is significant for hypertension treated with metoprolol.

On physical examination, temperature is 39.0 °C (102.2 °F); other vital signs are normal. The patient is alert but lethargic and answers questions with one-word responses. She is oriented to person only. Passive flexion of the neck elicits mild nuchal rigidity. Remaining physical examination findings are unremarkable.

Lumbar puncture is performed. Opening pressure is 21 mm H_2O. The cerebrospinal fluid (CSF) leukocyte count is 147/microliter (147×10^6/L) with 77% lymphocytes. CSF glucose and protein levels are normal. An MRI of the brain is normal.

Treatment with empiric acyclovir, 10 mg/kg intravenously every 8 hours, is initiated. By hospital day 3, the patient's fever has resolved and her mental status has normalized. Results of a CSF herpes simplex virus (HSV) polymerase chain reaction (PCR) performed at admission are negative.

Which of the following is the most appropriate management of this patient's acyclovir therapy?

(A) Change intravenous acyclovir to oral acyclovir to complete a 14-day course

(B) Continue intravenous acyclovir pending results of repeat HSV PCR

(C) Continue intravenous acyclovir to complete a 14-day course

(D) Discontinue intravenous acyclovir

Item 62

A 35-year-old man is evaluated in the emergency department for redness and pus that developed near a scratch on his left forearm.

On physical examination, temperature is 37.4 °C (99.4 °F), blood pressure is 140/80 mm Hg, pulse rate is 80/min, and respiration rate is 14/min. A 3 × 2-cm erythematous, warm patch is present over the left forearm with some associated purulent exudate but no fluctuance, drainable abscess, or lymphadenopathy.

Laboratory studies indicate a leukocyte count of 10,000/μL (10×10^9/L) with 70% neutrophils and 30% lymphocytes.

Which of the following is the most appropriate outpatient therapy?

(A) Amoxicillin

(B) Cephalexin

(C) Dicloxacillin

(D) Trimethoprim-sulfamethoxazole

Item 63

A 25-year-old man is evaluated for a 2-week history of purulent drainage from a small opening in a previously healed right lower extremity wound; this was preceded by about 10 days of tenderness and redness at the wound site. Six months ago, the patient had a motorcycle accident in which he sustained an open comminuted fracture of the proximal tibia. Management consisted of surgical debridement and lavage followed by open reduction and internal fixation with a metal plate and screws as well as empiric antibiotic therapy. Culture results during and after surgery were negative.

On physical examination, the patient appears well. Temperature is 37.2 °C (98.9 °F), blood pressure is 120/75 mm Hg, and respiration rate is 12/min. There is a well-healed surgical incision overlying the right tibia except for a 2-mm opening at the distal margin with minimal surrounding erythema and slight purulent drainage. The remainder of the examination is normal.

Swab samples obtained from the wound are sent to the microbiology laboratory for aerobic and anaerobic culture and sensitivity testing. *Proteus mirabilis* and an enterococcal species are isolated from the culture, both susceptible to all antibiotics tested.

Which of the following is the most appropriate next step in management?

(A) Bone biopsy cultures

(B) Intravenous ampicillin-sulbactam

(C) Oral ciprofloxacin and amoxicillin

(D) Technetium 99m–labeled bone scan

Item 64

A 28-year-old man is admitted to the hospital for 3 weeks of increasing dyspnea on exertion, dry cough, pleuritic chest pain, and fever. The patient has been in a monogamous ationship with a male partner for the past 3 years but had ultiple partners of both sexes previously.

On physical examination, temperature is 38.6 °C 01.5 °F), blood pressure is 110/66 mm Hg, pulse rate is 2/min, and respiration rate is 24/min. The oropharynx monstrates scattered white plaques. Lung auscultation closes diffuse crackles bilaterally. The remainder of the amination is normal.

Arterial blood gas levels with the patient breathing mbient air show a pH of 7.48, Pco$_2$ of 30 mm Hg (4.0 a), and Po$_2$ of 62 mm Hg (8.2 kPa). A rapid HIV test is sitive. Sputum Gram stain shows few neutrophils, eudohyphae, and mixed bacteria. A chest radiograph ows bilateral diffuse reticular infiltrates.

hich of the following is the most likely diagnosis?

) Cytomegalovirus pneumonia
) *Mycobacterium avium* complex infection
) *Pneumocystis jirovecii* pneumonia
) Pulmonary candidiasis

em 65

40-year-old man is admitted to the emergency depart-ent with a 1-day history of headache and epistaxis. He has d type 1 diabetes mellitus requiring insulin for 30 years d two episodes of ketoacidosis in the past year.

On physical examination, temperature is 36.0 °C 6.8 °F), blood pressure is 100/70 mm Hg, pulse rate is 0/min, and respiration rate is 22/min. There is mild optosis of the right eye with periorbital edema and a black char on the inferior turbinate of the right nostril. Skin amination shows no other lesions. The remainder of the amination is normal.

Laboratory studies are consistent with diabetic ketoaci->sis. Blood cultures are negative. A chest radiograph is rmal.

CT of the head reveals mild proptosis of the right eye d right ethmoid and maxillary sinusitis with bony erosion. travenous amphotericin B is instituted.

addition to treatment of this patient's diabetic toacidosis and institution of antifungal therapy, hich of the following is the most important next step treatment?

) Add piperacillin-tazobactam
) Add posaconazole
) Administer hyperbaric oxygen treatment
) Perform surgical debridement

em 66

35-year-old man is evaluated in the emergency depart-ent following the acute onset of bilateral lower extremity ralysis. The patient has a history of injection drug use. He is well until 5 days ago, when he developed severe pain in e middle of his back that was not relieved by topical heat ibuprofen. Today, he was unable to walk and was ought to the hospital by ambulance.

On physical examination, temperature is 37.8 °C (100.0 °F), blood pressure is 120/74 mm Hg, pulse rate is 98/min, and respiration rate is 14/min. Neurologic examination findings show 0/5 motor strength in both lower extremities and absent sensation below the level of the umbilicus.

Emergent MRI of the spine reveals evidence of osteomyelitis involving the lower half of the T10 vertebral body and the upper half of the T11 vertebral body, diskitis at the T10-T11 disk space, and an epidural mass compress-ing the spinal cord.

Blood cultures are obtained.

Which of the following is the most appropriate next step in management?

(A) Antimicrobial therapy
(B) CT-guided bone biopsy
(C) Emergent radiation therapy
(D) Emergent surgical decompression

Item 67

A 64-year-old woman is hospitalized for a 24-hour history of diffuse erythroderma, nausea, vomiting, and a rapidly progressive left lower leg soft tissue infection associated with fever, tachycardia, and hypotension.

An emergent MRI of the left lower leg is compatible with superficial fascial necrosis. Empiric broad-spectrum antibiotics are initiated, and emergent surgical débridement and fasciotomy are performed.

Gram stain reveals gram-positive cocci in short chains ultimately identified as *Streptococcus pyogenes*.

Which of the following precautions is most appropri-ate for this patient to prevent spread of this organism?

(A) Airborne precautions
(B) Contact precautions
(C) Droplet precautions
(D) Standard precautions only

Item 68

A 35-year-old man is evaluated during a routine follow-up visit. He was diagnosed with HIV infection 2 years ago. He started combination antiretroviral therapy with tenofovir, emtricitabine, and efavirenz and within 4 months had an undetectable HIV RNA viral load and a normal CD4 cell count. The patient has been adherent to his medication reg-imen. He is presently asymptomatic, feeling well, and hav-ing no problems with his medications.

The physical examination is normal.

Laboratory studies show an HIV RNA viral load of 275 copies/mL, with repeated results indicating 710 copies/mL. The CD4 cell count is normal. The remaining laboratory tests, including complete blood count, serum chemistries, and liver enzymes, are normal.

Which of the following is the most appropriate next step in the management of this patient?

(A) Continue present medication regimen and follow up in 4 weeks

(B) Discontinue present medication regimen and perform resistance testing in 1 week

(C) Discontinue present medication regimen and repeat CD4 cell count and HIV RNA viral load in 4 weeks

(D) Perform viral resistance testing and continue present medication regimen pending results

Item 69

A 20-year-old man is evaluated for a scratch on his right arm from a pet kitten that occurred 3 weeks ago. The patient now has a skin lesion at the inoculation site and painful swelling in the ipsilateral axillary area. He is also experiencing malaise. Medical history is unremarkable.

On physical examination, temperature is 37.2 °C (99.0 °F), blood pressure is 120/80 mm Hg, pulse rate is 80/min, and respiration rate is 14/min. A red papule is present on the biceps area of the right arm, and tender right axillary lymphadenopathy with overlying erythema is noted. The remainder of the examination is normal.

Laboratory studies indicate a leukocyte count of 11,500/μL (11.5×10^9/L) with 83% neutrophils and 17% lymphocytes and a normal metabolic panel.

Which of the following is the most appropriate treatment?

(A) Azithromycin

(B) Dicloxacillin

(C) Itraconazole

(D) Linezolid

Item 70

A 72-year-old man is evaluated for fatigue and weakness of 8 months' duration. The patient is a retired businessman who is an avid gardener and recalls many tick attachments over the past several years. He lives in Texas but has traveled extensively throughout the United States.

The patient was seen in a walk-in clinic 1 week ago and had laboratory testing for Lyme disease. An enzyme-linked immunosorbent assay for *Borrelia burgdorferi* was positive. A Western blot assay was negative for IgG antibodies and positive for IgM antibodies.

On physical examination today, vital signs are normal. Remaining physical examination findings are unremarkable.

An electrocardiogram is normal.

Which of the following is the most appropriate management?

(A) Initiate additional evaluation for fatigue and weakness

(B) Repeat serologic testing for *Borrelia burgdorferi* in 1 month

(C) Treat with ceftriaxone

(D) Treat with doxycycline

Item 71

A 32-year-old woman is evaluated for a 2-day history dysuria and urinary urgency and frequency and a 1-day h tory of fever. She has had no nausea or vomiting.

On physical examination, temperature is 38.5 (101.3 °F), blood pressure is 120/70 mm Hg, pulse rat 90/min, and respiration rate is 12/min. There is right fla tenderness on palpation.

A urinalysis shows more than 20 leukocytes/hpf a 4+ bacteria. A pregnancy test is negative.

In addition to obtaining a urine culture, which of t following is the most appropriate empiric treatmen

(A) Ampicillin

(B) Ciprofloxacin

(C) Nitrofurantoin

(D) Trimethoprim-sulfamethoxazole

Item 72

A 55-year-old man undergoes follow-up evaluation worsened cholesterol levels. He has a history of multidru resistant HIV infection, but he has been responding well his current antiretroviral regimen for the past 6 mont The patient follows a healthy diet and exercise regimen. currently smokes cigarettes and has no family history of p mature coronary artery disease. Medications are tenofo emtricitabine, raltegravir, and ritonavir-boosted darunav

Physical examination is unremarkable.

Laboratory studies:

Alanine aminotransferase	26 units/L
Aspartate aminotransferase	34 units/L
Cholesterol	
Total	264 mg/dL (6.8 mmol/
LDL	170 mg/dL (4.4 mmol/
HDL	46 mg/dL (1.2 mmol/L
Triglycerides	240 mg/dL (2.7 mmol/I

Which of the following is the most appropriate ma agement?

(A) Encourage strict dietary lipid restriction and reche lipid panel in 6 months

(B) Start atorvastatin

(C) Start fenofibrate

(D) Start simvastatin

Item 73

A 55-year-old man is evaluated for a 2-day history of fev headache, and confusion. Medical history is significant type 2 diabetes mellitus treated with metformin. T patient has no known drug allergies.

On physical examination, temperature is 39.2 (102.6 °F), blood pressure is 100/60 mm Hg, pulse rat 118/min, and respiration rate is 24/min. He is confus but responds to vigorous stimulation. There are no rash Neurologic examination findings are nonfocal.

Laboratory studies show a leukocyte count 22,000/μL (22×10^9/L) with 40% band forms.

A CT scan of the head without contrast is normal.

Lumbar puncture is performed. Cerebrospinal fluid (CSF) leukocyte count is 1500/μL (1500 × 10⁶/L) with [?]% neutrophils, glucose level is 26 mg/dL (1.4 mmol/L), [an]d protein level is 200 mg/dL (2000 mg/L). A CSF [g]ram stain is shown.

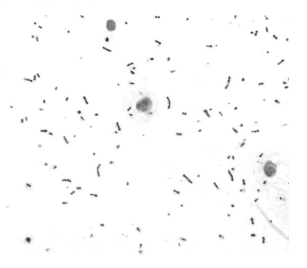

[In] addition to adjunctive dexamethasone, which of the [fo]llowing antimicrobial regimens should be initiated at [th]is time?

(A) Ampicillin and ceftriaxone
(B) Ceftriaxone
(C) Levofloxacin
(D) Vancomycin and ceftriaxone
(E) Vancomycin and gentamicin

[It]em 74

[A] 27-year-old man is hospitalized for fatigue, fever, and chills [th]at developed 48 hours ago after his return from a camping [tri]p in New Mexico. On the day of admission, he developed [sh]ortness of breath, pleuritic chest pain, and a productive [co]ugh with blood-streaked sputum. His medical history is [ot]herwise unremarkable, and he takes no medications.

On physical examination, he is in moderate respiratory [di]stress. Temperature is 38.6 °C (101.5 °F), blood pressure [is] 110/65 mm Hg, and pulse rate is 110/min. Oxygen sat[ur]ation with the patient breathing ambient air is 85%. Car[di]opulmonary examination discloses diffuse crackles bilat[er]ally and tachycardia. The remainder of the physical [ex]amination is normal.

Laboratory studies indicate a leukocyte count of [17],500/μL (17.5 × 10⁹/L) with 75% band forms and nor[m]al serum electrolyte levels and kidney and liver chemistry [re]sults. A chest radiograph shows diffuse infiltrates bilaterally.

Microscopic examination of the blood obtained on [ad]mission reveals gram-negative bipolar-staining bacilli.

[W]hich of the following is the most likely infectious [ag]ent?

(A) *Legionella pneumophila*
(B) *Pseudomonas aeruginosa*

(C) *Salmonella enteritidis*
(D) *Yersinia pestis*

Item 75

A 22-year-old woman is evaluated for an 8-day history of escalating fever, abdominal pain, headache, sore throat, dry cough, and initial constipation followed by frequent loose, watery stools. She returned 2 weeks ago from rural India where she spent the month of July. In preparation for travel, she took atovaquone-proguanil for malaria prophy-laxis and had ciprofloxacin in the event of a diarrheal ill-ness. Two weeks before her trip, she received a tetanus, diphtheria, and acellular pertussis vaccination and live oral vaccine for typhoid fever. She has received a complete hepatitis A and B virus vaccine series. She is otherwise healthy and takes no medications.

On physical examination, temperature is 39.5 °C (103.1 °F), blood pressure is 106/72 mm Hg, pulse rate is 64/min, and respiration rate is 16/min. She has a faint salmon-colored maculopapular rash on the trunk. Car-diopulmonary examination is normal. Splenomegaly but no palpable tenderness is noted on abdominal examination.

Laboratory studies:

Hemoglobin	10.5 g/dL (105 g/L)
Leukocyte count	3150/μL (3.15 × 10⁹/L) with 55% neutrophils, 42% lymphocytes, and 3% monocytes
Platelet count	106,000/μL (106 x 10⁹/L)
Alanine aminotransferase	167 units/L
Aspartate aminotransferase	98 units/L
Total bilirubin	2.4 mg/dL (41.0 μmol/L)
Sodium	130 meq/L (130 mmol/L)

Which of the following is the most likely diagnosis?

(A) Brucellosis
(B) Leishmaniasis
(C) Malaria
(D) Typhoid fever

Item 76

A 42-year-old man is evaluated in the emergency depart-ment for a 3-day history of dyspnea and dizziness. He is training for a marathon and initially attributed his symptoms to overexertion and dehydration. Despite refraining from training and increasing his fluid intake, his symptoms have persisted. He has no chest pain, fever, or cough. Medical history is unremarkable. The patient is a college professor in Rhode Island. He has not noted any tick attachments or antecedent rash.

On physical examination, he appears well. Temperature is normal, blood pressure is 100/60 mm Hg, and pulse rate is 35/min. Other than bradycardia, the remaining physical examination findings are unremarkable.

Results of initial laboratory studies show a normal com-plete blood count, metabolic panel, and cardiac enzyme

CONT.

measurements. The admission electrocardiographic rhythm strip is shown.

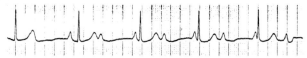

Serologic testing for *Borrelia burgdorferi* is performed. Both the initial enzyme-linked immunosorbent assay and a confirmatory Western blot assay are positive.

Which of the following is the most appropriate initial treatment?

(A) Intravenous ceftriaxone
(B) Oral cefuroxime
(C) Oral doxycycline
(D) Placement of a permanent pacemaker
(E) Observation

Item 77

A 25-year-old woman is evaluated for redness that developed over her right leg at the site of a mosquito bite. She is otherwise healthy and takes no medications.

On physical examination, temperature is 37.2 °C (99.0 °F), blood pressure is 120/70 mm Hg, pulse rate is 70/min, and respiration rate is 14/min. There is an erythematous 3 × 3-cm patch on the right thigh. The area is warm to the touch with no evidence of purulence, fluctuance, crepitus, or lymphadenopathy.

Which of the following is the most appropriate empiric outpatient therapy?

(A) Cephalexin
(B) Doxycycline
(C) Fluconazole
(D) Metronidazole
(E) Trimethoprim-sulfamethoxazole

Item 78

A 46-year-old woman is evaluated before undergoing a dental cleaning procedure involving deep scaling. She has a history of mitral valve prolapse without regurgitation and also had methicillin-resistant *Staphylococcus aureus* (MRSA) aortic valve endocarditis 10 years ago treated successfully with antibiotics. The patient notes an allergy to penicillin characterized by hypotension, hives, and wheezing. The remainder of the history is noncontributory.

On physical examination, vital signs are normal. Cardiopulmonary examination discloses a late systolic click. The remainder of the examination is normal.

Which of the following is the most appropriate prophylactic regimen for this patient before her dental procedure?

(A) Amoxicillin
(B) Cephalexin
(C) Clindamycin
(D) Vancomycin
(E) No prophylaxis

Item 79

A 36-year-old man is admitted to the emergency departme for a 1-week history of fever, chills, and cough productive yellow sputum and a 2-day history of progressive dyspnea

The patient experiences progressive respiratory distre in the emergency department and is intubated and plac on mechanical ventilation. Two sets of blood cultures a obtained, and empiric antibiotic therapy is begun.

On physical examination, temperature is 38.8 ° (101.8 °F), blood pressure is 85/50 mm Hg, pulse rate 130/min, and respiration rate is 28/min. BMI is 28. Bronch breath sounds are heard over the left and right lower lung fiel

Laboratory studies indicate a hemoglobin level of 1C g/dL (107 g/L), a leukocyte count of 4000/μL (4.0 10⁹/L), and a platelet count of 97,000/μL (97 × 10⁹/I

A chest radiograph shows findings consistent wi consolidation in the left and right lower lobes and patc airspace opacity in the right middle lobe.

In addition to Gram stain and culture of an endotr cheal aspirate, which of the following is the mc appropriate next step in the evaluation?

(A) Bronchoscopy with quantitative cultures
(B) *Legionella* and *Streptococcus pneumoniae* urine anti-gen assays
(C) *Legionella* serologic testing
(D) No further testing

Item 80

A 65-year-old man is evaluated for a 1-day history of l arm and left leg weakness. His wife has also noted sor asymmetry of his face. Medical history is significant hypertension and type 2 diabetes mellitus. Medications lisinopril and metformin.

On physical examination, temperature is 37.2 ° (99.0 °F), blood pressure is 170/100 mm Hg, pulse rate 90/min, and respiration rate is 14/min. Neurologic exa ination findings include a central cranial nerve VII palsy the left, 2/5 motor strength of the left upper extremity, a 4/5 motor strength of the left lower extremity. There a no sensory deficits. Hyperreflexia of the left arm and leg noted, and the left plantar response is positive.

Laboratory studies indicate a normal complete blo count and serum chemistry studies, including liver che istry studies and kidney function tests.

MRI of the brain with contrast shows a 3-cm rir enhancing lesion in the right parietal region with su rounding edema and a midline shift to the left.

Which of the following diagnostic studies should performed next?

(A) Stereotactic CT-guided aspiration of the lesion
(B) CT scan of the chest, abdomen, and pelvis
(C) Lumbar puncture
(D) Whole-body PET scan

Item 81

A 61-year-old man undergoes preoperative evaluation before coronary artery bypass surgery and aortic valve replacement surgery, both scheduled for tomorrow. He has been hospitalized in the cardiac intensive care unit (ICU) for 4 days after collapsing and experiencing cardiogenic shock. He was intubated in the field with a standard, non-silver-coated endotracheal tube and placed on mechanical ventilation in the ICU. He is being treated with both paralytic and sedating medications, in addition to a proton pump inhibitor and intravenous nitroglycerin.

On physical examination, the patient's condition has stabilized and he is afebrile. No attempts are made to wean him from the ventilator because of his impending surgery and his heart condition.

Which of the following is the most appropriate measure to prevent ventilator-associated pneumonia in this patient?

(A) Bathe patient daily in chlorhexidine
(B) Begin preoperative antimicrobial prophylaxis immediately and continue until extubation
(C) Maintain the head of bed above a 30° angle
(D) Perform tracheotomy and remove endotracheal tube
(E) Replace endotracheal tube with a silver-coated endotracheal tube

Item 82

A 55-year-old woman is evaluated for a 1-day history of diarrhea. She has had four liquid stools in the past 24 hours without visible mucus or blood. The patient does not have fever, nausea, vomiting, abdominal pain, or cramping. She returned yesterday from a 2-week trip to Guatemala, where she traveled to rural areas, swam in a local river, and brushed her teeth with tap water.

On physical examination, she is thin and in no acute distress. Vital signs, including temperature, are normal. She has no rash. Her mucous membranes are moist. Bowel sounds are mildly hyperactive, but no focal abdominal tenderness or peritoneal signs are present. Rectal examination is nontender with heme-negative brown stool in the vault.

Which of the following stool studies should be done next?

(A) Culture for bacteria
(B) Culture for viruses
(C) Examination for ova and parasites
(D) Testing for fecal leukocytes
(E) No diagnostic testing is indicated

Item 83

A 26-year-old man is admitted to the emergency department with a 3-day history of dysuria with yellow urethral discharge.

On physical examination, temperature is 37.3 °C (99.1 °F), blood pressure is 120/70 mm Hg, pulse rate is 80/min, and respiration rate is 12/min. There are purulent secretions noted at the urethral meatus. No tenderness of the epididymis, spermatic cords, or testes is noted.

A Gram stain of the urethral discharge is shown.

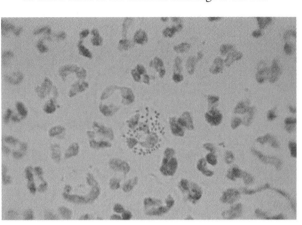

Which of the following is the most appropriate treatment?

(A) Azithromycin
(B) Cefoxitin
(C) Ceftriaxone and azithromycin
(D) Ciprofloxacin and azithromycin

Item 84

A 30-year-old woman is evaluated in the emergency department for a right lower extremity skin infection. She works in a nursing facility where she experienced a minor laceration of the right shin 3 days ago. She initially applied a topical sterile dressing but developed purulent drainage from her wound with increasing surrounding tenderness and a fever over the past 24 hours.

On physical examination, temperature is 38.5 °C (101.3 °F), blood pressure is 125/75 mm Hg, pulse rate is 90/min, and respiration rate is 18/min. An area of purulent cellulitis measuring approximately 4 × 5 cm is present over the right lower extremity surrounding a 1.5-cm laceration. There is no fluctuance. Cardiopulmonary examination is normal. No costovertebral angle tenderness or signs of meningeal irritation are present.

Laboratory studies indicate a leukocyte count of 14,000/µL (14 × 10⁹/L) with 90% neutrophils and 10% lymphocytes. Urinalysis is normal. A radiograph of the right lower extremity shows only soft tissue swelling.

Which of the following β-lactam antibiotics is most appropriate for treatment of this infection?

(A) Ceftaroline
(B) Ceftriaxone
(C) Meropenem
(D) Oxacillin

Item 85

A 65-year-old man undergoes a routine examination. He feels well. He has a history of hypertension treated with lisinopril. The remainder of the history is noncontributory.

On physical examination, temperature is 37.2 °C (99.0 °F), blood pressure is 124/84 mm Hg, pulse rate is 86/min, and respiration rate is 22/min. Physical examination is notable for a soft, nontender enlarged prostate without nodules.

As part of a health insurance evaluation, urinalysis and culture are performed. Urinalysis shows 1+ protein and trace leukocyte esterase, and the urine culture grows more than 10^5 colony-forming units of *Escherichia coli* susceptible to ciprofloxacin and trimethoprim-sulfamethoxazole.

Which of the following is the most appropriate management?

(A) Ciprofloxacin
(B) Kidney ultrasound
(C) Repeat urinalysis and urine culture
(D) Trimethoprim-sulfamethoxazole
(E) No further evaluation or treatment necessary

Item 86

A 25-year-old woman is evaluated in the emergency department for anaphylaxis following a transfusion of packed red blood cells after trauma resulting from a motor vehicle collision 3 weeks ago. She was diagnosed with systemic lupus erythematosus after a pregnancy 2 years ago. She has a history of eczema since childhood as well as a history of recurrent sinopulmonary and urinary tract infections. Six months ago, she was diagnosed with chronic, unexplained diarrhea.

On physical examination, temperature is 37.5 °C (99.5 °F), blood pressure is 112/60 mm Hg, pulse rate is 80/min, and respiration rate is 14/min. The skin is pruritic and red with poorly demarcated, eczematous, crusted, papulovesicular plaques and excoriations located in the antecubital and popliteal fossae. The remainder of her physical examination is normal.

Laboratory studies show a leukocyte count of 8000/µL (8.0×10^9/L).

A chest radiograph is normal.

Which of the following is the most likely diagnosis?

(A) C1-inhibitor deficiency
(B) Terminal complement deficiency
(C) Properdin deficiency
(D) Selective IgA deficiency

Item 87

A 56-year-old woman is evaluated in the emergency department in May for a 2-day history of fever, myalgia, and headache. She works as a horse trainer on a farm in Oklahoma and recalls removing at least three ticks from her skin in the past 2 weeks.

On physical examination, the patient appears ill. Temperature is 39.3 °C (102.7 °F); other vital signs are normal. There is no nuchal rigidity, lymphadenopathy, or rash. Remaining physical examination findings are nonfocal.

Laboratory studies:

Leukocyte count	14,600/µL (14.6×10^9/ with 87% neutrophils
Platelet count	136,000/µL (136×10^9,
Alanine aminotransferase	177 units/L
Aspartate aminotransferase	211 units/L
Alkaline phosphatase	114 units/L
Creatinine	1.4 mg/dL (123.7 µmol/

Serologic testing *for Rickettsia rickettsii, Anaplas phagocytophilum*, and *Ehrlichia chaffeensis* is performed

Which of the following is the most appropriate n step in the management of this patient?

(A) Begin empiric amoxicillin
(B) Begin empiric doxycycline
(C) Withhold antibiotics unless a petechial skin rash develops
(D) Withhold antibiotics while awaiting serologic resul

Item 88

A 28-year-old woman who is 3 months pregnant unc goes evaluation in September. She is a nurse and work a local hospital. There is an influenza A virus outbreak the community, and she wants to prevent infection dur her pregnancy.

On physical examination, temperature is 36.5 (97.7 °F), blood pressure is 110/70 mm Hg, pulse rat 88/min, and respiration rate is 14/min. The remainder the examination is normal.

Which of the following is the most appropri influenza virus prophylaxis for this patient?

(A) Amantadine
(B) Live attenuated intranasal influenza vaccine
(C) Oseltamivir
(D) Trivalent inactivated influenza vaccine

Item 89

A 22-year-old man is evaluated for a 1-day history of fe rash, and abdominal pain. He has a 5-year history of rec rent episodes of these symptoms plus occasional joint p in the knee or hip that resolves spontaneously after sev days.

On physical examination, temperature is 38.6 (101.5 °F), blood pressure is 120/70 mm Hg, pulse rat 70/min, and respiration rate is 14/min. A sharply dem cated, tender, raised, erythematous, warm rash is pres over the dorsa of both feet and both anterior legs t extends approximately 10 cm in diameter. There is inguinal lymphadenopathy or fluctuance, ulcer, or pu lence. Abdominal examination discloses normal bo sounds and minimal tenderness to palpation. Distal pu are normal.

Laboratory studies indicate a leukocyte count 13,000/µL (13×10^9/L) with 80% neutrophils, 17% ly phocytes, and 3% monocytes and a platelet count 400,000/µL (400×10^9/L).

Which of the following is the most likely diagnosis?

) Erythromelalgia
) Familial Mediterranean fever
) Staphylococcal cellulitis
•) Sweet syndrome

em 90

32-year-old woman who is 41 weeks pregnant is admit-
d to the hospital for an elective cesarean delivery. The
oman is a known carrier of group B *Streptococcus* as evi-
nced by a vaginal/rectal surveillance culture obtained at
stational week 36. She has gestational diabetes that has
en well controlled throughout pregnancy with diet only.
e also has a 10-pack-year smoking history and continues
smoke approximately 5 cigarettes daily. Her only med-
tion is a daily prenatal vitamin.

Physical examination, including vital signs, is normal.

hich of the following is the most appropriate mea-
re for preventing surgical site infection in this
tient?

) Decolonization of group B *Streptococcus* vaginal/rec-
tal carriage before surgery
) Prophylactic antibiotics for 72 hours after incision
:) Shaving of the surgical field
)) Surgical antimicrobial prophylaxis 30 to 60 minutes
before initial incision

em 91

32-year-old man undergoes follow-up evaluation for recur-
nt genital herpes simplex virus infection. His most recent
tbreak was the third episode within 8 months and con-
ted of painful vesicles on the penile shaft and perianal area.
e lesions resolved after acyclovir therapy, which is consis-
nt with his response to treatment of previous episodes. He
as diagnosed with HIV infection 10 years ago and discon-
ued antiretroviral therapy (ART) 1 year ago because of
verse effects. His last CD4 cell count was 30/μL. His only
edication is trimethoprim-sulfamethoxazole.

On physical examination, temperature is normal, blood
essure is 130/70 mm Hg, pulse rate is 80/min, and res-
ration rate is 14/min. He presently has no active lesions.

addition to encouraging this patient to restart his
tiretroviral therapy, which of the following is the
ost appropriate therapy to prevent symptomatic gen-
I herpes simplex virus reactivation?

) Acyclovir
) Cidofovir
:) Foscarnet
)) Valganciclovir

em 92

50-year-old woman is admitted to the emergency depart-
nt for a 2-day history of fever and chills, dyspnea,

hemoptysis, and left-sided pleuritic chest pain. She
underwent allogeneic hematopoietic stem cell transplantation for myelodysplastic syndrome 6 months ago; until
2 days ago she had been doing well. Her medications are
trimethoprim-sulfamethoxazole, acyclovir, prednisone, and
cyclosporine.

On physical examination, temperature is 39.3 °C
(102.7 °F), blood pressure is 110/68 mm Hg, pulse rate is
122/min, and respiration rate is 24/min. Dullness to percussion, crackles, and egophony are heard at the left lung
base. The remainder of the examination is normal.

Laboratory studies show a leukocyte count of
4400/μL (4.4×10^9/L), a platelet count of 155,000/μL
(155×10^9/L), and a hematocrit of 30%.

Chest radiograph shows a dense infiltrate in the left
lower lobe.

**Infection with which of the following is the most likely
diagnosis?**

(A) *Candida krusei*
(B) Cytomegalovirus
(C) *Pneumocystis jirovecii*
(D) *Streptococcus pneumoniae*

Item 93

A 27-year-old man is evaluated in the emergency department
for a 2-day history of fever, weakness, and dark-colored urine.
The patient returned yesterday from a 2-week camping trip
to Cape Cod, Massachusetts. While there, he developed a
target-shaped lesion on his thigh. He was evaluated at a walk-
in clinic, where early-stage Lyme disease was diagnosed. He
is currently on day 10 of a 14-day course of doxycycline.

On physical examination, temperature is 38.5 °C
(101.3 °F), blood pressure is 122/66 mm Hg, and pulse
rate is 118/min. The previously noted lesion on the thigh
has resolved. He is jaundiced. The liver is tender and is palpable 5 cm below the costophrenic margin.

Laboratory studies:

Hemoglobin	8.4 g/dL (84 g/L)
Reticulocyte count	10%
Leukocyte count	12,600/μL (12.6×10^9/L)
Platelet count	110,000/μL (110×10^9/L)
Lactate dehydrogenase	675 units/L
Total bilirubin	8.3 mg/dL (145.3 μmol/L)

**Which of the following pathogens is most likely caus-
ing this patient's current findings?**

(A) *Anaplasma phagocytophilum*
(B) *Babesia microti*
(C) *Borrelia burgdorferi*
(D) *Rickettsia rickettsii*
(E) West Nile virus

Item 94

A 58-year-old man is admitted to the emergency department with a 2-day history of fever, chills, cough, progressively worsening dyspnea, and left-sided pleuritic chest

pain. He has no other medical problems and takes no medications.

Pneumonia is diagnosed, and two sets of blood cultures and a urine sample for pneumococcal and *Legionella* antigens are obtained. Treatment with cefotaxime and azithromycin is begun. The patient is admitted to the medical ward.

On physical examination, temperature is 38.2 °C (100.8 °F), blood pressure is 130/80 mm Hg, pulse rate is 115/min, and respiration rate is 28/min. Oxygen saturation is 87% with the patient breathing ambient air. Markedly diminished breath sounds are heard in the left lung base with dullness to percussion.

Chest radiograph shows consolidation of the left lower lobe and lingula with a pleural effusion to the midpoint of the left hemithorax on upright images.

Which of the following is the most appropriate management of this patient?

(A) Add metronidazole to ceftriaxone and azithromycin
(B) Change antimicrobial therapy to cefepime and vancomycin
(C) Diagnostic ultrasound-guided thoracentesis if no improvement within 24 to 48 hours
(D) Immediate ultrasound-guided thoracentesis

Item 95

A 33-year-old woman undergoes routine evaluation. She feels well but inquires about HIV screening because she has had several lifetime partners, but within monogamous relationships and always using condoms. She has had no known sex partners with HIV infection and reports that none of her partners were known injection drug users or men who have sex with men. She has no history of sexually transmitted infections, has never been pregnant, and is sexually active only with her husband of 8 years. Her husband is healthy but has never been tested for HIV infection. Her only medication is an oral contraceptive.

Physical examination is normal.

Which of the following is the most appropriate next step in the management of this patient?

(A) HIV antibody enzyme immunoassay
(B) HIV antibody Western blot assay
(C) HIV nucleic acid amplification test
(D) No testing indicated

Item 96

A 36-year-old woman is evaluated for fever and headache 7 days after undergoing a craniotomy for removal of a mass lesion in her right frontal lobe. Pathologic examination demonstrated a malignant astrocytoma. The patient had been doing well before development of the current symptoms.

On physical examination, temperature is 38.9 °C (102.0 °F); other vital signs are normal. Her neck is stiff. The remaining physical examination findings are normal.

Laboratory studies show a leukocyte count of 9600/µL (9.6×10^9/L) with a normal differential.

MRI of the brain reveals postoperative changes b only minimal cerebral edema in the area of the surge Lumbar puncture is performed.

Cerebrospinal fluid analysis:
Leukocyte count   450/µL (450×10^6/L)
Erythrocyte count   100/µL (100×10^6/L)
Glucose   45 mg/dL (2.5 mmol/L)
Protein   500 mg/dL (5000 mg/L)
Gram stain   Negative

In addition to vancomycin, which of the followi empiric antimicrobial agents should be administer now?

(A) Ceftriaxone
(B) Gentamicin
(C) Meropenem
(D) Metronidazole
(E) Trimethoprim-sulfamethoxazole

Item 97

A 70-year-old woman undergoes evaluation. She will traveling to Mexico for vacation, visiting several Mexic villages with accommodations at local inns. In preparati for her travel, she has received the full hepatitis A vacci series and has been instructed on protection against m quitoes and other biting insects. She is current with all ag appropriate recommended vaccinations. Medical history significant for intermittent flares of inflammatory bowel d ease for which she takes 5-aminosalicylic acid. She is othe wise healthy and takes no other medications.

Physical examination, including vital signs, is norma

Because of her underlying gastrointestinal conditic the patient is concerned about developing a diarrheal illn during her travel.

Which of the following will be most helpful in redu ing this patient's risk for travelers' diarrhea?

(A) Avoidance of tap water
(B) Prophylactic bismuth subsalicylate
(C) Prophylactic *Lactobacillus* probiotic
(D) Prophylactic loperamide
(E) Prophylactic rifaximin

Item 98

A 22-year-old man is evaluated for diarrhea and weight lc The patient has a 3-week history of foul-smelling, large-v ume, watery stools associated with abdominal bloatir There is no visible blood or mucus in the stools. He repo a 4.5-kg (10-lb) weight loss, which he attributes to a pc appetite. One month before symptoms developed, he to a 2-week hiking trip along the Appalachian Trail, where slept in primitive camp sites without running water. His gi friend, who accompanied him on the trip, is well.

On physical examination, the patient appears thin bu in no acute distress. Vital signs are normal. Abdominal exa ination discloses high-pitched, increased bowel sounds a diffuse tenderness to palpation, without peritoneal signs.

Results of a stool examination are negative for occult blood and fecal leukocytes.

Which of the following stool studies is most likely to be diagnostic?

(A) Stool assay for *Giardia* antigen
(B) Stool culture for bacteria
(C) Stool examination for ova and parasites
(D) Stool sample for modified acid-fast staining for *Cryptosporidium*

Item 99

A 19-year-old man is evaluated in the emergency department for a 10-day history of fever, cervical lymphadenopathy, malaise and fatigue, sore throat, headache, and nausea, but no vomiting, diarrhea, abdominal pain, nasal congestion, or cough. He had a rash a few days ago that has resolved. He is sexually active with both men and women and does not use condoms.

On physical examination, temperature is 38.1 °C (100.6 °F), blood pressure is 110/88 mm Hg, pulse rate is 96/min, and respiration rate is 16/min. He appears uncomfortable but is not in distress. Significant lymphadenopathy is noted in the cervical, axillary, and inguinal regions. The oropharynx is erythematous with mildly enlarged tonsils but no exudate. Sclerae and conjunctivae are clear, and the skin is without rash. The remainder of the examination, including cardiac, joint, abdominal, and genital findings, is unremarkable.

Results of the heterophile antibody test, rapid streptococcal antigen test, HIV enzyme immunoassay, and rapid plasma reagin test are negative.

Which of the following is the most appropriate diagnostic test to perform next?

(A) CD4 cell count
(B) HIV nucleic acid amplification test
(C) HIV Western blot assay
(D) Repeat HIV enzyme immunoassay

Item 100

A 32-year-old woman who is 5 months pregnant undergoes evaluation before international travel. The patient is a photojournalist, and in 3 weeks, she will be traveling to a rural area in Kenya, Africa, on assignment for 10 days. The patient takes a prenatal vitamin.

Physical examination, including vital signs, is normal. The patient is given advice on mosquito bite avoidance and insect repellent (DEET).

Which of the following is the most appropriate malaria chemoprophylaxis of this patient?

(A) Atovaquone-proguanil
(B) Chloroquine
(C) Doxycycline
(D) Mefloquine

Item 101

A 36-year-old man who was admitted to the intensive care unit for treatment of multiple traumatic injuries sustained in a motor vehicle accident is diagnosed with ventilator-associated pneumonia.

On physical examination, temperature is 38.3 °C (101.0 °F), blood pressure is 130/88 mm Hg, pulse rate is 108/min, and respiration rate is 22/min. Breath sounds reveal bilateral basilar crackles. The remainder of the physical examination, consistent with his history of multiple trauma-related injuries, is otherwise noncontributory.

A chest radiograph reveals bilateral lower lobe infiltrates. A quantitative bronchoalveolar lavage culture grows methicillin-resistant *Staphylococcus aureus* with susceptibilities to vancomycin, daptomycin, linezolid, rifampin, and tigecycline. Two sets of blood cultures are negative.

Vancomycin is initiated, and on hospital day 3, the patient develops an urticarial rash. The patient's clinical status has remained unchanged.

In addition to discontinuing vancomycin, which of the following is the most appropriate treatment?

(A) Daptomycin
(B) Linezolid
(C) Rifampin
(D) Tigecycline

Item 102

A 60-year-old man is evaluated in the emergency department for swelling and erythema of the right leg with associated fever.

On physical examination, temperature is 38.1 °C (100.6 °F), blood pressure is 135/85 mm Hg, pulse rate is 99/min, and respiration rate is 16/min. BMI is 28. An area of cellulitis measuring 4 × 3 cm is present on the distal right lower extremity with associated tenderness, warmth, and edema but without necrosis, purulent exudate, fluctuance, or lymphadenopathy. Tinea pedis infection is found between several toes of both feet. The remainder of the physical examination is normal.

Laboratory studies indicate a leukocyte count of 12,000/µL (12 × 10⁹/L) with 80% neutrophils, 18% lymphocytes, and 2% monocytes. A metabolic panel is normal. Topical clotrimazole is prescribed for the tinea pedis infection.

The patient refuses hospital admission.

Which of the following is the most appropriate outpatient therapy?

(A) Clindamycin
(B) Doxycycline
(C) Rifampin
(D) Trimethoprim-sulfamethoxazole

Item 103

A 68-year-old man is admitted to the emergency department for a 3-day history of cough and increasing dyspnea. He was previously healthy and takes no medications.

On physical examination, temperature is 38.6 °C (101.5 °F), blood pressure is 145/90 mm Hg, pulse rate is 100/min, and respiration rate is 30/min. Oxygen saturation is 95% with the patient breathing ambient air. There are crackles in the right lower posterior lung field. The remainder of the physical examination is normal.

Laboratory studies:

Hemoglobin	12.2 g/dL (122 g/L)
Leukocyte count	10,700/μL (10.7 × 10⁹/L)
Platelet count	210,000/μL (210 × 10⁹/L)
Blood urea nitrogen	25 mg/dL (8.9 mmol/L)
Creatinine	1.0 mg/dL (88.4 μmol/L)
Glucose	110 mg/dL (6.1 mmol/L)
Electrolytes	Normal

Chest radiograph shows right lower lobe airspace disease.

Results of blood cultures, sputum Gram stain, and pneumococcal urine antigen assays are pending.

Which of the following is the most appropriate management of this patient?

(A) Administer a single dose of empiric intravenous antibiotic therapy and discharge on oral antibiotic therapy
(B) Begin empiric antibiotic therapy and admit to the intensive care unit
(C) Begin empiric antibiotic therapy and admit to the medical ward
(D) Discharge and prescribe oral antibiotic therapy

Item 104

A 30-year-old man is evaluated for a 3-month history of fever, night sweats, and headache. The patient has a history of injection drug use and is currently incarcerated.

On physical examination, temperature is 38.3 °C (101.0 °F), blood pressure is 110/65 mm Hg, pulse rate is 95/min, and respiration rate is 20/min. He is oriented but lethargic. Cardiopulmonary and neurologic examinations are normal.

The leukocyte count is 15,000/μL (15 × 10⁹/L) with 70% neutrophils, 20% lymphocytes, and 10% monocytes, and the serum albumin level is 2.3 g/dL (23 g/L). The remaining metabolic panel and results of urinalysis are normal.

Lumbar puncture is performed. Opening pressure is 250 mm H₂O. Cerebrospinal fluid (CSF) examination shows a cell count of 400/μL (400 × 10⁶/L) with 95% lymphocytes, a protein level of 200 mg/dL (2000 mg/L), and a glucose level of 20 mg/dL (1.1 mmol/L). CSF polymerase chain reaction is positive for *Mycobacterium tuberculosis*, and CSF culture grows *M. tuberculosis*. Blood culture specimens show no growth. A CT scan of the head reveals basilar meningeal enhancement.

Treatment with isoniazid, rifampin, pyrazinamide, and ethambutol and corticosteroids is begun. Mycobacteria are fully susceptible to all four antituberculous agents.

Which of the following is the most appropriate treatment duration?

(A) 4 to 6 months
(B) 9 to 12 months
(C) 15 to 18 months
(D) 24 months

Item 105

A 29-year-old man is evaluated in the hospital 2 weeks af[ter] allogeneic hematopoietic stem cell transplantation for acu[te] myeloid leukemia. He has had a dry cough and persiste[nt] fever for 3 days despite taking antibiotic agents. The patie[nt] and donor were both seropositive for cytomegalovirus. H[is] medications are imipenem, ciprofloxacin, vancomycin, ac[y]clovir, and fluconazole.

On physical examination, temperature is 38.5 °[C] (101.3 °F), blood pressure is 122/74 mm Hg, pulse ra[te] is 98/min, and respiration rate is 18/min. Skin examina[tion] shows some petechiae but no lesions or rash. Ca[r]diopulmonary and abdominal examinations are norm[al.] The intravenous catheter site is without erythema [or] drainage.

Laboratory studies show a hematocrit of 24%, a leuk[o]cyte count of 100/μL (0.10 × 10⁹/L), and a platelet cou[nt] of 15,000/μL (15 × 10⁹/L). Chest radiograph disclos[es] scattered opacities. A noncontrast CT scan of the che[st] demonstrates nodular infiltrates without cavitation.

Which of the following is the most likely infectio[us] cause of this patient's fever?

(A) *Aspergillus*
(B) Cytomegalovirus
(C) Mucormycosis (zygomycosis)
(D) *Pneumocystis jirovecii*

Item 106

A 26-year-old woman undergoes follow-up evaluation af[ter] completing an appropriate antibiotic course for a urina[ry] tract infection (UTI) diagnosed 3 days ago; she is curren[tly] asymptomatic. She has had five similar episodes in the pa[st] year, the symptoms for all of which began after sexual inte[r]course and responded well to antibiotic treatment. She h[as] increased her fluid intake and routinely voids after sex[ual] intercourse. She is sexually active with one partner and do[es] not use spermicides. Her only form of birth control is [an] intrauterine device, which has been in place for 6 mont[hs.] She is otherwise healthy, with no medical problems and [no] history of sexually transmitted infections. She curren[tly] takes no medications.

Physical examination, including vital signs, is norma[l.]

Which of the following is the most appropriate ne[xt] step to reduce this patient's risk for UTIs?

(A) Chronic suppressive therapy with trimethoprim-sul[-]famethoxazole
(B) Drinking cranberry juice
(C) Postcoital antimicrobial prophylaxis

) Removal of intrauterine device

) Using a spermicide prior to intercourse

em 107

28-year-old man undergoes follow-up evaluation and
iew of his most recent routine laboratory studies. He has
mptomatic HIV infection and is adherent to his anti-
roviral therapy regimen. He has had two sexual partners
hin the past 6 months. Although he has communicated
 HIV status to both partners, he still has not used con-
ms consistently. His only medication is efavirenz-emtric-
oine-tenofovir. He has no medication allergies.

Physical examination is normal with the exception of
otty axillary and inguinal lymphadenopathy, unchanged
m previous examinations. His neurologic examination is
rmal.

A comprehensive metabolic profile is normal. The
04 cell count is 680 cells/μL, HIV RNA viral load is
detectable, and the serum rapid plasma reagin titer is
 6 compared with negative results 6 months ago. Results
 serum fluorescent treponemal antibody absorption test-
 are positive.

hich of the following is the most appropriate treat-
nt?

) Aqueous crystalline penicillin G intravenously for 10
   days

) Intramuscular benzathine penicillin G weekly for
   three doses

) Oral doxycycline for 14 days

) Single-dose intramuscular benzathine penicillin G

em 108

27-year-old woman is evaluated for a 2-day history of
er, hemoptysis, and chest pain. She was recently diag-
sed with acute myeloid leukemia and completed her last
urse of chemotherapy 2 weeks ago. Her course has been

complicated by profound neutropenia, thrombocytopenia,
and fever that initially resolved after treatment with
cefepime and vancomycin.

On physical examination, temperature is 38.9 °C
(102.0 °F), blood pressure is 110/70 mm Hg, pulse rate is
100/min, and respiration rate is 20/min. A friction rub is
heard at the left posterior lung base.

Laboratory studies indicate a leukocyte count of
100/μL (0.10×10^9/L). Serum galactomannan antigen
immunoassay results are positive, consistent with a diagnosis of invasive pulmonary aspergillosis.

A chest radiograph shows a pleural-based nodular density at the left lung base.

A CT scan of the chest is shown.

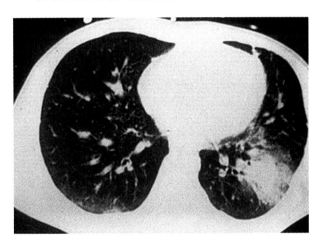

**Which of the following is the most appropriate treat-
ment?**

(A) Itraconazole

(B) Liposomal amphotericin B

(C) Micafungin

(D) Voriconazole

Answers and Critiques

Item 1   Answer: C

Educational Objective: Diagnose common variable immunodeficiency.

Serum levels of IgG, IgA, and IgM should be measured. There is a high probability that this patient has common variable immunodeficiency (CVID). The onset is usually between 15 and 25 years of age, and a history of recurrent respiratory tract infections with encapsulated organisms such as *Streptococcus pneumoniae* and *Haemophilus influenzae* is common; giardiasis can also occur. Patients with CVID have a higher incidence of autoimmune disorders, particularly autoimmune hemolytic anemia and thrombocytopenia, pernicious anemia, and rheumatoid arthritis, as well as disorders of the gastrointestinal tract leading to diarrhea and malabsorption. This patient's anemia and high mean corpuscular volume are suggestive of vitamin B_{12} deficiency. There is a familial predisposition to selective IgA deficiency and malignancies. A higher incidence of CVID exists in those of northern European ancestry.

If serum IgG and IgA or IgM levels are low, the antibody response to protein- and polysaccharide-based vaccines should then be assessed. If IgG levels are very low (<200 mg/dL [2.0 g/L]) or undetectable, assessment of vaccine response is not necessary because antibody levels are predictably absent. Therefore, the first step in the evaluation of patients with suspected CVID is measurement of serum immunoglobulin levels.

A low CD4 cell count may occur in patients with CVID; however, measurement of the CD4 cell count would not contribute to the diagnosis. Involvement of cellular immunity in CVID is variable. T-cell numbers, including CD4 cells or T-cell function, can be normal in nearly 50% of patients.

Total hemolytic complement should be checked whenever a complement deficiency is suspected. A low total hemolytic complement level is seen with classical and terminal complement pathway deficiencies. Complement deficiencies involving the early components of the complement system are associated with autoimmune disorders, most specifically systemic lupus erythematosus. These patients may experience recurrent infections caused by encapsulated organisms such as *Streptococcus pneumoniae* or disseminated neisserial infections. Deficiencies in the terminal components of the complement system are associated with recurrent neisserial infections including meningitis and disseminated gonorrheal infection. The patient's clinical presentation is most compatible with CVID, not deficiencies in the early or terminal complement system.

> **KEY POINT**
>
> - Patients with common variable immunodeficiency frequently develop sinopulmonary infections, autoimmune disorders, malabsorption, and lymphoma, and their response to vaccination is poor.

Bibliography

Chapel H, Cunningham-Rundles C. Update in understanding common variable immunodeficiency disorders (CVIDs) and the management of patients with these conditions. Br J Haematol. 2009;145(6):709-727. [PMID: 19344423]

Item 2   Answer: A

Educational Objective: Manage an immunocompromised patient who has been exposed to a close contact with active tuberculosis.

Isoniazid and pyridoxine should be started for treatment of latent tuberculosis infection (LTBI). This patient has HIV infection and was recently exposed to a close contact with active tuberculosis. Patients with HIV infection or other serious immunocompromising conditions who are close contacts of persons with active tuberculosis should be treated for LTBI regardless of the results of a tuberculin skin test or interferon-γ release assay (IGRA) once active disease has been excluded. This patient is asymptomatic and has a normal chest radiograph, which exclude active disease. Patients with LTBI are typically treated with a 9-month regimen of isoniazid. Pyridoxine may also be given to certain patients at risk for developing peripheral neuropathy secondary to isoniazid. These include patients with HIV infection, diabetes mellitus, uremia, alcoholism, malnutrition, and seizure disorders, as well as pregnant women. In this patient, the tuberculin skin test or IGRA should be repeated 8 to 10 weeks after the most recent exposure. If results are still negative, isoniazid and pyridoxine can be discontinued. However, some experts recommend a complete course of treatment for LTBI in patients with HIV infection, who may not be able to mount a positive tuberculin skin test or IGRA response because of anergy.

Isoniazid, rifampin, pyrazinamide, pyridoxine, and ethambutol are used to treat active tuberculosis. This patient is asymptomatic and has a normal chest radiograph, making active disease highly unlikely.

The use of rifampin and pyrazinamide for treatment of LTBI is not recommended by the Centers for Disease Control and Prevention and the American Thoracic Society because of associated hepatic toxicity, which results in increased rates of hospitalization and death.

This patient with HIV infection and a recent exposure to a close contact with active tuberculosis requires treatment for latent tuberculosis infection, regardless of the results of a tuberculin skin test or IGRA; providing no further evaluation or treatment would not be appropriate.

- **Regardless of their response to a tuberculin skin test or interferon-γ release assay, patients with HIV infection who have had a known recent exposure to a close contact with active tuberculosis should receive treatment for latent tuberculosis infection after active disease has been excluded.**

Bibliography

National Tuberculosis Controllers Association; Centers for Disease Control and Prevention (CDC). Guidelines for the investigation of contacts of persons with infectious tuberculosis: Recommendations from the National Tuberculosis Controllers Association and CDC. MMWR Recomm Rep. 2005;54(RR-15):1-47. [PMID: 16357823]

Item 3   Answer: A

Educational Objective: Treat life-threatening candidemia.

This patient should be treated with caspofungin. She has fungemia, which is most likely caused by *Candida* species. The most likely source is the central venous catheter, the site of which shows obvious signs of infection including erythema and purulent drainage. She has multiple risk factors for candidemia, including exposure to broad-spectrum antibiotics and having received parenteral nutrition via a central venous catheter. In addition to catheter removal, it is essential that antifungal therapy be instituted promptly. Because she is severely ill, the therapy of choice is an echinocandin agent. The Infectious Diseases Society of America guidelines do not distinguish among the echinocandins; therefore, any of them (caspofungin, anidulafungin, or micafungin) would be appropriate.

Amphotericin B or a lipid formulation of amphotericin B is an alternative choice if there is intolerance to or limited availability of other antifungal agents. This patient has kidney failure, which would be exacerbated by either formulation of amphotericin B.

Fluconazole is recommended for patients who are less critically ill than this patient and who have had no recent exposure to azole antifungal agents. When this patient becomes clinically stable, she can be transitioned from receiving an echinocandin to fluconazole if the isolate is likely to be susceptible to fluconazole.

Voriconazole is effective for the treatment of candidemia, but it offers little advantage over fluconazole and is recommended as step-down oral therapy for selected patients with candidiasis caused by *Candida krusei* or voriconazole-susceptible *Candida glabrata*.

- **Antifungal therapy with an echinocandin agent (caspofungin, anidulafungin, or micafungin) is the treatment of choice for critically ill patients with candidemia.**

Bibliography

Pappas PG, Kauffman CA, Andes D, et al; Infectious Diseases Society of America. Clinical practice guidelines for the management of candidiasis: 2009 update by the Infectious Diseases Society of America. Clin Infect Dis. 2009;48(5):503-535. [PMID: 19191635]

Item 4   Answer: A

Educational Objective: Treat recurrent mild to moderate *Clostridium difficile* infection.

This patient has recurrent mild to moderate *Clostridium difficile* infection (CDI) and requires a repeat course of oral metronidazole for 14 days. The most appropriate treatment regimen for both the initial episode and the first recurrence of CDI is determined by the severity of the illness. Severe CDI is characterized by leukocytosis, defined as a leukocyte count greater than 15,000/microliter (15 × 10^9/L), and a significant decrease in kidney function, defined as an increase in the serum creatinine level greater than 1.5 times the baseline level. Patients without clinical or laboratory findings consistent with severe disease are at low risk for complications, and the recommended treatment is metronidazole for 10 to 14 days. Despite appropriate initial therapy, CDI recurs in approximately 20% of patients. The choice of therapy for the first recurrence does not decrease the probability of a second recurrence, and treatment is determined by the severity of illness in the same way as for the initial presentation.

Prolonged courses of metronidazole, such as a taper over 42 days, are not recommended because neurotoxicity can develop.

Oral vancomycin for 10 to 14 days is indicated for patients meeting the criteria for severe CDI, which this patient does not have.

Combination therapy with oral vancomycin and parenteral metronidazole is reserved for patients in whom enteral antimicrobial agents may not reach the distal colon, such as those with ileus or megacolon.

Patients who have a second recurrence of CDI of any degree of severity should be treated with a prolonged vancomycin taper over 4 to 8 weeks.

- **In patients with *Clostridium difficile* infection, the most appropriate treatment regimen for both the initial episode and the first recurrence is determined by the severity of the illness.**

Bibliography

Cohen SH, Gerding DN, Johnson S, et al; Society for Healthcare Epidemiology of America; Infectious Diseases Society of America

Clinical practice guidelines for Clostridium difficile infection in adults: 2010 update by the Society for Healthcare Epidemiology of America (SHEA) and the Infectious Diseases Society of America (IDSA). Infect Control Hosp Epidemiol. 2010;31(5):431-455. [PMID: 20307191]

Item 5   Answer: A

Educational Objective: Treat primary genital herpes simplex virus infection.

The most appropriate treatment is acyclovir. This patient's clinical examination findings are consistent with herpes simplex virus (HSV) infection. Because she has several lesions accompanied by systemic symptoms (malaise, fever), she most likely has a primary infection. Both HSV-1 and HSV-2 can cause primary genital infection; the incidence of primary infection from HSV-1 has increased in recent years. HSV-1 genital infections are less likely to be associated with recurrences and subclinical viral shedding. Although the clinical presentation is consistent with HSV infection, the diagnosis should be confirmed by viral culture or polymerase chain reaction testing; direct fluorescence antibody testing is a much less sensitive diagnostic modality. Pending the results of diagnostic testing, the patient should begin receiving antiviral therapy to reduce the severity and duration of symptoms. Acyclovir, valacyclovir, and famciclovir are all recommended for the treatment of primary HSV infections; acyclovir is available generically and therefore is the least-expensive treatment option. Valacyclovir has the advantage of twice-daily dosing compared with thrice-daily dosing of acyclovir or famciclovir. Regardless of the regimen chosen, the patient should be treated for 7 to 10 days. Patients with newly diagnosed genital HSV infection must be counseled regarding the risks of recurrence and transmission. Women and men with genital HSV infection should be educated regarding the risk of neonatal infection. Chronic therapy with valacyclovir has been shown to reduce the risk of transmission of infection to sexual partners.

Benzathine penicillin G is the appropriate treatment choice for primary syphilis. Syphilis is characterized by chancres, which are usually single painless lesions with a clean base (unless secondarily infected), although multiple lesions can also occur.

Ceftriaxone plus azithromycin is appropriate treatment for mucopurulent cervicitis. HSV infection can cause cervicitis, but the presentation would be characterized by ulcerative lesions on the cervix.

Single-dose fluconazole is the appropriate treatment for candidal vaginitis, which may include fissures and excoriations from pruritus, but ulcerative lesions would not be typical.

KEY POINT

- Pending the results of diagnostic testing, patients with suspected primary herpes simplex virus infection should begin receiving empiric antiviral therapy with acyclovir, valacyclovir, or famciclovir to reduce the severity and duration of symptoms.

Bibliography

Workowski KA, Berman S; Centers for Disease Control and Prevention (CDC). Sexually transmitted diseases treatment guidelines, 2010. MMWR Recomm Rep. 2010;59(RR-12):1-110. [PMID: 21160459]

Item 6   Answer: D

Educational Objective: Diagnose acute pulmonary histoplasmosis.

This patient's recent travel history and clinical symptoms are most consistent with acute pulmonary histoplasmosis (also known as "Ohio Valley fever"). *Histoplasma capsulatum*, a dimorphic fungal organism that is particularly endemic to the southeastern United States, is found in high concentrations in soil contaminated with bird or bat droppings. The infection is acquired through inhalation of the fungus in its mold form. Although most acute infections are asymptomatic, some persons develop a flu-like syndrome (fever, myalgia, malaise) and pulmonary symptoms (dyspnea, cough, chest discomfort). In a few patients, histoplasmosis may become disseminated, causing bone marrow involvement and pancytopenia, as well as involvement of the meninges, adrenal glands, and other organs. Persons who have a weakened immune system such as from AIDS or immunosuppressive therapy for autoimmune conditions, neoplasms, or transplantation are at higher risk for disseminated histoplasmosis. This patient's travel history and symptoms are suspicious for histoplasmosis, and diagnosis may be confirmed by laboratory testing.

Symptoms caused by acute infection with *Blastomyces dermatitidis*, which is also a dimorphic fungus, are very similar to those caused by *H. capsulatum*. In addition, the endemic geographic distribution of *Blastomyces* and *Histoplasma* overlap. However, acute pulmonary blastomycosis is rarely associated with hilar lymphadenopathy, a common finding in acute pulmonary histoplasmosis. Furthermore, acute blastomycosis is more often associated with exposure to soil containing decaying vegetation and wood products, not bat caves.

This patient's clinical-epidemiologic scenario is not consistent with that of acute pulmonary coccidioidomycosis because *Coccidioides immitis* is endemic to the southwestern United States (Arizona, New Mexico, California, and west Texas).

Infection caused by *Cryptococcus neoformans* typically affects immunocompromised persons and most often causes localized pulmonary lesions.

- *Histoplasma capsulatum* is a dimorphic fungal organism endemic to the southeastern United States; is found in soil contaminated with bird or bat droppings; and is characterized by a flu-like syndrome and dyspnea, cough, and chest discomfort.

Bibliography

Dylewski J. Acute pulmonary histoplasmosis. CMAJ. 2011;183(14): E1090. [PMID: 21810958]

Item 7   Answer: B

Educational Objective: Manage a patient with a prosthetic joint infection.

The most appropriate management of this patient who has requested no further surgery is to retain her prosthesis and administer lifelong therapy with trimethoprim-sulfamethoxazole. This patient most likely has chronic osteomyelitis in her tibia with a chronically infected prosthetic joint. Ideally, removal of all the hardware and debridement of the necrotic bone tissue, followed by a prolonged course of a pathogen-directed parenteral or oral antimicrobial treatment regimen, would occur. However, the patient has refused a surgical management option. In patients with no systemic or severe local signs of infection and in whom the prosthesis is not loose or in whom surgery is not possible or desired, lifelong oral antimicrobial therapy may be considered in an attempt to suppress the infection and retain usefulness of the total joint replacement. The success of this treatment modality partly depends on the relative virulence of the causative microorganism and its sensitivity to an orally absorbed antimicrobial drug. Assuming no known allergies to sulfa-containing medications, trimethoprim-sulfamethoxazole would be an acceptable choice.

The use of rifampin alone in treating methicillin-resistant *Staphylococcus aureus* infections often leads to the development of organism resistance to this drug and is not recommended.

Repeating an antimicrobial regimen to eradicate this chronic bone-joint infection with retained hardware would unnecessarily expose the patient to the risks associated with lengthy parenteral antimicrobial treatment and would provide only a minimal chance of eradication of the infectious process.

Careful observation with symptomatic relief but no antimicrobial treatment would confer a risk for local extension of the septic process and possible systemic spread of the infection.

- In patients with prosthetic joint infection with no systemic or severe local signs of infection and in whom the prosthesis is not loose or surgery is not possible or desired, lifelong oral antimicrobial therapy may be considered to suppress the infection and retain usefulness of the total joint replacement.

Bibliography

Cobo J, Del Pozo JL. Prosthetic joint infection: diagnosis and management. Expert Rev Anti Infect Ther. 2011;9(9):787-80 [PMID: 21905787]

Item 8   Answer: C

Educational Objective: Identify infectious cause of hemorrhagic colitis.

The most likely pathogen is Shiga toxin–producing *Escherichia coli* (STEC). The presence of visible blood the stool is diagnostic of hemorrhagic colitis, and the STE strain *E. coli* O157:H7 is the most common cause of th condition in the United States. Both *E. coli* O157:H7 ar the newly described *E. coli* O104:H4 (which caused a larg outbreak of hemorrhagic gastroenteritis in Europe in 201 induce vascular damage by producing a Shiga toxin. Gro blood is found in stool samples in more than 60% patients with *E. coli* O157:H7 infection, and a history visible blood in the stool can be elicited in more than 90 of patients. STEC organisms are typically foodbor pathogens, and clusters or outbreaks of disease may develc in persons who have eaten contaminated foods. Other cli ical findings suggestive of STEC infection include abdor inal tenderness and leukocytosis. Fever is relatively uncor mon and develops in only one third of patients.

Bacillus cereus and *Staphylococcus aureus* are both assc ciated with foodborne gastrointestinal disease caused by preformed toxin. Therefore, symptoms occur less than 2 hours after ingestion rather than after several days as STEC infection and are characterized by nausea and vom iting rather than by diarrhea.

Campylobacter jejuni and *Yersinia enterocolitica* als cause foodborne gastroenteritis, but grossly bloody stoc are uncommon, and fever occurs in most patients.

- The presence of visible blood in the stool is diagnostic of hemorrhagic colitis, which in the United States is most often caused by Shiga toxin–producing *Escherichia coli*.

Bibliography

Guerrant RL, Van Gilder T, Steiner TS, et al; Infectious Diseases Soc ety of America. Practice guidelines for the management of infectio diarrhea. Clin Infect Dis. 2001;32(3):331-351. [PMI 11170940]

Item 9   Answer: B

Educational Objective: Treat shigellosis.

This patient has shigellosis, and even though her symptoms have resolved, she requires treatment with ciprofloxacin. *Shigella* organisms are extremely infectious even at a low inoculum, and outbreaks of disease in day care settings and nursing homes are well described. The spectrum of clinical disease ranges from a mild, self-limited gastrointestinal illness to dysentery associated with bloody diarrhea and fever. While culture results are pending, empiric therapy with ciprofloxacin is indicated for patients with severe symptoms who have a high clinical suspicion for shigellosis and also for those with milder disease such as the elderly, immunocompromised, and those working in food services and child care centers because treatment shortens the duration of fever, diarrhea, and shedding of the organism by about 48 hours. Otherwise, in patients with milder symptoms, obtaining culture results before beginning treatment is a reasonable approach. However, once a microbiologic diagnosis is established, treatment is generally indicated even if the illness has resolved to hasten clearance of fecal shedding of bacteria and reduce the risk of secondary spread to other persons. Use of a fluoroquinolone is appropriate because most *Shigella* organisms have not developed resistance to these agents. Treatment is usually for 3 days in immunocompetent individuals; conversion of stools to negative generally requires at least 48 hours of antibiotic treatment, and patients at high risk of spreading the disease should avoid exposure during that period.

Azithromycin is the recommended empiric therapy for *Campylobacter* infection because of the high rates of fluoroquinolone resistance in these organisms.

Metronidazole is not active against aerobic bacteria and is not effective therapy for *Shigella* infection.

KEY POINT

- **In a patient with shigellosis confirmed by microbiologic diagnosis, ciprofloxacin is indicated to hasten clearance of fecal shedding of bacteria and reduce the risk of secondary spread to other persons even if the illness has resolved.**

Bibliography

Guerrant RL, Van Gilder T, Steiner TS, et al; Infectious Diseases Society of America. Practice guidelines for the management of infectious diarrhea. Clin Infect Dis. 2001;32(3):331-351. [PMID: 11170940]

Item 10   Answer: A

Educational Objective: Manage a patient with bloodstream infection due to vancomycin-intermediate methicillin-resistant *Staphylococcus aureus*.

In this patient, vancomycin should be discontinued and daptomycin should be initiated. The causative pathogen is a vancomycin-intermediate *Staphylococcus aureus* (VISA), which has a minimal inhibitory concentration (MIC) of 4 micrograms/mL to vancomycin. Although vancomycin is a reasonable initial choice for empiric therapy for treating a possible methicillin-resistant *S. aureus* (MRSA) bloodstream infection, daptomycin is recommended as an alternative to vancomycin for treatment of bloodstream infection caused by vancomycin-intermediate *S. aureus*, particularly in patients treated with vancomycin who do not appear to be responding to treatment. Daptomycin is a bactericidal agent, which has been studied extensively for treatment of bloodstream infections due to *S. aureus*, including MRSA. Daptomycin retains activity against many strains of *S. aureus* with elevated MICs to vancomycin (≥ 2 micrograms/mL).

Linezolid has activity against *S. aureus* but is not indicated for the treatment of bloodstream infection.

Recently, trimethoprim-sulfamethoxazole has been used more frequently for treatment of MRSA skin infection, but it is not recommended as a primary agent for the treatment of bloodstream infection.

Because of the intermediate sensitivity of the identified organism to vancomycin, optimal pharmacodynamic targets may not be possible by increasing the vancomycin dose. To avoid treatment-related toxicity, the use of an alternative agent is preferred versus increasing the vancomycin dose.

KEY POINT

- **Daptomycin is recommended for treatment of bloodstream infections caused by methicillin-resistant *Staphylococcus aureus* when the minimal inhibitory concentration to vancomycin is more than 2 micrograms/mL.**

Bibliography

Liu C, Bayer A, Cosgrove SE, et al. Clinical practice guidelines by the Infectious Diseases Society of America for the treatment of methicillin-resistant *Staphylococcus aureus* infections in adults and children: executive summary. Clin Infect Dis. 2011;52(3):285-292. [PMID: 21217178]

Item 11   Answer: C

Educational Objective: Treat cervicitis.

The most appropriate treatment is ceftriaxone plus azithromycin. The findings on pelvic examination confirm that the patient's vaginal discharge is due to mucopurulent cervicitis, which is most commonly caused by *Neisseria gonorrhoeae* and *Chlamydia trachomatis* infection. The presence of leukocytes, an elevated pH level, and a negative whiff test are consistent with this diagnosis. The patient should be treated with a single-dose regimen that will provide coverage against the two most common pathogens. The preferred treatment of cervicitis is ceftriaxone, 250 mg intramuscularly in a single dose, plus azithromycin, 1 g orally in a single dose. Ceftriaxone provides coverage against *N. gonorrhoeae*, and azithromycin has activity against *C. trachomatis*. Reports of decreased susceptibility to cephalosporins have led to the recommendation that all infections (cervicitis, urethritis, pharyngitis, and proctitis) be treated with a 250-mg dose, rather than a 125-mg dose of ceftriaxone, as was recommended previously.

Cefixime is an alternative to ceftriaxone for the management of cervicitis or urethritis (although parenteral therapy with ceftriaxone is preferred); however, all patients should also be treated for possible chlamydial disease with a single dose of azithromycin or 7 days of doxycycline.

Fluoroquinolones such as ciprofloxacin are no longer recommended for treatment of the gonorrheal component of cervicitis because of the emergence of resistance to these agents.

The combination of cefoxitin (or cefotetan) plus doxycycline would be appropriate therapy for a patient with pelvic inflammatory disease. However, the absence of uterine, adnexal, and cervical motion tenderness in this patient makes such a diagnosis unlikely.

> **KEY POINT**
> - **The preferred treatment of cervicitis is ceftriaxone, 250 mg intramuscularly in a single dose, plus azithromycin, 1 g orally in a single dose.**

Bibliography

Centers for Disease Control and Prevention (CDC). Cephalosporin susceptibility among Neisseria gonorrhoeae isolates—United States, 2000-2010. MMWR Morb Mortal Wkly Rep. 2011;60(26):873-877. [PMID: 21734634]

Item 12   Answer: B

Educational Objective: Evaluate for *Mycobacterium tuberculosis* infection in a patient who received bacillus Calmette-Guérin cancer therapy.

In this physician who has a history of bladder cancer treated with bacillus Calmette-Guérin (BCG), tuberculosis screening using an interferon-γ release assay (IGRA) is preferred. Either an IGRA or a tuberculin skin test (TST) can be used to diagnose tuberculosis, although neither can distinguish between latent tuberculosis infection and active disease. However, an IGRA is preferred for two groups of patients: those who have received BCG as a vaccine or as cancer therapy and those who are unlikely to return for interpretation of the TST. Conversely, the TST is preferred for testing children who are younger than 5 years of age.

If the IGRA result is positive, active disease should be excluded by determining whether associated signs and symptoms are present (fever, chills, night sweats, weight loss, cough), obtaining a chest radiograph, and possibly obtaining microbiologic examination of sputum (or other involved fluids or tissues) when appropriate. When active disease has been ruled out, a diagnosis of latent tuberculosis infection is made.

A two-step tuberculin test is sometimes done patients who will be undergoing serial testing (such as physician) to establish a baseline result for future testin This is particularly useful in individuals with a remote exp sure to tuberculin antigens (BCG, previous infection, atypical mycobacterial infection) because their immu response to these antigens may have waned. The initial te "boosts" the immune response, possibly improving the re ability of the subsequent test. However, this test would n be desirable in this patient with recent BCG treatment.

> **KEY POINT**
> - **The interferon-γ release assay is preferred over the tuberculin skin test for tuberculosis screening when patients have received bacillus Calmette-Guérin either as a vaccine or as cancer therapy.**

Bibliography

Mazurek GH, Jereb J, Vernon A, et al; IGRA Expert Committee; Ce ters for Disease Control and Prevention (CDC). Updated guid lines for using interferon gamma release assays to detect Mycob terium tuberculosis infection - United States, 2010. MMW Recomm Rep. 2010;59(RR-5):1-25. [PMID: 20577159]

Item 13   Answer: B

Educational Objective: Manage a patient with a clenched-fist injury who is allergic to penicillin.

The most appropriate treatment is clindamycin and mo floxacin. This patient, who is allergic to penicillin, has clenched-fist injury to the left hand and requires imme ate prophylaxis with clindamycin and moxifloxaci Clenched-fist injuries result unintentionally when a pers punches the mouth of another person. Initial evaluati and management are similar to that for human and anim bites. Patients with clenched-fist injuries are at increas risk for infection involving deep structures, including te dons, joints, and bones. The Infectious Diseases Society America practice guidelines for skin and soft tissue infe tions recommend that all patients with human bite woun should receive prompt prophylaxis. Infection is caused human oral flora and typically involves a mixture of aerob organisms, including α-hemolytic streptococci, staphyl cocci, *Haemophilus* species, and *Eikenella corrodens*, a anaerobic organisms, many of which produce β-lactamas Although amoxicillin-clavulanate is an oral agent that pr vides such coverage, it should not be given to a patient wi a history of a hypersensitivity reaction to penicillin. Instea the combination of clindamycin and moxifloxacin provid the polymicrobial coverage needed for human bi wound–associated prophylaxis in patients with a type 1 lactam allergy. Moxifloxacin is effective against *E. corrode* and clindamycin is active against anaerobes, staphylococ and streptococci. Clindamycin is a pregnancy risk catego B drug and moxifloxacin a category C (risk cannot be rul out) drug.

Cephalexin is active against streptococci and staphylococci but not *E. corrodens* and gram-negative anaerobes. This agent also should not be given to a patient who has an IgE-mediated penicillin allergy.

This patient does not require tetanus immunization because she was vaccinated 4 years ago, and the vaccine is effective for 10 years.

Trimethoprim-sulfamethoxazole, which can be given to patients who are allergic to penicillin, provides good coverage for aerobic bacteria but has limited activity against anaerobes. Adding an anaerobic antimicrobial agent such as metronidazole to trimethoprim-sulfamethoxazole would provide adequate coverage.

Observation is inappropriate because patients with clenched-fist injuries are at high risk for developing an infection and require immediate antimicrobial prophylaxis.

KEY POINT

- **The combination of clindamycin and moxifloxacin is the recommended antimicrobial prophylactic regimen for a patient with a clenched-fist injury who is allergic to penicillin.**

Bibliography

Stevens DL, Bisno AL, Chambers HF, et al; Infectious Diseases Society of America. Practice guidelines for the diagnosis and management of skin and soft tissue infections. Clin Infect Dis. 2005;41(10):1373-1406. [PMID: 16231249]

Item 14   Answer: C

Educational Objective: Prevent varicella infection in a patient with leukemia.

This patient should receive varicella-zoster immune globulin (VZIG) if it can be procured. He is severely immunocompromised and at high risk for serious complications of varicella virus infection. However, the production of VZIG has been discontinued by the manufacturer, and an investigational varicella-zoster immune globulin product (VariZIG™) is available under a compassionate-use protocol. If a VZIG product cannot be obtained, the Centers for Disease Control and Prevention suggest the use of intravenous immune globulin. Susceptible persons who are immunocompromised or pregnant should receive a VZIG product or intravenous immune globulin within 96 hours of exposure, and this patient should be treated because his exposure was within this time frame. Patients who receive a VZIG preparation should be monitored for development of varicella for 28 days after exposure because the immune globulin may prolong the incubation period.

Treating immunocompromised persons with acyclovir for postexposure prophylaxis of varicella virus has not been studied; however, treatment of active varicella infection in this immunocompromised host is indicated.

The varicella vaccine is a live virus vaccine and is contraindicated for use in immunocompromised patients. However, because of the infection's association with high morbidity and the excellent efficacy of the vaccine, the vaccine is used in selected groups of immunocompromised persons such as those with leukemia who are in remission. Nonetheless, the varicella vaccine would not be an option for this patient with active leukemia under treatment.

Withholding treatment is not appropriate because the varicella virus causes significant morbidity and mortality in immunocompromised hosts.

KEY POINT

- **Varicella-zoster immune globulin (VZIG) or investigational VZIG (VariZIG™) or intravenous immune globulin (if a VZIG product is unavailable) should be used in immunocompromised or pregnant persons within 96 hours of exposure to the varicella virus to prevent infection.**

Bibliography

Fisher JP, Bate J, Hambleton S. Preventing varicella in children with malignancies: what is the evidence? Curr Opin Infect Dis. 2011;24(3):203-211. [PMID: 21455062]

Item 15   Answer: B

Educational Objective: Understand the goals of antimicrobial stewardship and de-escalation of empiric antimicrobial therapy in the clinical setting.

In this patient, piperacillin-tazobactam should be discontinued and ampicillin begun. The primary reason for this recommendation is to reduce the likelihood of induction of resistance to broad-spectrum antibiotics used in empiric therapy. The early use of aggressive antibiotic treatment is widely accepted for critically ill patients before confirmation of a specific diagnosis. In this patient, treatment with a broad-spectrum antibiotic with activity against the likely infecting organism identified in the urine by the presence of gram-negative rods was indicated. However, once a specific organism is isolated and its sensitivities to available antibiotics known, it is beneficial to focus or "de-escalate" therapy to avoid the selection of organisms resistant to currently effective broad-spectrum antibiotics. Willingness to de-escalate therapy can be challenging in a patient who has responded well to broad-spectrum antibiotic coverage. However, failure to curtail excess antibiotic use is an ecologic hazard for the patient and the medical unit as a whole. Ampicillin is a narrow-spectrum agent with activity against this infectious pathogen and is a good choice for de-escalation.

Nitrofurantoin is also a narrow-spectrum agent but is not significantly absorbed into the bloodstream and thus would not be an appropriate therapeutic choice for bloodstream infection.

Piperacillin-tazobactam, imipenem, and ciprofloxacin are each active against this infectious pathogen but provide unnecessarily broad-spectrum coverage, which can promote the emergence of antimicrobial resistance.

- Antimicrobial stewardship is a growing quality-based movement focused on optimizing antimicrobial prescribing and limiting unnecessary prescribing.

Bibliography

Dellit TH, Owens RC, McGowan JE Jr, et al. Infectious Diseases Society of America; Society for Healthcare Epidemiology of America. Infectious Diseases Society of America and the Society for Healthcare Epidemiology of America guidelines for developing an institutional program to enhance antimicrobial stewardship. Clin Infect Dis. 2007;44(2):159-177. [PMID: 17173212]

Item 16   Answer: D

Educational Objective: Diagnose *Vibrio vulnificus*–associated necrotizing fasciitis.

This patient most likely has necrotizing fasciitis secondary to *Vibrio vulnificus* infection. He has hemochromatosis with evidence of portal hypertension (ascites). *V. vulnificus* infection should always be considered in a patient with liver disease who presents with sepsis and cutaneous manifestations of hemorrhagic bullae after possible exposure to this waterborne, gram-negative rod. Increased iron availability has been shown to enhance the virulence and growth of *V. vulnificus*, which perhaps explains why patients with hemochromatosis are more likely to develop infection in addition to their having the decreased opsonization and serum bactericidal activity found in patients with liver disease. Septicemia occurs after ingestion of raw or undercooked shellfish, usually oysters. Patients may also develop wound-associated *V. vulnificus* infection when the pathogen is inoculated through traumatized skin. This organism thrives in warm brackish or salt water, such as the Gulf of Mexico, and most infections occur during the summer months, when seawater temperatures facilitate its growth.

Babesia microti is the pathogen responsible for babesiosis, a tick-associated infection that occurs in the coastal northeastern and upper midwestern United States. Flu-like symptoms develop about 1 week after tick exposure, and the diagnosis is typically established by evaluation of a peripheral blood smear that shows intraerythrocytic parasites. Rash is not a typical feature of babesiosis. Patients with decreased splenic function are more likely to develop serious complications.

Capnocytophaga canimorsus is a gram-negative rod that can cause cellulitis and overwhelming sepsis in patients with decreased splenic function who have been bitten by a dog or cat.

Rickettsia rickettsii is a tick-associated pathogen responsible for Rocky Mountain spotted fever (RMSF). Although liver chemistry studies can be abnormal in patients with both RMSF and *V. vulnificus* infection, the rash in RMSF characteristically begins on the palms, soles, wrists, and ankles before moving centripetally to involve the trunk. The rash is initially maculopapular but eventually becomes petechial. Aseptic meningitis may also develop. RMSF is unlikely in this patient with hemorrhagic bullae.

- Patients with liver disease are at increased risk for developing necrotizing fasciitis secondary to *Vibrio vulnificus* infection after eating raw or undercooked shellfish or following exposure of traumatized skin to contaminated sea water.

Bibliography

Bross MH, Soch K, Morales R, Mitchell RB. Vibrio vulnificus infection: diagnosis and treatment. Am Fam Physician. 2007;76(4):53 544. [PMID: 17853628]

Item 17   Answer: C

Educational Objective: Manage a health care provider with exposure to suspected smallpox.

The most appropriate intervention for this patient's nur is smallpox vaccine. This patient most likely has active small pox (variola) infection, to which his nurse has likely experienced unprotected respiratory exposure. Smallpox infecti is initially asymptomatic, with respiratory tract infection an viremia occurring during a 7- to 17-day incubation perio High fever, headache, vomiting, and backache follow, lasting 2 to 4 days. The smallpox rash first appears on the buccal and pharyngeal mucosa and most often spreads to the hands and face before spreading to the trunk, arms, leg and feet. The centrifugally distributed skin lesions evolve synchronously (same stage of maturation on any one are of the body) from macules to papules to vesicles to pustul and eventually become crusted. Patients remain contagiou until all scabs and crusts are shed. Presumably, the soldier infection was acquired through exposure to an intention spread of smallpox virus through an act of bioterroris because smallpox was eradicated in 1979, and no know naturally occurring case has been reported in more than decades. Vaccination with the live virus preparation, va cinia, made from a distinct and separate related pox viru provides immunity to smallpox. When given within 3 da of exposure, this active vaccine can prevent or significant lessen the severity of smallpox symptoms in most peop and is indicated in all exposed persons.

Chickenpox is the viral exanthem infection most like to be confused with smallpox. The varicella-zoster vir infection differs from smallpox in the former's centripet mode of rash distribution, which is most concentrated the torso, with fewest lesions on the hands and feet, as we as the presence of various stages of lesions (papules, vesicle and crusts) existing simultaneously. Acyclovir is not a appropriate prophylactic agent for either chickenpox smallpox.

Cidofovir, an intravenous antiviral agent demonstrating in vitro antiviral activity against the smallpox virus, m theoretically be clinically useful in the event of a widesprea

allpox outbreak or to treat severe vaccine-related reac-
ns; however, it currently is not indicated to prevent or
at smallpox.

Considering the patient's signs and symptoms and
tential occupational exposure to smallpox through an act
bioterrorism, providing no intervention to his nurse,
o was exposed to this patient within the past few days,
uld not be prudent.

EY POINT

- Vaccination with the live virus preparation, vaccinia, provides immunity to smallpox, and,
  when given within 3 days of exposure, can prevent or significantly lessen the severity of smallpox symptoms in most people.

bliography

haroy R, Panzik R, Noviasky JA, et al. Smallpox: clinical features,
  prevention, and management. Ann Pharmacother.
  2004;38(3):440-447. [PMID: 14755066]

em 18   Answer: D

lucational Objective: Diagnose tacrolimus
phrotoxicity in a patient following kidney
insplantation.

is patient has tacrolimus toxicity resulting in acute kid-
y injury. The most common manifestation of tacrolimus
phrotoxicity is an acute increase in the serum creatinine
d blood urea nitrogen levels; other manifestations of
phropathy include tubular disorders and a hemolytic-ure-
c syndrome. Patients may also have hypertension, neu-
oxicity, and metabolic abnormalities, including hyper-
cemia, hyperkalemia, and hypomagnesemia. Many of the
munosuppressive agents are associated with significant
g interactions. Interactions affecting drug metabolism
cur when cyclosporine, tacrolimus, or sirolimus is com-
ned with macrolide antibiotics or azole antifungal agents,
e interaction of which results in increased levels of one or
th drugs. Tacrolimus metabolism by hepatic cytochrome
450 enzymes is significantly inhibited by the macrolide
ibiotic clarithromycin, and the interaction between these
o agents leads to several-fold increases in tacrolimus lev-
, resulting in toxicity. If a macrolide antibiotic must be
ed in a transplant recipient, azithromycin, which is not a
nificant inhibitor of the cytochrome P-450 enzyme sys-
n, should be chosen.

The most common side effects of mycophenolate
ofetil are gastrointestinal (nausea, diarrhea, and cramp-
g) and bone marrow suppression but not acute kidney
ury. Antibiotics have no effect on mycophenolate mofetil
g levels.

Acute interstitial nephritis is most commonly caused by
hypersensitivity reaction to a medication and may mani-
t as fever, rash, and eosinophilia. Urine findings may
lude leukocyte casts, eosinophils, and a urine protein-
atinine ratio usually less than 2.5 mg/mg. There are no

findings to suggest acute interstitial nephritis in this patient,
and clarithromycin is an exceedingly rare cause of drug-
induced interstitial nephritis.

Organ rejection could cause acute kidney injury; however, this patient's condition has been stable, with no medical problems for 7 months following transplantation.
Therefore, her current symptoms and findings are more
likely attributable to toxicity from a known drug interaction
between clarithromycin and tacrolimus than rejection.

KEY POINT

- Drug toxicity can occur when cyclosporine,
  tacrolimus, or sirolimus is combined with
  macrolide antibiotics or azole antifungal agents.

Bibliography

Spriet I, Meersseman W, de Hoon J, von Winckelmann S, Wilmer A,
  Willems L. Mini-series: II. Clinical aspects. Clinically relevant
  CYP450-mediated drug interactions in the ICU. Intensive Care
  Med. 2009;35(4):603-612. [PMID: 19132344]

Item 19   Answer: D

Educational Objective: Diagnose West Nile virus
myelitis.

This patient presents with the acute onset of asymmetric
flaccid paralysis consistent with West Nile virus (WNV)
myelitis, and a WNV IgM antibody assay should be performed to confirm the diagnosis. WNV has been identified
as an important cause of encephalitis throughout the continental United States. Birds are the main reservoir of this
virus in nature. Several species of mosquitoes can acquire
the virus after biting a bird with high-level viremia and
transmit the infection to humans. A poliomyelitis-like syndrome has been described in as many as 12% of patients
with WNV neuroinvasive disease. Neuromuscular symptoms range in severity from mild unilateral weakness to
quadriplegia with respiratory failure. WNV myelitis may
occur in isolation or may be part of an overlap syndrome
with encephalitis or meningitis. WNV IgM antibody is
detectable in the cerebrospinal fluid (CSF) in greater than
90% of patients with WNV neuroinvasive disease at the time
of presentation. Because WNV viremia is of brief duration,
CSF viral cultures are positive in less than 10% of patients,
and results of WNV polymerase chain reaction are positive
in less than 60% of patients.

Cytomegalovirus may cause a polyradiculopathy, but
this occurs almost exclusively in patients with advanced
HIV infection and is characterized by sensory loss and urinary retention.

Although ehrlichiosis may cause a febrile illness that is
variably associated with meningoencephalitis, this infection
is not associated with focal paralysis.

Neurologic manifestations of *Borrelia burgdorferi*, the
causative agent of Lyme disease, typically occur more than
a month after infection. Early disseminated Lyme disease
may present as aseptic meningitis, cranial neuropathy, or

CONT.

radiculopathy. Encephalopathy or encephalomyelitis has been reported in late disease.

> **KEY POINT**
>
> - **West Nile virus (WNV) IgM antibody is detectable in the cerebrospinal fluid in greater than 90% of patients with WNV neuroinvasive disease at the time of presentation.**

Bibliography

Sejvar JJ, Bode AV, Marfin AA, et al. West Nile virus-associated flaccid paralysis. Emerg Infect Dis. 2005;11(7):1021-1027. [PMID: 16022775]

Item 20   Answer: C

Educational Objective: Diagnose *Mycobacterium avium* complex lung disease.

This patient requires a repeat acid-fast bacilli smear and culture before treatment is initiated. Nontuberculous mycobacteria (NTM), also referred to as atypical mycobacteria, when acting as invasive pathogens most often involve the lungs. Because NTM species are readily recovered from the environment (especially tap water and soil), when they are isolated from nonsterile human sites, results must be interpreted within the context of the patient's clinical syndrome to avoid treating for colonization alone. *Mycobacterium avium* complex (MAC) is the most frequently recognized NTM causing pulmonary disease and develops after inhalation of the organism. Although the classic presentation of pulmonary MAC disease is a subacute to chronic illness occurring in persons with a history of underlying pulmonary disease, MAC has also been increasingly recognized in middle-aged to elderly women with no pre-existing lung disease. The more indolent clinical course in this latter group of patients consists mainly of chronic cough. Systemic symptoms are generally absent. Discrete pulmonary nodules best visualized on CT scan of the lungs are very commonly found.

Because of the significant frequency of positive sputum cultures for MAC in persons without active disease, it is often difficult to differentiate colonization from actual active lung disease. The isolation of MAC from a single sputum culture has a low predictive value and therefore is not proof of infection with NTM. To avoid unnecessary, lengthy, multidrug antimicrobial therapy, clinicians can follow specific diagnostic criteria to define a clinical case of MAC lung disease. Along with her symptoms and chest CT scan abnormalities, this patient would require a second positive MAC sputum culture obtained through a routine sputum culture, a bronchial wash or lavage, or a histopathologic specimen for a diagnosis to be established. Because the patient is clinically stable, isolating the organism from a second sputum sample would be the least-invasive and lowest-risk method for confirming the diagnosis. If a repeat culture were negative for MAC, then more aggressive interventions, such as bronchoalveolar lavage or lung biopsy, to

assess for the presence of the infection or other poten causes of her symptoms would be indicated.

Initiating treatment before confirming the diagn would be premature.

Instituting no further evaluation would not be prud given the potential significance of her clinical sympto and radiographic findings.

> **KEY POINT**
>
> - ***Mycobacteria avium* complex infection occurs frequently in middle-aged to elderly women with no preexisting lung disease and most ofte consists of chronic cough, the absence of systemic symptoms, and discrete pulmonary nodules commonly located in the middle lobe or lingular areas and best visualized by CT.**

Bibliography

Kasperbauer SH, Daley CL. Diagnosis and treatment of infections to Mycobacterium avium complex. Semin Respir Crit Care M 2008;29(5):569-576. [PMID: 18810690]

Item 21   Answer: A

Educational Objective: Diagnose cryptococcal meningitis in a patient with HIV infection and immune reconstitution inflammatory syndrome.

The most likely diagnosis is *Cryptococcus neoformans* in tion. This patient with AIDS has developed symptoms meningitis after initiation of antiretroviral treatment, wh is consistent with immune reconstitution inflammatory s drome (IRIS), most likely from cryptococcal mening With the initiation of combination antiretroviral thera viral load levels decrease sharply, CD4 cell counts incre and immune responses improve. In the presence of opportunistic infection, which may not have been clinic recognized previously, this process can lead to drama inflammatory responses as the newly revived immune tem reacts to high burdens of antigens. IRIS usually occ a few weeks to a few months after initiation of antiretro rals in the setting of various opportunistic infections, m commonly mycobacterial or disseminated fungal in tions, including cryptococcal meningitis. This patie prolonged duration of symptoms, including headac mental status changes, and cranial nerve involvement, typical of cryptococcal meningitis as are the lumbar pu ture results showing evidence of inflammation. Fungal tures of cerebrospinal fluid may eventually grow the org ism, but results of cryptococcal serum or cerebrospinal f antigen testing will be available more quickly and hav sensitivity of more than 95%. Acute treatment consist intravenous amphotericin B followed by long-term oral conazole, with special attention to management increased intracranial pressure.

Cytomegalovirus infection can cause encephalitis, it is much less common, especially in patients with CD4 unts greater than 100/microliter; the MRI would also ely show periventricular involvement.

Histoplasmosis is caused by *Histoplasma capsulatum*, thermal dimorphic fungus endemic to the midwestern tes of the Ohio and Mississippi river valleys. Patients may ve acute or chronic pulmonary disease, and immuno-mpromised patients, especially, may present with dissem-ated disease. Central nervous system involvement can cur, but usually as part of obvious dissemination includ-g pulmonary disease, which is not consistent with this tient's presentation.

Toxoplasmosis can cause encephalitis in patients with DS, usually in those with CD4 cell counts less than 0/microliter and headache, mental status changes, and cal deficits. But the MRI findings in affected patients uld show the characteristic multiple ring-enhancing ions of the toxoplasmic abscesses, which are not present this patient.

EY POINT

- In patients with HIV infection, immune recon-stitution inflammatory syndrome can occur a few weeks to a few months after initiation of antiretroviral therapy and results in a dramatic inflammatory response to opportunistic infections.

bliography
endre SL, Ellis RJ, Everall I, Ances B, Bharti A, McCutchan JA. Neurologic complications of HIV disease and their treatment. Top HIV Med. 2009;17(2):46-56. [PMID: 19401607]

em 22   Answer: D

ucational Objective: Diagnose aseptic menin-cis caused by herpes simplex virus type 2 infection.

is patient's clinical illness and cerebrospinal fluid (CSF) dings are most consistent with aseptic meningitis caused herpes simplex virus (HSV). Aseptic meningitis is fined as meningeal inflammation without a known bac-ial or fungal cause. Most cases are caused by viruses, hough aseptic meningitis may also be associated with dif-ult-to-identify infectious agents, inflammation triggered medications, malignancy, and other systemic inflamma-ry conditions. Although HSV-1 is typically associated th encephalitis, overt viral meningitis is much more com-on with HSV-2. The genital lesions of HSV-2 usually pre-de or accompany the onset of meningitis.

Typical CSF findings of acute bacterial meningitis clude a leukocyte count of 1000 to 5000/microliter 000 to 5000 × 10⁶/L), a predominance of neutrophils, glucose level of less than or equal to 40 mg/dL (2.2 nol/L), a CSF-to-plasma glucose ratio of less than or ual to 0.4, and Gram stain positivity of 60% to 90%.

The differential diagnosis of HSV aseptic meningitis cludes illnesses with concurrent genital or perineal ulcer-ons and central nervous system involvement, such as

other viral causes, Behçet disease, porphyria, collagen vas-cular diseases, and inflammatory bowel disease. Patients with Behçet disease have recurrent painful oral and genital aphthous ulcerations, skin lesions, and uveitis; this disease is relatively rare in the United States. Neurologic manifes-tations are seen in up to 25% of patients. When Behçet dis-ease causes aseptic meningitis, the level of pleocytosis is usu-ally less than 100 cells/microliter. Additionally, the lack of history or findings of other manifestations of this uncom-mon condition makes this an unlikely diagnosis.

Acute retroviral infection may present with a syndrome characterized by fatigue, fever, pharyngitis, and lym-phadenopathy. A small percentage of patients may have central nervous system involvement, including meningitis. The rash associated with acute HIV infection tends to be a diffuse, maculopapular eruption across the chest, back, face, and upper extremities; it may affect the palms and soles and is generally not painful or pruritic. Although it should be considered that this patient is at risk for acute HIV infec-tion, her presentation is less consistent with this diagnosis.

KEY POINT

- Aseptic meningitis is commonly associated with genital infection from herpes simplex virus 2 and is characterized by recurrent episodes of fever, headache, vomiting, and photosensitivity.

Bibliography
Davis LE. Acute and recurrent viral meningitis. Curr Treat Options Neurol. 2008;10(3):168-177. [PMID: 18579020]

Item 23   Answer: C

Educational Objective: Manage a patient with an erythema migrans skin lesion.

The skin lesion shown is consistent with erythema migrans, and oral doxycycline should be started immediately. Ery-thema migrans may be due to either early localized Lyme disease or Southern tick–associated rash illness. Although these two infections are caused by specific tick vectors with relatively distinct geographic distributions, both ticks are endemic to Virginia. Geographic location is therefore of lit-tle value in differentiating between these two syndromes in this patient. However, empiric doxycycline is the recom-mended treatment for erythema migrans regardless of the cause. Treatment should be given based on the clinical find-ing of an expansile, target-like skin lesion, particularly at the site of a known tick attachment.

Borrelia burgdorferi polymerase chain reaction testing is not indicated. Although *B. burgdorferi* may be amplified from erythema migrans skin biopsy specimens if the diag-nosis is uncertain, this study is generally not needed because the presence of the characteristic erythema migrans rash, such as is seen in this patient, dictates treatment.

Intravenous ceftriaxone is reserved for patients with cardiac or neurologic manifestations of disseminated Lyme disease.

Serologic testing for *B. burgdorferi* is not recommended because false-negative antibody assay results may occur in patients with early localized Lyme disease and would be negative in patients with Southern tick–associated rash illness.

KEY POINT

- Empiric oral doxycycline is the recommended treatment for erythema migrans regardless of the cause.

Bibliography

Stonehouse A, Studdiford JS, Henry CA. An update on the diagnosis and treatment of early Lyme disease: "focusing on the bull's eye, you may miss the mark". J Emerg Med. 2010;39(5):e147-151. [PMID: 17945460]

Item 24   Answer: C

Educational Objective: Diagnose herpes simplex virus type 2–induced benign recurrent lymphocytic meningitis.

This patient most likely has benign recurrent lymphocytic meningitis, and the most appropriate study to confirm the diagnosis is cerebrospinal fluid (CSF) polymerase chain reaction for herpes simplex virus type 2 (HSV-2). Benign recurrent lymphocytic meningitis, formerly known as Mollaret meningitis, is most often caused by HSV-2, although some cases have been associated with HSV-1 and Epstein-Barr virus. Patients usually experience 2 to 3 to at least 10 episodes of meningitis (most often characterized by headache, fever, and stiff neck) that last for 2 to 5 days and are followed by spontaneous recovery. About 50% of patients may also have transient neurologic manifestations, such as seizures, hallucinations, diplopia, cranial nerve palsies, or an altered level of consciousness. Disease occurs in patients without symptoms or signs of genital or cutaneous infection. Nucleic acid amplification tests, such as CSF polymerase chain reaction to detect the DNA of HSV-2, will establish the diagnosis. Patients usually recover without therapy; it is not clear whether antiviral agents alter the course of mild infection.

Given the recurrent nature of this patient's illness, it is unlikely to be caused by a malignancy. Cytologic studies are therefore unnecessary at this time. Cytology may reveal Mollaret cells, which are large atypical monocytes, but they are not seen in all cases, and their presence does not establish the etiologic diagnosis.

The recurrent episodes that this patient has experienced also make West Nile virus infection unlikely.

MRI of the brain would be appropriate if the patient had the clinical presentation of encephalitis (fever, hemicranial headache, language and behavioral abnormalities, memory impairment, cranial nerve deficits, and seizures), which is most often caused by HSV-1 rather than HSV-2.

KEY POINT

- Herpes simplex virus type 2 is the most common cause of benign recurrent lymphocytic meningitis, and the diagnosis is established by cerebrospinal fluid polymerase chain reaction.

Bibliography

Shalabi M, Whitley RJ. Recurrent benign lymphocytic meningitis. Infect Dis. 2006;43(9):1194-1197. [PMID: 17029141]

Item 25   Answer: A

Educational Objective: Treat cryptococcal meningitis in a patient with AIDS.

This patient should be treated with conventional amphotericin B and flucytosine. He has AIDS and disseminated cryptococcosis, including cryptococcal meningitis. Headache and alterations in mental status are the most common symptoms. The skin lesions, which are molluscum-like, are characteristic of disseminated cryptococcosis. The cerebrospinal fluid (CSF) profile, including the paucity of leukocytes, is consistent with cryptococcal meningitis in the setting of AIDS. Control of CSF pressure is crucial to a successful outcome in patients with cryptococcal meningoencephalitis. If the CSF pressure is greater than or equal to 250 mm H₂O and there are symptoms of increased intracranial pressure, the pressure should be relieved by CSF drainage. The treatment of cryptococcal meningoencephalitis in HIV-infected patients consists of three stages: (1) induction, (2) consolidation, and (3) maintenance (suppression). The induction therapy of choice in patients with normal kidney function is conventional amphotericin B plus flucytosine for at least 2 weeks. The 2-week induction course is followed by oral fluconazole for a minimum of 8 weeks. Lipid formulations of amphotericin B are reserved for those with or predisposed to kidney dysfunction.

Echinocandins such as caspofungin have no role in the treatment of cryptococcal meningoencephalitis because they lack activity against cryptococci and have poor penetration into the CSF.

Other regimens for induction therapy in patients with cryptococcal meningoencephalitis include amphotericin B plus fluconazole, high-dose fluconazole plus flucytosine, high-dose fluconazole alone, and itraconazole alone, although itraconazole is discouraged because of poor penetration into the CSF.

KEY POINT

- Conventional amphotericin B plus flucytosine is the preferred treatment for cryptococcal meningitis in a patient with AIDS.

Bibliography

Perfect JR, Dismukes WE, Dromer F, et al. Clinical practice guidelines for the management of cryptococcal diseases: 2010 update by the Infectious Diseases Society of America. Clin Infect Dis. 2010;50(3):291-322. [PMID: 20047480]

Item 26   Answer: C

Educational Objective: Treat pelvic inflammatory disease in an outpatient.

This patient has pelvic inflammatory disease (PID) and requires a single dose of parenteral ceftriaxone followed by 14 days of oral doxycycline. This regimen may be given with or without oral metronidazole. The patient has evidence of cervicitis; however, the presence of uterine tenderness should prompt a diagnosis of PID. The clinical diagnosis of PID is imprecise. Because of the potential serious sequelae of untreated PID, including tubal scarring that can lead to infertility, ectopic pregnancy, and chronic pelvic pain syndromes, an approach using a very low threshold for diagnosis is recommended. The Centers for Disease Control and Prevention (CDC) guidelines recommend that women who present with abdominal or pelvic pain and have cervical motion tenderness, adnexal tenderness, or uterine tenderness be treated for PID. This infection is always considered to be polymicrobial. Antimicrobial regimens for PID must include coverage of *Neisseria gonorrhoeae*, *Chlamydia trachomatis*, aerobic gram-negative rods, and anaerobes that may be found in the vaginal flora. Early follow up (within 72 hours) must be arranged, and hospitalization is required for patients who do not respond to treatment with oral therapy or who cannot take oral therapy owing to nausea and vomiting. Male partners of women with PID who have had sexual contact in the past 60 days should be referred for evaluation and treatment.

The combination of clindamycin and gentamicin is an acceptable parenteral treatment for PID. However, this patient does not have signs of systemic toxicity, so outpatient treatment is appropriate.

Ciprofloxacin can no longer be used for the treatment of infections that may be due to *N. gonorrhoeae* because of increasing fluoroquinolone resistance.

Single-dose intramuscular ceftriaxone plus single-dose oral azithromycin is appropriate management for cervicitis, but single-dose therapy would not be sufficient for the treatment of PID.

KEY POINT

- Women with abdominal or pelvic pain and cervical motion tenderness, adnexal tenderness, or uterine tenderness who can tolerate outpatient therapy should be treated for pelvic inflammatory disease, with single-dose intramuscular ceftriaxone and oral doxycycline for 14 days.

Bibliography

Workowski KA, Berman S; Centers for Disease Control and Prevention (CDC). Sexually transmitted diseases treatment guidelines, 2010. MMWR Recomm Rep. 2010;59(RR-12):1-110. [PMID: 21160459]

Item 27   Answer: A

Educational Objective: Diagnose genital herpes simplex virus infection.

The most appropriate diagnostic test to perform next is herpes simplex virus (HSV) polymerase chain reaction (PCR) assay of the fissure. The patient has a history of recurrent genital symptoms consisting of itching and burning, which is a very characteristic prodrome of recurrent genital HSV infection. Although the patient reports no history of genital lesions, serologic surveys have shown that most patients with serologic evidence of HSV-2 infection do not have a history of symptomatic genital ulcer disease. The presence of a fissure is well described as an atypical presentation of genital HSV-2 infection. PCR is the most sensitive diagnostic methodology for confirming that the lesion is due to HSV; alternatively, a viral culture can be obtained. Viral cultures are less expensive than HSV PCR but are less sensitive.

Lymphogranuloma venereum (LGV) is a genital ulcer disease caused by the L1, L2, and L3 serovars of *Chlamydia trachomatis*. Classic LGV presents as a painless papule or ulcer at the site of inoculation that resolves without treatment and is followed by painful unilateral inguinal lymphadenopathy accompanied by fever and malaise. This patient's symptoms are not compatible with LGV, and serologic testing for this infection is not indicated.

A Tzanck smear for HSV is limited by low sensitivity and specificity and is only helpful when results are positive.

Patients with candidal vulvovaginitis may have vaginal pruritus and burning associated with fissures, but evidence of vaginal discharge and small erythematous papular lesions (satellite lesions) should be visible, peripheral to the involved area. Consequently, wet mount of vaginal secretions with the addition of potassium hydroxide is not necessary.

KEY POINT

- Polymerase chain reaction is the most sensitive and specific diagnostic test for confirming a diagnosis of herpes simplex virus infection.

Bibliography

Van Wagoner NJ, Hook EW 3rd. Herpes diagnostic tests and their use. Curr Infect Dis Rep. 2012;14(2):175-184. [PMID: 22311664]

Item 28   Answer: D

Educational Objective: Diagnose primary syphilis.

This patient's clinical presentation and examination findings are most consistent with a syphilitic chancre. Chancres are most frequently single lesions, but multiple lesions can occur, and the lesions are generally painless. The ulcer's border is raised and has a firm, cartilaginous consistency. The incidence of primary and secondary syphilis in the United States has increased among certain populations, especially young men who have sex with men, particularly those who are members of racial and ethnic minorities. A recent epidemiologic study from New York City found that men who have sex with men are at a 140-fold higher risk of newly diagnosed syphilis compared with heterosexual men. Factors such as drug use and the perception that unprotected oral sex is "safer" than anal intercourse are believed to be contributing to this increase. Because the methodology needed to demonstrate *Treponema pallidum* organisms in clinical specimens is not available in most settings, the clinical diagnosis can be confirmed by serologic testing; however, the serum rapid plasma reagin titer is frequently negative in primary syphilis. This patient should be offered HIV testing, screening for gonorrhea and chlamydia infection, and risk reduction counseling. In addition to syphilis, the differential diagnosis of genital ulcer disease includes chancroid and herpes simplex virus infection. Bacterial secondary infection of traumatic genital lesions can also have the appearance of an ulcer.

Chancroid causes single or multiple painful ulcers with a ragged border; the ulcer's base has a granulomatous appearance, frequently with a purulent exudate. This patient does not have chancroid.

Herpes simplex virus infection generally presents with multiple painful ulcers that were initially vesicular on an erythematous base.

Human papillomavirus infection causes genital warts, not ulcerative lesions.

KEY POINT

- Syphilitic chancres are most frequently single, painless lesions, with a raised border and a firm cartilaginous consistency; multiple lesions can also occur.

Bibliography

Su JR, Beltrami JF, Zaidi AA, Weinstock HS. Primary and secondary syphilis among black and Hispanic men who have sex with men: case report data from 27 States. Ann Intern Med. 2011;155(3):145-151. [PMID: 21810707]

Item 29   Answer: D

Educational Objective: Diagnose disseminated gonococcal infection.

The most appropriate next step in diagnosis is a nucleic acid amplification urine test for *Neisseria gonorrhoeae*. This is a noninvasive, sensitive test for diagnosing gonorrhea in men that provides rapid results (within hours) and can help guide therapy pending return of blood and synovial fluid culture results. Mucosal cultures, including of the throat, anus, urethra, or cervix, may also be helpful in establishing the diagnosis because they tend to have a higher diagnostic yield than blood and synovial fluid cultures in patients with disseminated gonococcal infection (DGI).

Although this young patient may have an autoimmune inflammatory arthritis such as systemic lupus erythematosus

or rheumatoid arthritis, he has evidence of an arthritis-d matitis syndrome and should be evaluated for DGI. In co trast to nongonococcal septic arthritis, patients with D present with migratory joint symptoms and often ha involvement of several joints with tenosynovitis rather th involvement of just a single joint. Asymmetric joint involv ment helps distinguish DGI from autoimmune disease–ass ciated polyarthritis, which is typically symmetric. Skin lesic are found in more than 75% of patients with DGI but m be few in number; consequently, a careful examination the skin must be performed. Lesions are most likely to found on the extremities. The classic lesion is characteriz by a small number of necrotic vesicopustules on an eryth matous base. Organisms are rarely cultured from the sk lesions of DGI, although they may be demonstrat through nucleic acid amplification techniques.

The prevalence of HLA B27 in patients with reacti arthritis is only 50%; consequently, HLA B27 testing is n very useful in establishing a diagnosis. In addition, reacti arthritis tends to present as a symmetric oligoarthritis, a this patient's arthritis is asymmetric. The associated ra keratoderma blennorrhagica, consists of hyperkerato lesions on the palms and soles, which are not present in t patient. Patients with reactive arthritis may also have co junctivitis, urethritis, oral ulcers, and circinate balanitis.

KEY POINT

- To confirm a presumptive diagnosis of disseminated gonococcal infection, in addition to blood and synovial fluid cultures, specimens should be obtained from mucosal surfaces, including the throat, anus, and urethra, or cervix, which can be tested via nucleic acid amplification tests or culture.

Bibliography

García-De La Torre I, Nava-Zavala A. Gonococcal and nongonoc cal arthritis. Rheum Dis Clin North Am. 2009;35(1):63-[PMID: 19480997]

Item 30   Answer: D

Educational Objective: Manage mild pneumoni. caused by *Histoplasma capsulatum* in a healthy host.

This patient has mild pulmonary histoplasmosis, which self-limiting and requires no treatment in a healthy host. those who become ill, the incubation period is 7 to 21 da and most have symptoms by day 14. Histoplasmosis is co mon in states bordering the Ohio river valley and the low Mississippi river. Infection may be asymptomatic, but t diagnosis should be considered in any patient with pu monary and systemic symptoms following potential exp sure in a geographically endemic area. In most symptoma patients, disease is mild and resolves without therapy with 1 month. In a few patients, particularly those wi immunocompromise (such as HIV infection) or other co current illnesses, severe pneumonia with respiratory failu

y result. Histoplasmosis may also cause chronic infec-
n, including pulmonary and mediastinal masses, cavitary
ons, central nervous system involvement, pericarditis,
d arthritis and arthralgia. Antifungal treatment is indi-
ed for severe or moderately severe acute pulmonary,
onic pulmonary, disseminated, and central nervous sys-
n histoplasmosis or for those patients whose symptoms
not improve within 1 month. Evidence of effectiveness,
wever, is lacking to support this recommendation.

If treatment is indicated for acute pulmonary histo-
smosis, the treatment of choice is itraconazole. Lipid for-
lations of amphotericin B are indicated for more severe
ms of pulmonary histoplasmosis. Fluconazole has been
ed for treatment of histoplasmosis, but it is less effective
n itraconazole. Fluconazole resistance has also been
ted in some patients who have not responded to therapy.

EY POINT

- Mild forms of histoplasmosis do not require
  treatment, whereas more severe forms may be
  treated with amphotericin B or one of the
  newer triazole antifungal agents.

bliography

eat LJ, Freifeld AG, Kleiman MB, et al; Infectious Diseases Society of America. Clinical practice guidelines for the management of
patients with histoplasmosis: 2007 update by the Infectious Diseases
Society of America. Clin Infect Dis. 2007;45(7):807-825. [PMID:
17806045]

em 31   Answer: B

ducational Objective: Prevent catheter-associ-
ed urinary tract infection.

is patient's urine-collecting bag should be maintained
low the level of the bladder to avoid catheter-associated
nary tract infection (CAUTI). The most effective way to
event UTIs is to decrease catheter use. Devices should be
ed for specific indications. Examples include (1) to diag-
se pathologic findings in the lower urinary tract or the
use of urinary retention, (2) to monitor fluid status in
utely ill patients when this directly impacts medical treat-
nt, and (3) to manage patients with stage 3 or 4 pressure
ers on the buttocks. However, urinary catheters often
e used for convenience, which significantly increases the
k of UTIs. If the catheter is needed, measures are
quired to decrease the risk of bacteriuria and subsequent
ection. These include hand washing, using an aseptic
chnique and sterile equipment for catheter insertion and
re, securing the catheter properly, and maintaining unob-
ucted urine flow and closed sterile drainage. Finally, to
event the backflow of stagnating, contaminated urine, it
important to keep the collecting bag below the level of
e bladder at all times.

There is no proven preventive benefit associated with
ansing the meatal area of the catheter with antiseptics.

Although removing the catheter at the first possible
opportunity is an important measure in preventing
CAUTI, routine exchange of urinary catheters is not necessary or effective.

Screening and treatment of asymptomatic bacteriuria
does not improve patient outcomes in nonpregnant
patients and does not prevent CAUTI.

Using antiseptic-coated catheters has not yet been
demonstrated to significantly affect the incidence of
CAUTI, although it significantly reduces colonization rates
and colonization densities of urinary catheters.

KEY POINT

- **Maintaining the urine-collecting bag below the
  level of the bladder is an established measure
  for preventing catheter-associated urinary tract
  infections.**

Bibliography

Chenoweth CE, Saint S. Urinary Tract Infections. Infect Dis Clin
North Am. 2011;25(1):103-115. [PMID: 21315996]

Item 32   Answer: D

Educational Objective: Diagnose catheter-associated urinary tract infection.

A urine culture demonstrating more than 10^3 colony-forming units (CFU)/mL will establish the diagnosis of
catheter-associated urinary tract infection (CAUTI).
CAUTI can be difficult to diagnose, and it may be difficult
to distinguish colonization in a patient with a bladder
catheter from true infection. The Infectious Diseases Society of American (IDSA) has suggested criteria to aid in the
diagnosis of CAUTI. In patients with indwelling urethral,
indwelling suprapubic, or intermittent catheterization,
CAUTI is defined by the presence of symptoms or signs
compatible with UTI with no other identified source of
infection and 10^3 or more CFU/mL of one or more bacterial species in a single catheter urine specimen. Signs and
symptoms compatible with CAUTI include new-onset or
worsening of fever, rigors, altered mental status, malaise, or
lethargy with no other identified cause; flank pain; costovertebral angle tenderness; acute hematuria; and pelvic
discomfort. In patients with spinal cord injury, increased
spasticity, autonomic dysreflexia, or sense of unease are also
compatible with CAUTI.

The cloudiness of the urine or detection of organisms
on urine Gram stain is not adequate for establishing a diagnosis of CAUTI. Cloudy appearance of urine is not diagnostic of UTI and is not part of the IDSA UTI definition.

The presence of positive leukocyte esterase on a dipstick urinalysis is consistent with the presence of leukocytes
in the urine. Although the absence of evidence of leukocytes in the urine has a high negative predictive value for
UTI, in a patient with an indwelling catheter in which colonization and concentration of normal urinary contents

CONT.

may occur, the presence of urinary leukocytes is not sufficient to make a diagnosis of CAUTI.

> **KEY POINT**
>
> - Catheter-associated urinary tract infection is defined by the presence of symptoms or signs compatible with urinary tract infection with no other identified source of infection and 10^3 or more colony-forming units/mL of one or more bacterial species in a single catheter urine specimen.

Bibliography

Hooton TM, Bradley SF, Cardenas DD, et al; Infectious Diseases Society of America. Diagnosis, prevention, and treatment of catheter-associated urinary tract infection in adults: 2009 International Clinical Practice Guidelines from the Infectious Diseases Society of America. Clin Infect Dis. 2010;50(5):625-663. [PMID: 20175247]

Item 33   Answer: A

Educational Objective: Manage newly diagnosed HIV infection.

The most appropriate management is treatment with tenofovir, emtricitabine, and efavirenz now. Because of the benefits associated with earlier initiation of combination antiretroviral therapy and the diminished complexity of and greater tolerance to these regimens, indications for when to begin therapy have expanded. The Department of Health and Human Services 2011 guidelines recommend initiation of antiretroviral therapy for patients with a history of an AIDS-defining opportunistic infection or malignancy, the presence of symptoms, a CD4 cell count less than 500/microliter, HIV-associated nephropathy, active co-infection with hepatitis B virus infection, and pregnancy (to prevent perinatal transmission). In addition, the International AIDS Society–USA Panel recommends treatment of those with active hepatitis C virus co-infection and those who are at high risk for or have active cardiovascular disease, regardless of CD4 cell count. Whether to start treatment in all patients with HIV infection is controversial and remains under investigation as of this writing.

Based on accumulating data from cohort studies showing better outcomes in those patients who initiate treatment earlier, recent guidelines have raised the CD4 cell count threshold from 350/microliter to 500/microliter, below which antiretroviral treatment should be started.

Because the CD4 cell count is a better indicator of risk for progression and disease than is HIV RNA viral load, recent guidelines have removed viral load levels as an indicator of need for initiation of antiretroviral therapy.

Because this patient's CD4 cell count is less than 500/microliter, he should initiate HIV treatment regardless of whether symptoms are present.

> **KEY POINT**
>
> - Initiating combination antiretroviral therapy is appropriate in patients with HIV infection and a CD4 cell count less than 500/microliter, regardless of whether symptoms are present.

Bibliography

Panel on Antiretroviral Guidelines for Adults and Adolescents. Guidelines for the use of antiretroviral agents in HIV-1-infected ad and adolescents. Department of Health and Human Servi October 14, 2011;1-167. Available at: www.aidsinfo.nih.go ContentFiles/AdultandAdolescentGL.pdf. Accessed December 2011.

Item 34   Answer: B

Educational Objective: Treat community-acquired pneumonia in an outpatient.

This patient should be treated with azithromycin. H clinical presentation and radiographic findings are cons tent with community-acquired pneumonia (CAP). outpatients, risk factors for drug-resistant *Streptococ pneumoniae* infection influence the selection of empi therapy. These risk factors include age greater than years, recent (within the past 3 months) β-lactam thera medical comorbidities, immunocompromising conditic and immunosuppressive therapy, alcoholism, and exp sure to a child in day care. This patient is a young, healt man with no risk factors for drug-resistant *S. pneumon* infection; therefore, treatment with a macrolide age such as azithromycin, will provide adequate coverage the likely pathogens, including drug-sensitive *S. pneum niae*, *Haemophilus influenzae*, *Mycoplasma*, and *Chlar dophila* species.

Amoxicillin would not provide coverage for the aty cal pathogens such as *Mycoplasma* or *Chlamydophila* a would not cover all *H. influenzae* strains because increasing number of strains are β-lactamase producir Although very few studies exist on the microbiology CAP in outpatients, *Mycoplasma* and *Chlamydophila* mc likely cause pneumonia in ambulatory patients. High-dc amoxicillin combined with a macrolide is an alternative patients with risk factors for drug-resistant *S. pneumon* infection.

Cefuroxime will provide coverage for drug-sensitive *pneumoniae* and *H. influenza*e but not for atypic pathogens. A respiratory fluoroquinolone such as mo floxacin or levofloxacin provides appropriate coverage the likely pathogens associated with CAP but is unnece sarily broad for this indication. A respiratory fluor quinolone would be appropriate if this patient had risk f tors for infection with drug-resistant *S. pneumoniae*.

Ciprofloxacin has very poor activity against *S. pne moniae* and should never be used as empiric therapy CAP.

KEY POINT

• In previously healthy patients with pneumonia but no risk factors for drug-resistant *Streptococcus pneumoniae* infection, treatment with a macrolide agent, such as azithromycin, will provide adequate coverage for the likely pathogens.

Bibliography

andell LA, Wunderink RG, Anzueto A, et al; Infectious Diseases Society of America; American Thoracic Society. Infectious Diseases Society of America/American Thoracic Society consensus guidelines on the management of community-acquired pneumonia in adults. Clin Infect Dis. 2007;44(suppl 2):S27-72. [PMID: 17278083]

Item 35   Answer: B

Educational Objective: Diagnose acute coccidioidomycosis.

his patient has the acute form of coccidioidomycosis infection. Coccidioidomycosis is endemic to the desert regions of the southwestern United States and to Central and South America. It is estimated that only half of patients infected acutely come to medical attention. Those who do frequently present with what is known as "valley fever," a subacute respiratory illness with systemic symptoms, such as fever and fatigue, which persist for weeks to months. Some symptomatic patients also note joint symptoms, a presentation frequently described as "desert rheumatism." Erythema nodosum (painful nodules on the extensor surfaces of the extremities) is also a common manifestation of acute coccidioidomycosis infection. Although uncommon in immunocompetent persons, complicated disease may occur, particularly in those with impaired cell-mediated immunity. Persons of American Indian, African, or Filipino descent are also more likely to develop serious infection. Routine laboratory findings are usually normal except for an increased erythrocyte sedimentation rate. Because the manifestations of early coccidioidal infections are nonspecific, epidemiologic clues are important when deciding to perform specific laboratory testing. The incubation period is 1 to 3 weeks. Culture is the most sensitive means of establishing the diagnosis, but identification of spherules by direct examination is more rapid. Serologic studies are also available for diagnosing coccidioidomycosis infection.

Although blastomycosis and histoplasmosis can also cause pneumonia and erythema nodosum, blastomycosis is endemic to the Mississippi river and Ohio river basins and around the Great Lakes. The diagnosis may be confirmed by the appearance of characteristic broad-based budding organisms in sputum or tissue samples by potassium hydroxide (KOH) preparation or cytohistologic methods. Histoplasmosis is also endemic to the states bordering the Ohio river valley and the lower Mississippi River. It does not produce spherules, and the yeast forms seen in clinical specimens are relatively small.

Sporotrichosis is a very rare cause of pneumonia and very rarely has been associated with erythema nodosum. Symptoms and signs of pulmonary sporotrichosis include productive cough, lung nodules and cavitations, fibrosis, and hilar lymphadenopathy. It is a chronic disease with slow progression. It does not form spherules.

KEY POINT

• Coccidioidomycosis is a common pulmonary fungal infection endemic to the desert regions of the southwestern United States and to Central and South America, is frequently asymptomatic, and may present with a subclinical pulmonary infection, systemic symptoms, joint pain, and erythema nodosum.

Bibliography

Ampel NM. New perspectives on coccidioidomycosis. Proc Am Thorac Soc. 2010;7(3):181-185. [PMID: 20463246]

Item 36   Answer: D

Educational Objective: Manage acute, uncomplicated cystitis in a woman.

This patient has acute, uncomplicated cystitis, and she should be given nitrofurantoin for 5 days. Nitrofurantoin is a first-line agent for uncomplicated cystitis owing to its efficacy, current minimal resistance, and minimal propensity to select drug-resistant organisms. A 3-day regimen of nitrofurantoin is not as effective as a 3-day regimen of trimethoprim-sulfamethoxazole or fluoroquinolone agents. Nitrofurantoin should not be used if early pyelonephritis is suspected. If the patient had not been allergic to sulfa drugs, a 3-day course of trimethoprim-sulfamethoxazole would have been appropriate if local resistance rates of urinary tract pathogens did not exceed 20% or if the infecting organism was known to be susceptible.

Amoxicillin or ampicillin should not be used unless the infecting organism is known to be susceptible because of the relatively high frequency of *Escherichia coli* species resistant to these agents among patients with community-acquired urinary tract infections.

Fosfomycin is another alternative first-line agent for uncomplicated cystitis if it is available, but it has inferior efficacy compared with other short-course, first-line agents. It should not be used if early pyelonephritis is suspected.

Fluoroquinolone agents, such as levofloxacin, are alternatives for patients who are allergic to or intolerant of first-line agents or live in areas where resistance to trimethoprim-sulfamethoxazole is higher than 20%. Fluoroquinolones are highly effective agents, and 3-day regimens are equivalent in efficacy to longer treatment courses. They should be reserved for more serious infections than acute cystitis.

KEY POINT

- Nitrofurantoin or trimethoprim-sulfamethoxazole is the preferred management strategy for acute, uncomplicated cystitis in nonpregnant young women.

Bibliography

Gupta K, Hooton TM, Naber KG, et al; Infectious Diseases Society of America; European Society for Microbiology and Infectious Diseases. International clinical practice guidelines for the treatment of acute uncomplicated cystitis and pyelonephritis in women: a 2010 update by the Infectious Diseases Society of America and the European Society for Microbiology and Infectious Diseases. Clin Infect Dis. 2011;52(5):e103-120. [PMID: 21292654]

Item 37   Answer: C

Educational Objective: Treat tuberculous pericarditis.

The most appropriate treatment at this time is prednisone. This patient has tuberculous pericarditis resulting in cardiac tamponade and requiring pericardiocentesis. In addition to antituberculous therapy for at least 6 months, consensus guidelines of the American Thoracic Society, Centers for Disease Control and Prevention, and the Infectious Diseases Society of America recommend use of adjunctive corticosteroid therapy. Specifically, adults with tuberculous pericarditis should receive prednisone for the first 11 weeks of therapy. The following doses and duration of prednisone are recommended: 60 mg/d for 4 weeks, then 30 mg/d for 4 weeks, then 15 mg/d for 2 weeks, and finally 5 mg/d for the last week. The use of corticosteroids appears to be associated with improved survival and decreased need for pericardiectomy.

NSAIDs, such as indomethacin, and colchicine can be considered for patients with acute idiopathic or viral pericarditis. These agents are helpful in resolving acute inflammation and symptoms and in preventing recurrences. However, this patient has known tuberculous pericarditis, and the role of NSAIDs and colchicine in the treatment of this disorder in lieu of prednisone is not supported by current guidelines.

At this point, the patient has no indications for more invasive treatment of his tamponade, including pericardial window or pericardiectomy, and he is likely to respond to antituberculous therapy. Indications for more invasive treatment include recurrent pericardial effusions, loculated effusion, or diagnostic need for pericardial biopsy.

KEY POINT

- In addition to rifampin, isoniazid, pyrazinamide, and ethambutol therapy, adjunctive corticosteroids are recommended for the treatment of patients with tuberculous pericarditis.

Bibliography

American Thoracic Society, CDC, Infectious Diseases Society of America. Treatment of tuberculosis. MMWR Recomm Rep. 2003;52(RR-11):1-77. [PMID: 12836625]

Item 38   Answer: B

Educational Objective: Prevent transmission of hospital-acquired infection.

Hand hygiene is the single most important measure to prevent infections, including from multidrug-resistant organisms. Hand hygiene, enacted before and after patient contact, consists of hand washing with soap and water for least 15 to 30 seconds; alcohol-based hand disinfectants a acceptable alternatives to soap and water. In addition hand hygiene, standard precautions include the use barrier protection, including wearing gloves and person protective equipment for the mouth, nose, and eye appropriate handling of patient care equipment and instr ments/devices (avoiding exposure to skin and using appr priate cleaning techniques); and proper handling, tran porting, and processing of used/contaminated linen.

Bleach has an important role in cleaning the rooms patients with *Clostridium difficile* infection but has n proved helpful in controlling patient-to-patient transmi sion of infection with *Acinetobacter baumannii*.

Prophylactically treating the roommate for *Acinet bacter* infection is not nearly as effective or safe as prop hand hygiene. Furthermore, improper use of antibiotics this fashion is likely to quickly lead to antibiotic resistanc

Removing the contaminated catheters and drains fro a source patient has not been demonstrated to reduce t risk for spread of pathogens to other patients.

KEY POINT

- Hand hygiene is the single most important measure to prevent spread of hospital-acquired infections.

Bibliography

Burke JP. Infection control - a problem for patient safety. N Eng Med. 2003;348(7):651-656. [PMID: 12584377]

Item 39   Answer: A

Educational Objective: Evaluate a patient with osteomyelitis.

The next study that should be performed is a CT scan of t foot. The clinical hallmarks of acute osteomyelitis are loc pain and fever, particularly in patients with acute hematog nous osteomyelitis, but these symptoms may be absent patients with chronic and contiguous osteomyelitis.

Given the limitations of physical examination finding in the diagnosis of osteomyelitis, radiologic studies are fr quently used. In patients in whom radiographic results a negative but clinical suspicion for osteomyelitis remai high, MRI is indicated. MRI scans show changes of acu osteomyelitis within days of infection and are superior and more sensitive (90%) and specific (80%) than plain filn and CT scans; can detect soft tissue abscesses and epidur paravertebral, or psoas abscesses possibly requiring surgic drainage; and can delineate anatomy before surgery. Nonetheless, false-positive MRI results may occur in patients with noninfectious conditions such as fractures, tumors, and healed osteomyelitis. In patients with a pacemaker or metal hardware precluding MRI or in those in whom MRI results are inconclusive, CT scans or (if metal hardware is likely to impair CT imaging) nuclear studies may be used instead of MRI. CT reveals excellent anatomic imaging details, and it is the imaging study of choice for patients with osteomyelitis when MRI cannot be obtained.

Nuclear imaging studies can reliably detect the presence of inflammation related to acute infection. However, such visualized abnormalities, which may be caused by bone turnover or inflammation, can also be from other noninfectious causes, including trauma, neoplasm, and degenerative joint disease. Gallium scanning, once a gold standard for cancer diagnosis, may still be used to visualize inflammation and chronic infections, partly because gallium binds to the membranes of neutrophils recruited to a site of infection. However, leukocyte-labeled nuclear scans have almost entirely replaced this imaging technique. Except in the setting of diminished blood flow to the affected area, a negative three-phase bone scan confers a high negative predictive value for osteomyelitis.

KEY POINT

- CT scan is the imaging study of choice for suspected osteomyelitis when MRI cannot be performed.

Bibliography
Mihara S, Segreti J. Osteomyelitis. Dis Mon. 2010;56(1):5-31. [PMID: 19995624]

Item 40   Answer: A

Educational Objective: Diagnose a returning traveler with malaria.

The most likely malaria species against which treatment should be directed is *Plasmodium falciparum*. Malaria should be considered the most likely cause of fever in any traveler returning from a malaria-endemic area of the world. After Africa, Asia is the geographic destination with the highest risk of imported malaria. *P. falciparum* causes most malaria cases diagnosed in the United States following travel. Although mostly all cases occur in travelers who did not take any chemoprophylaxis or who were not adherent to it, infection can still be contracted despite compliance with all medical and preventive measures. In this instance, the patient spent time in Thailand, one of the rare malaria-infested zones where mefloquine-resistant *P. falciparum* has been reported.

There are no pathognomonic clinical signs or symptoms of malaria. In general, the signs and symptoms of uncomplicated malaria are nonspecific and infrequently occur before 1 to 4 weeks after return from travel. Fever, present in 100% of patients, may have a recurring cyclical pattern every 48 or 72

hours, varying according to the specific *Plasmodium* species and corresponding to the synchrony of organism replication. However, classic periodic malarial fever is most often absent in imported cases. Other common symptoms include myalgia, headache, and gastrointestinal discomfort. The degree of anemia depends on the duration of disease and degree of parasitemia. Although leukocyte counts may be variable, thrombocytopenia is present in greater than 50% of patients. Kidney impairment may also occur, the pathogenesis of which likely relates to hemolysis and erythrocyte sequestration within the kidney circulation. The term "blackwater fever" is given to the very dark urine secondary to significant hemoglobinuria sometimes observed in patients with severe *falciparum* malaria. Moreover, overwhelming disease may occur in patients who have anatomic or functional asplenia. The standard for malaria diagnosis is the Giemsa-stained blood smear by light microscopy. *P. falciparum* can involve erythrocytes of any size and are characterized by ring forms, some of which may be multiple, positioned along the periphery of the erythrocyte against the inner surface of its membrane. Classic "banana-shaped" gametocytes, if detected, can help to distinguish *falciparum* malaria species from the other potential *Plasmodium* species.

Infection with *Plasmodium malariae* should be considered if the paroxysms of fever occur every 72 hours and when the parasitized erythrocytes demonstrate the characteristic band form trophozoite, neither of which is consistent with this patient's clinical scenario.

Infection with *Plasmodium ovale* and *Plasmodium vivax* may show trophozoite and schizont forms on the peripheral blood smear with Schüffner dots inside of enlarged erythrocytes, inconsistent with this patient's peripheral blood smear findings.

KEY POINT

- A diagnosis of malaria should be considered in the differential diagnosis of travelers returning from malaria-endemic areas who present with fever and a peripheral smear indicating *Plasmodium* organisms in the erythrocytes.

Bibliography
Taylor SM, Molyneux ME, Simel DL, et al. Does this patient have malaria? JAMA. 2010;304(18):2048-2056. [PMID: 21057136]

Item 41   Answer: D

Educational Objective: Manage a patient with active tuberculosis who has discontinued her medications.

This patient's therapy for active tuberculosis should be restarted from the beginning. She is infected with a strain of *Mycobacterium tuberculosis* that is sensitive to all first-line antituberculous agents, but she interrupted her initial 2-month phase of treatment. Interruptions in treatment are not uncommon. Decisions regarding subsequent therapy are based on the duration of treatment and when the medications were discontinued. Consensus guidelines recommend that an interruption of 2 or more weeks during the initial 2-month phase of therapy requires restarting the same regimen from the beginning.

When the lapse is less than 2 weeks, recommendations are that the initial regimen should be continued until the planned total number of doses is taken, provided that all doses are taken within 3 months.

Regardless of whether results of a sputum smear are negative for acid-fast bacilli, the recommended treatment regimen for a pulmonary infection caused by a fully susceptible strain of *M. tuberculosis* includes an initial 2-month phase followed by a continuation phase of at least 4 months' duration.

Because all of this patient's medications were discontinued at the same time, there is no indication that the strain of tuberculosis has developed resistance; therefore, there is no need to restart a different treatment regimen.

> **KEY POINT**
> - When a patient with active tuberculosis being treated with initial-phase antituberculous agents discontinues treatment for 2 weeks or longer, the same antituberculous regimen should be restarted from the beginning.

Bibliography

American Thoracic Society; CDC; Infectious Diseases Society of America. Treatment of tuberculosis. MMWR Recomm Rep. 2003;52(RR-11):1-77. [PMID: 12836625]

Item 42   Answer: C

Educational Objective: Treat mild disseminated extrapulmonary blastomycosis in a healthy host.

This patient, who is a healthy host, has mild disseminated extrapulmonary blastomycosis and should be treated with oral itraconazole for 6 to 12 months or until all signs and symptoms of the disease have abated. Up to 40% of those infected with blastomycosis develop extrapulmonary infection, which is usually cutaneous (most commonly), genitourinary, osteoarticular, or central nervous system (CNS) disease. Two types of cutaneous lesions (verrucous and ulcerative) occur frequently in the absence of clinically active pulmonary disease and are the most common extrapulmonary manifestation of blastomycosis. Verrucous lesions usually are found on exposed skin. Over time, lesions may undergo central clearing, scar formation, and depigmentation. Both verrucous and ulcerative lesions may occur in the same patient. Definitive diagnosis requires growth of the organism in culture. A presumptive diagnosis is made by visualizing the characteristic yeast with broad-based buds in pus, secretions, or tissue. Because of toxicity, conventional amphotericin B and amphotericin B lipid formulations are reserved for patients with moderately severe to severe pulmonary, disseminated, and CNS

blastomycosis, whereas itraconazole is the drug of choice for the treatment of non–life-threatening, non–CNS blastomycosis. Itraconazole drug levels should be measured during the first month of treatment in patients with disseminated or pulmonary blastomycosis.

Fluconazole has a very limited role in the treatment of blastomycosis. Results from one study using low to standard doses were disappointing, whereas higher doses were more efficacious.

Because the response to antifungal therapy is very good, there is no role for surgical excision of skin lesions caused by blastomycosis.

> **KEY POINT**
> - Mild to moderate disseminated extrapulmonary blastomycosis can be effectively treated with oral itraconazole.

Bibliography

Chapman SW, Dismukes WE, Proia LA, et al; Infectious Diseases Society of America. Clinical practice guidelines for the management of blastomycosis: 2008 update by the Infectious Diseases Society of America. Clin Infect Dis. 2008;46(12):1801-1812. [PMID: 18462107]

Item 43   Answer: E

Educational Objective: Manage influenza virus infection during an outbreak in the community.

This patient has classic symptoms of influenza occurring during a confirmed outbreak of influenza A (H1N1) virus infection in the community. She has mild illness and is otherwise healthy; therefore, she does not need treatment with an antiviral medication. The Advisory Committee on Immunization Practices (ACIP) recommends early antiviral treatment of suspected or confirmed influenza for hospitalized patients; those with severe, complicated, or progressive illness; and those at high risk for influenza complications. Other high-risk medical conditions include cardiovascular disease (except isolated hypertension), active cancer, chronic kidney disease, chronic liver disease, hemoglobinopathies, immunocompromise (including HIV disease), and neurologic diseases that impair handling of respiratory secretions. When treatment is indicated, it should be started within the first 2 days of symptom onset to reduce the duration of illness and decrease the risk for serious complications. Oseltamivir or zanamivir is indicated for those with influenza A (H1N1), influenza A (H3N2), or influenza B virus infection or for those in whom the influenza virus type or influenza A virus subtype is unknown. Oseltamivir and zanamivir differ in pharmacokinetics, safety profile, route of administration, approved age groups, and recommended dosages. Zanamivir is administered by an inhaler device and is not recommended for persons with underlying airways disease such as asthma or COPD.

Amantadine and rimantadine are related antiviral medications in the adamantane class that are active against fluenza A viruses but not influenza B viruses. In recent ars, widespread adamantane resistance among influenza (H3N2 and H1N1) strains has been noted. These agents e not recommended for antiviral treatment or chemo-ophylaxis of currently circulating influenza A strains.

- **Antiviral therapy is not indicated for mild influenza in healthy persons.**

Bibliography

ore AE, Fry A, Shay D, Gubareva L, Bresee JS, Uyeki TM; Centers for Disease Control and Prevention (CDC). Antiviral agents for the treatment and chemoprophylaxis of influenza — recommendations of the Advisory Committee on Immunization Practices (ACIP). MMWR Recomm Rep. 2011;60(1):1-24. [PMID: 21248682]

Item 44   Answer: C

Educational Objective: Understand the potential de effects associated with first-line drugs used to eat tuberculosis.

razinamide is most likely responsible for causing an acute tack of gout in this patient who is being treated for active berculosis. Pyrazinamide can cause hyperuricemia and out by inhibiting renal tubular excretion of uric acid. ther potential side effects include hepatitis, rash, and strointestinal upset. Pyrazinamide is contraindicated for e in patients with active gout and should be used with ution in those with a known history of chronic gout.

Amlodipine is commonly associated with nausea, flush-g, palpitations, dizziness, peripheral edema, and muscle in; however, it does not increase uric acid levels, and its e is not contraindicated in patients with gout.

Side effects of isoniazid use include hepatitis, rash, ripheral neuropathy, and a lupus-like syndrome, but not peruricemia.

Rifampin can cause rash, hepatitis, gastrointestinal set, and orange-coloring of body fluids. Of note, ampin enhances kidney excretion of uric acid.

- **Pyrazinamide use is associated with hyper-uricemia, which can result in gouty arthritis.**

Bibliography

nerican Thoracic Society; CDC; Infectious Diseases Society of America. Treatment of tuberculosis. MMWR Recomm Rep. 2003;52(RR-11):1-77 [PMID: 12836625]

Item 45   Answer: A

Educational Objective: Treat extensively drug-sistant *Pseudomonas aeruginosa.*

his patient requires treatment with intravenous colistin. tensively drug-resistant *Pseudomonas aeruginosa* is a eatment challenge. This organism frequently colonizes clinical settings, such as intensive care units, and is the most common cause of widely resistant gram-negative health care–acquired pneumonia. Patients with burns also appear to be particularly susceptible to pseudomonal infection, which confers a poor prognosis, even with aggressive treatment. This resistance pattern and susceptibility in this patient make selection of adequate antibiotic therapy difficult. Colistin (polymyxin E) is an older antimicrobial agent that historically was used infrequently owing to high rates of nephrotoxicity. Recently, colistin has been used more frequently because it is one of the few agents with reliable activity against resistant gram-negative bacilli, such as extensively drug-resistant *P. aeruginosa*, and it is the only agent of the options listed that that is effective in this setting and achieves adequate systemic drug levels.

Minocycline and rifampin, which are older antimicrobial agents, lack reliable pseudomonal activity and are therefore inappropriate for use in this situation.

Tigecycline, a newer glycylcycline agent, has no pseudomonal activity.

- **Colistin is one of the only available options for treatment of extensively drug-resistant *Pseudomonas aeruginosa* infection.**

Bibliography

Pogue JM, Marchaim D, Kaye D, Kaye DS. Revisiting "older" antimicrobials in the era of multidrug resistance. Pharmacotherapy. 2011;31(9):912-921. [PMID: 21923592]

Item 46   Answer: C

Educational Objective: Manage a hospitalized patient with bacteremic pneumococcal pneumonia.

This patient with bacteremic pneumococcal pneumonia should be discharged on oral amoxicillin to complete 7 days of therapy. His physical examination findings on hospital day 3 (afebrile, pulse rate ≤100/min, respiration rate ≤24/min, and systolic blood pressure ≥90 mm Hg) plus normal oxygen saturation while breathing ambient air indicate that he is clinically stable and should be considered for discharge. In addition, patients considered stable for discharge should have a normal (or baseline) mental status and be able to tolerate oral therapy. The presence of pneumococcal bacteremia does not warrant a more prolonged course of intravenous therapy. Once patients are clinically stable, they are at very low risk for subsequent clinical deterioration and can be safely discharged from the hospital.

Levofloxacin would provide unnecessarily broad-spectrum coverage for this patient's penicillin-susceptible pneumonia, and levofloxacin would be a more expensive treatment option.

Seven days of therapy is sufficient for treatment of community-acquired pneumonia in most patients, especially those who have a prompt clinical response to treatment, even in the setting of bacteremic infection. A 14-day treatment regimen would be unnecessarily long for this patient.

Studies have shown that continued observation after switching from intravenous to oral therapy is not necessary.

KEY POINT

- Hospitalized patients with bacteremic community-acquired pneumonia who respond promptly to therapy do not require a more prolonged course of intravenous therapy and can be discharged home on oral medication when they are clinically stable.

Bibliography

Weinstein MP, Klugman KP, Jones RN. Rationale for revised penicillin susceptibility breakpoints versus Streptococcus pneumoniae: coping with antimicrobial susceptibility in an era of resistance. Clin Infect Dis. 2009;48(11):1596-1600. [PMID: 19400744]

Item 47   Answer: A

Educational Objective: Diagnose anthrax infection.

The most likely infectious agent is *Bacillus anthracis*. This patient most likely has inhalational anthrax, a form of disease previously diagnosed only in persons having potential occupational exposure to this bacillus. The spores of *B. anthracis* lie dormant in soil. Disease may follow infection with spores acquired through cutaneous contact, ingestion, or inhalation. The rapid development of a septic state following a nonspecific prodromal flu-like syndrome is characteristic of inhalational anthrax. Although anthrax does not generally manifest as pneumonitis, migration of inhaled spores to the mediastinal lymph nodes leads to tissue destruction and hemorrhage, resulting in the classic widening of the mediastinum and occasional bloody pleural effusions demonstrated on chest radiograph or CT imaging. The diagnosis is confirmed by isolation of the organism (commonly from blood cultures with inhalational disease) or by detection of its presence in tissue or fluid through polymerase chain reaction testing.

Erysipelothrix rhusiopathiae, another infrequently encountered gram-positive bacillus recognized as a pathogen in animals and a colonizer in fish, is most commonly associated with human infection in persons with occupational exposure to contaminated meat or fish. Most infections are cutaneous; the rarely occurring invasive form develops primarily as infective endocarditis.

Although *Listeria monocytogenes* is often acquired through ingestion of contaminated foods or unpasteurized milk products, severe disease most often occurs in the very young, elderly, or those who have an underlying state of immunocompromise. Generally, *L. monocytogenes* presents as a diarrheal illness, but it may lead to sepsis and central nervous system involvement. This patient's constellation of signs and symptoms is not consistent with *L. monocytogenes*.

Nocardia infections can manifest as cutaneous, ly phocutaneous, pulmonary, or central nervous system c ease. Nodular and cavitary lesions are predominan observed when the lungs are involved. Bacteremia with t weakly staining gram-positive bacillus is rare.

KEY POINT

- The rapid development of a septic state following a nonspecific prodromal flu-like syndrome and widening of the mediastinum is characteristic of inhalational anthrax.

Bibliography

Inglesby TV, O'Toole T, Henderson DA, et al. Anthrax as a biolc weapon, 2002: updated recommendations for management. JAM 2002;287(17):2236-2252. [PMID: 11980524]

Item 48   Answer: D

Educational Objective: Manage a patient with stool samples containing *Blastocystis* species.

Asymptomatic patients in whom *Blastocystis* species found in stool samples do not require therapy or additio studies to document eradication of the organisms. *Blas cystis* species are protozoal parasites that are frequen found in human stool samples submitted for microsco examination. However, their clinical significance is unc tain. Epidemiologic studies have found no significant c ference in the prevalence of *Blastocystis* species in stool sa ples of patients with diarrheal illnesses compared w asymptomatic control patients. Fecal carriage may pers for many months in the absence of symptoms. Studies ev uating treatment of symptomatic patients have provid conflicting reports regarding resolution of gastrointesti symptoms. Most authorities recommend reserving tre ment only for patients with diarrhea lasting longer than days in whom other infectious or noninfectious causes ha been excluded.

Ciprofloxacin is not active against *Blastocystis* specie

Treatment regimens reported to be effective agai *Blastocystis* species include metronidazole, trimethopri sulfamethoxazole, and nitazoxanide. Controversy exists to whether resolution of symptoms with one of th agents is attributable to eradication of *Blastocystis* organis or to treatment of another undiagnosed pathogen.

There is controversy regarding obtaining stool stud in patients with diarrhea. Clinically meaningful resu occur in an estimated 2% to 6% of stool cultures, and m episodes of mild to moderate diarrhea are self-limit Additionally, positive culture results may be difficult interpret, particularly in patients whose symptoms ha resolved. Thus, for cases of mild to moderate diarrh symptomatic treatment for 48 to 72 hours is reasonal before cultures are obtained, whereas immediate studies generally recommended for patients with severe sympton significant comorbidities, the immunosuppressed, a those with public contact (such as food preparers or ch re workers) who may require negative stool studies to turn to work.

- Asymptomatic patients in whom *Blastocystis* species are found in stool samples do not require therapy or additional studies to document eradication of the organisms.

Bibliography

n KS, Mirza H, Teo JD, Wu B, Macary PA. Current Views on the Clinical Relevance of Blastocystis spp. Curr Infect Dis Rep. 2010;12(1):28-35. [PMID: 21308496]

em 49   Answer: C

ducational Objective: Diagnose sporadic reutzfeldt-Jakob disease.

his patient most likely has sporadic Creutzfeldt-Jakob sease (sCJD). All forms of CJD are associated with the cumulation of the prion protein in neural tissue, spongirm brain pathology without inflammation, normal cereospinal fluid (CSF), relentless symptomatic progression, d no specific treatment. The findings of rapidly proessive dementia and myoclonus, together with his age, and CSF findings, and a nondiagnostic neuroimaging idy, are most consistent with sCJD. The definitive diagsis of sCJD requires visualization of spongiform changes pathologic examination of brain tissue. Supportive findgs include evidence of 1- to 2-Hz periodic sharp waves an electroencephalogram or the presence of the 14-3-protein in a CSF sample, although the latter finding is nspecific.

Cryptococcal and *Mycobacterium tuberculosis* infecns of the central nervous system cause a subacute to ronic meningitis associated with CSF pleocytosis, adache, fever, and meningeal signs. Myoclonus is not a ture of these infections.

Tertiary neurosyphilis may cause dementia. However, s typically progresses over months to years rather than eks and is associated with CSF pleocytosis.

- Sporadic Creutzfeldt-Jakob disease is characterized by rapidly progressive dementia and myoclonus, bland cerebrospinal fluid findings, and nondiagnostic neuroimaging studies, but the definitive diagnosis requires finding spongiform changes on pathologic examination of brain tissue.

bliography

o C, Shi Q, Tian C, et al. The epidemiological, clinical, and laboratory features of sporadic Creutzfeldt-Jakob disease patients in China: surveillance data from 2006 to 2010. PLoS One. 2011;6(8):e24231. [PMID: 21904617]

Item 50   Answer: C

Educational Objective: Treat a patient with suspected community-associated methicillin-resistant *Staphylococcus aureus* pneumonia.

The most appropriate empiric treatment is ceftriaxone, azithromycin, and vancomycin. The patient has no risk factors for health care–associated pneumonia; therefore, initial empiric antibiotic therapy would include ceftriaxone (or cefotaxime) and azithromycin (or doxycycline) to provide coverage for the most common community-acquired pneumonia (CAP) pathogens, *Streptococcus pneumoniae, Haemophilus influenzae*, and the atypical pathogens. However, the presence of a cavitary infiltrate warrants consideration of additional pathogens. In this patient with no risk factors for aspiration pneumonia, involvement of *Staphylococcus aureus*, including possible community-associated methicillin-resistant *S. aureus* (CA-MRSA) infection, is a consideration. CA-MRSA pneumonia can occur following an influenza-like illness; the classic history is a viral syndrome that seems to be improving and then suddenly worsens. *S. aureus* is responsible for less than 10% of cases of CAP; however, the risk increases when pneumonia occurs after influenza infection. Because this patient with a cavitary infiltrate and influenza-like prodrome may have *S. aureus* infection, initial empiric antibiotics should include coverage for CA-MRSA. Consequently, vancomycin should be added to ceftriaxone and azithromycin.

Aztreonam provides coverage only for aerobic gram-negative rods. Although gram-negative pathogens can cause necrotizing pneumonia, initial empiric coverage should not be limited to only gram-negative organisms.

Moxifloxacin does not provide adequate coverage for CA-MRSA.

- **Community-associated methicillin-resistant *Staphylococcus aureus* pneumonia can occur following an influenza-like illness and requires initial empiric antibiotics with ceftriaxone or cefotaxime and azithromycin or doxycycline plus vancomycin.**

Bibliography

Taneja C, Haque N, Oster G, et al. Clinical and economic outcomes in patients with community-acquired Staphylococcus aureus pneumonia. J Hosp Med. 2010;5(9):528-534. [PMID: 20734457]

Item 51   Answer: A

Educational Objective: Diagnose botulism.

The most likely diagnosis is botulism. Ingestion of preformed toxin from exposure to home-canned foods, or in vivo toxin production after spore germination following ingestion (infant botulism with honey) or wound contamination, are the most common forms of botulism.

Distinguishing naturally occurring foodborne botulism from botulism contracted through deliberate contamination of foods with botulinum toxin may be difficult. Both modes of exposure would likely present within 1 to 5 days of toxin ingestion with a classic triad of symmetric, descending flaccid paralysis with prominent bulbar palsies; normal body temperature; and a clear sensorium. Bulbar signs include the "4 Ds": Diplopia, Dysarthria, Dysphonia, and Dysphagia. Respiratory dysfunction may result from upper airway obstruction or diaphragmatic weakness. A diagnosis can be confirmed by detection of toxin in serum, stool, gastric aspirate, or suspect foods. Treatment is mainly supportive and consists of passive immunization using trivalent equine antitoxin (A, B, and E) and close monitoring of the respiratory status. Antibiotics would be indicated only in patients with complications, such as nosocomial infections.

Guillain-Barré syndrome can clinically mimic botulism because it is characterized by oculomotor dysfunction; however, this condition is usually associated with a history of antecedent infection (gastroenteritis from *Campylobacter* infection), ascending paralysis, and paresthesias. This constellation of symptoms and findings is not consistent with that of this patient.

Paralytic shellfish poisoning is characterized by a history of ingestion of any type of filter-feeding molluscan shellfish (for example, clams, oysters, scallops, or mussels) in which a specific neurotoxin (saxitoxin) produced by microscopic algae has accumulated, particularly in temperate and tropical locations. Symptoms may begin a few minutes to hours after ingestion and commonly include tingling of the lips and tongue that progresses to paresthesias of the digits of the hands and feet, with loss of control of the arms and legs. Depending on the quantity of toxin ingested, muscles of the thorax and abdomen may become paralyzed, resulting in respiratory difficulties

Tick paralysis, associated with *Dermacentor* ticks and most often encountered in the United States Pacific Northwest, also produces an ascending paralysis, predominantly affecting proximal large muscles. This patient's recent travel itinerary and physical examination findings are not consistent with tick paralysis.

KEY POINT

- **Botulism presents with a classic triad of symmetric, descending flaccid paralysis with prominent bulbar palsies (diplopia, dysarthria, dysphonia, and dysphagia); normal body temperature; and a clear sensorium.**

Bibliography
Cherington M. Botulism: update and review. Semin Neurol. 2004;24(2):155-163. [PMID: 15257512]

Item 52   Answer: E
Educational Objective: Manage a patient with esophageal candidiasis.

This patient should be treated with oral fluconazole. Sh has evidence of oral candidiasis (thrush), with typical whi plaques on visual inspection and symptoms of dysphag indicating esophageal involvement. Although oral candic asis has been typically associated with advanced immun suppression in patients with HIV (CD4 cell coun <200/microliter), it may occur with higher CD4 c counts in the setting of other risk factors, such as inhal corticosteroids or broad-spectrum antibiotics.

Although isolated oral disease can be treated with to ical agents such as nystatin or clotrimazole, this patien swallowing symptoms suggest concurrent esophageal d ease. Esophageal candidiasis requires systemic therapy su as fluconazole, which can be administered orally as long the patient can swallow pills.

Although this patient's inhaled corticosteroids m have predisposed her to oral candidiasis, the most appr priate management is to treat the candidal disease and n to discontinue the inhaled corticosteroids, which are important part of the successful management of h asthma.

This patient has no history of previous treatment wi fluconazole and is therefore unlikely to have fluconazo resistant *Candida*.

Amphotericin B is an intravenous treatment, is asso ated with increased toxicity, and is not as convenient as o therapy; consequently, it is not warranted as initial trea ment of esophageal candidiasis.

KEY POINT

- **Oral candidiasis with esophageal involvement is characterized by whitish plaques on the oral mucosa and difficulty swallowing; treatment with a systemic agent such as fluconazole is required.**

Bibliography
Kaplan JE, Benson C, Holmes KH, Brooks JT, Pau A, Masur H; Ce ters for Disease Control and Prevention (CDC); National Institu of Health; HIV Medicine Association of the Infectious Disea Society of America. Guidelines for prevention and treatment opportunistic infections in HIV-infected adults and adolescer recommendations from CDC, the National Institutes of Heal and the HIV Medicine Association of the Infectious Diseases Sc ety of America. MMWR Recomm Rep. 2009;58(RR-4):1-2 [PMID: 19357635]

Item 53   Answer: D
Educational Objective: Empirically treat diabet mellitus–associated osteomyelitis.

The most appropriate empiric treatment of this patient vancomycin and meropenem. This patient is experienci a septic syndrome and limb-threatening foot infectio nb-threatening infections are characterized by extensive ⊏ading cellulitis, extending far beyond the wound or ⊏er, with systemic illness and possible sepsis with ulcers ⊏ending deep into the subcutaneous tissue, as well as tis- ⊏ ischemia. Limb-threatening infections are polymicro- ⊏l, including staphylococci, streptococci, enteric gram- ⊏gative rods, *Pseudomonas aeruginosa*, and anaerobes. ⊏ally, a biopsy of the affected bone and deep soft tissues ⊏uld be attempted before empiric antimicrobial therapy ⊏nitiated. However, in the setting of sepsis and a limb- ⊏eatening infection in a patient with diabetes mellitus, ⊏imicrobial therapy using agents directed at suspected ⊏hogens should urgently be administered. Surgical ⊏pridement will also be required. Patients with severe ⊏ections should receive parenteral therapy. Pending the ⊏ults of microbiologic cultures, vancomycin and ⊏ropenem would be an appropriate combination of ⊏nts, predictably supplying broad coverage against the ⊏tential pathogens of concern.

Because they are not active against gram-positive cocci, ⊏reonam and metronidazole would not provide coverage ⊏inst streptococci and staphylococci. Although metron- ⊏zole has excellent activity against anaerobic gram-nega- ⊏e bacilli, the narrow spectrum of activity of cefazolin ver- ⊏ many gram-negative bacilli, as well as its inactivity ⊏inst methicillin-resistant strains, may be inadequate.

Because of clindamycin's methicillin-resistant activity, ⊏s agent cannot reliably treat serious infections potentially ⊏olving staphylococci.

The use of gentamicin or other aminoglycosides to ⊏ovide coverage against aerobic gram-negative bacilli in ⊏piric antibiotic regimens for treatment of complex dia- ⊏ic foot infections is not currently recommended because ⊏the narrow toxicity-to-benefit ratio with such use. In ⊏dition, aminoglycosides may exhibit diminished antimi- ⊏bial activity in a necrotic, anaerobic environment.

⊏Y POINT

- ⊏ In the setting of sepsis and a limb-threatening infection in a patient with diabetes mellitus, antimicrobial therapy with agents directed at suspected pathogens should urgently be administered.

⊏liography

⊏lson AS, Coll AP. The treatment of diabetic foot infections. J ⊏antimicrob Chemother. 2010;65(suppl 3):iii3-9. [PMID: ⊏0876626]

⊏m 54   Answer: C

⊏ucational Objective: Manage HIV infection in ⊏egnancy.

⊏e most appropriate management of this pregnant patient ⊏immediate institution of antiretroviral therapy with ⊏ovudine, lamivudine, and lopinavir-ritonavir. About one ⊏four neonates born to women with HIV infection will acquire HIV infection perinatally if antiretroviral therapy is not given. Appropriate antiretroviral therapy can reduce the risk of HIV transmission to the newborn to less than 2%. This patient should receive antiretroviral therapy now, regardless of CD4 cell count, viral load, or presence or absence of symptoms.

Although about two thirds of perinatal HIV transmission occurs during delivery, one third occurs in utero; consequently, antiretroviral therapy should be started now and not withheld until the onset of labor to maximally reduce chances of perinatal transmission.

Efavirenz is contraindicated in women who are or who may be pregnant because of the risk for teratogenicity.

Withholding treatment until there is a decrease in CD4 cell count or onset of HIV symptoms would not be appropriate because all pregnant women with HIV infection should receive antiretroviral therapy to reduce the likelihood for perinatal transmission.

KEY POINT

- **In pregnant women with HIV infection, antiretroviral therapy with zidovudine, lamivudine, and lopinavir-ritonavir can reduce the risk of HIV transmission to the newborn to less than 2% and should be given regardless of CD4 cell count, viral load, or presence or absence of HIV symptoms.**

Bibliography

Panel on Treatment of HIV-Infected Pregnant Women and Prevention of Perinatal Transmission. Recommendations for use of antiretroviral drugs in pregnant HIV-1-infected women for maternal health and interventions to reduce perinatal HIV transmission in the United States. September 14, 2011;1-207. Available at: www.aidsinfo.nih.gov/ContentFiles/PerinatalGL.pdf. Accessed December 20, 2011.

Item 55   Answer: A

Educational Objective: Diagnose dengue fever.

Dengue fever, a flavivirus infection transmitted by the bite of the *Aedes aegypti* mosquito, is the most prevalent mosquito-borne viral illness in the world. Dengue is endemic to many parts of the world, especially Southeast Asia and tropical geographic areas. A significant rise in the incidence of dengue has occurred recently in the Caribbean islands and Latin America, resulting from the reestablishment of the *A. aegypti* vector in these areas. On several occasions, domestically acquired (autochthonous) cases in the United States, generally limited to the southern states, have been reported. Classic manifestations in symptomatic persons present after an incubation period of 4 to 7 days. Typically, patients experience abrupt fever with chills, severe frontal headache, retro-orbital pain, and musculoskeletal pain, characteristically severe in the lumbar spine, earning dengue the name "break-bone fever." A nonspecific macular or maculopapular rash, sparing the palms and soles, often develops within 3 to 4 days of onset of illness, tending to coincide with the resolution of fever. Referred to as a "saddle-back" pattern, a second episode of fever and symptoms may occur in some patients. Abnormal laboratory findings include leukopenia, neutropenia, thrombocytopenia, and mildly elevated liver aminotransferase concentrations, with the serum aspartate aminotransferase level often higher than the serum alanine aminotransferase level. The febrile illness may be followed by a prolonged episode of fatigue. Full recovery is expected in all infected persons. The diagnosis of dengue fever remains mainly clinical. During the early phase of illness, real-time reverse transcriptase polymerase chain reaction can be useful in detecting virus in the blood. However, acute and convalescent serologic testing is commonly used to confirm a diagnosis in returning travelers. Treatment of dengue fever involves symptomatic relief. Currently, no vaccine is clinically available to protect against infection.

Leptospirosis, caused by infection with pathogenic spirochetes belonging to the genus *Leptospira*, is endemic throughout the world. Infection occurs through direct or indirect contact with urine or tissues of infected animals, most often rodents and other small mammals. In most infected patients, a self-limited illness characterized by high fever, myalgia, abdominal pain, and conjunctival suffusion occurs, with a rash developing infrequently.

Malaria does not cause a rash and is not endemic to the Caribbean islands except for the Dominican Republic and Haiti.

Yellow fever, another flavivirus infection contracted through the bite of the *A. aegypti* mosquito, occurs mostly in areas of sub-Saharan Africa and South America, but is not endemic to the Caribbean islands.

KEY POINT

- Classic manifestations of dengue infection in symptomatic persons include fever with chills, severe frontal headache, retro-orbital pain, and musculoskeletal pain that is characteristically severe in the lumbar spine, as well as a nonspecific macular or maculopapular rash sparing the palms and soles.

Bibliography
Ross TM. Dengue virus. Clin Lab Med. 2010;30(1):149-160. [PMID: 20513545]

Item 56   Answer: E

Educational Objective: Treat a community-associated methicillin-resistant *Staphylococcus aureus* skin infection.

Trimethoprim-sulfamethoxazole (TMP-SMX) is an older antibiotic drug that has been used with increasing frequency for treatment of skin and soft tissue infections caused by community-associated methicillin-resistant

Staphylococcus aureus (CA-MRSA), and it has retain excellent activity against most strains of CA-MRSA. T patient presents with a cutaneous abscess that is larger th 5 cm with purulent drainage and associated cellulitis. Gram stain of the lesion aspirate is suggestive of *S. aure* which is consistent with CA-MRSA infection. Treatme with TMP-SMX is appropriate empiric therapy aft drainage of the lesion. Limitations of TMP-SMX inclu sulfa allergy (including Stevens-Johnson syndrom hyperkalemia, and possible kidney toxicity. Therapy m be further directed once culture and sensitivity results ha returned.

Amoxicillin-clavulanate is an expanded spectrum β-la tam antimicrobial agent, but it is not active against MRS

Azithromycin, a macrolide, has poor activity agai MRSA and should not be used for empiric treatment CA-MRSA.

Moxifloxacin, a fluoroquinolone, has increased activ against *S. aureus* compared with other fluoroquinolon but resistance to this agent has emerged among CA-MR strains; consequently, moxifloxacin is not a good empi choice.

Rifampin has activity against some strains of MRSA t should not be used as a single agent for treatment of inf tion because of the risk for rapid emergence of resistance

KEY POINT

- Trimethoprim-sulfamethoxazole is a first-line choice for treatment of skin and soft tissue infection due to suspected or confirmed community-associated methicillin-resistant *Staphylococcus aureus*.

Bibliography
Liu C, Bayer A, Cosgrove SE, et al. Clinical practice guidelines by Infectious Diseases Society of America for the treatment of met cillin-resistant Staphylococcus aureus infections in adults and c dren: executive summary. Clin Infect Dis. 2011;52(3):285-2 [PMID: 21217178]

Item 57   Answer: D

Educational Objective: Interpret a tuberculin skin test reaction in a patient who uses injection drugs.

No additional evaluation or treatment is indicated for a p son who uses injection drugs and has a tuberculin skin t reaction of less than 10 mm of induration.

Certain high-risk groups require a chest radiograph exclude active tuberculosis when their tuberculin skin t reaction is greater than or equal to 5 mm. These grou include recent contacts of patients with active tuberculo patients with HIV infection, persons with fibrotic chang on prior chest radiographs consistent with old healed tub culosis, and organ transplant recipients and patients w other immunocompromising conditions. High-risk perso who require a chest radiograph when their tuberculin sk t reaction is greater than or equal to 10 mm include ction drug users; persons from countries with a high evalence of tuberculosis who immigrated to the United ates less than 5 years ago; employees or residents of high-k congregate settings such as prisons, nursing homes, spitals, or homeless shelters; mycobacteriology labora-y workers; patients with clinical conditions that put them increased risk for active tuberculosis (for example, ronic kidney disease; diabetes mellitus; silicosis; lympho-oliferative disorders; cancer of the neck, head, or lung; strectomy or jejunoileal bypass and weight loss of ≥10% om ideal body weight); children who are younger than 4 ars of age; and adolescents, children, and infants who are posed to adults in high-risk categories. Asymptomatic rsons in either of these two groups who have a chest radi-raph that is normal or is inconsistent with active tuber-losis should receive treatment for latent tuberculosis ection because they are at increased risk for tuberculosis. eatment will substantially reduce the risk that latent berculosis will progress to active disease. Treatment of ent tuberculosis typically consists of isoniazid for 9 onths unless there is strong suspicion of infection with niazid-resistant mycobacteria (for example, exposure to person with known isoniazid-resistant tuberculosis). In is situation, rifampin for 4 months is a reasonable alter-tive. Recently, the Centers for Disease Control and Pre-ntion also included 3 months of directly observed, once-ekly rifapentine and isoniazid combination therapy for atment of latent tuberculosis.

Four-drug therapy with isoniazid, rifampin, pyrazi-mide, and ethambutol is used to treat active tuberculo-. There is no evidence that the asymptomatic person scribed here has active tuberculosis.

EY POINT

- A tuberculin skin test reaction of less than 10 mm in a person who uses injection drugs requires no additional evaluation or treatment.

bliography
nerican Thoracic Society. Targeted tuberculin testing and treatment of latent tuberculosis infection. MMWR Recomm Rep. 2000;49(RR-6):1-51. [PMID: 10881762]

em 58   Answer: A

ducational Objective: Diagnose cytomegalovirus fection after kidney transplantation.

his patient has cytomegalovirus (CMV) infection and dis-se presenting as the CMV syndrome, which typically curs in the first few months after transplantation. Typical dings include fever, cytopenias, and hepatitis and may clude pneumonitis or colitis. The onset of CMV in this tient was delayed by the prophylaxis given for the first few onths following transplantation. The periods following lid organ transplant during which opportunistic infections n occur are the early period (within the first month after

transplantation), the middle period (the first few months after transplantation), and the late period (more than a few months after transplantation). This patient is at higher risk for CMV infection because she was a seronegative recipient of an organ from a seropositive donor. Testing for CMV viremia should be performed, and treatment with intravenous ganci-clovir or oral valganciclovir should be started.

This patient is also at risk for Epstein-Barr virus reacti-vation and disease, and this would be the appropriate time frame (5 months posttransplantation) for this infection to occur; however, in transplant recipients, this infection usu-ally presents with lymphadenopathy as Epstein-Barr virus–associated posttransplant lymphoproliferative disease. Lymphadenopathy is absent in this patient.

Listeria monocytogenes infection may occur during this posttransplantation time frame but more often causes menin-goencephalitis with headache and mental status changes or neurologic deficits, which this patient does not have.

Polyoma BK virus infection is a late complication of transplantation. Kidney transplant recipients with BK virus infection may develop BK-related nephropathy, organ rejection, or ureteral strictures. Transplant recipients with BK-related nephropathy have decoy cells in the urine (cells with intranuclear inclusions), evidence of which is absent in this patient.

KEY POINT

- **Cytomegalovirus infection typically occurs in the first few months after solid organ trans-plantation (the middle period); is characterized by fever, malaise, leukopenia, and thrombocy-topenia; and may involve the lungs or gastro-intestinal tract.**

Bibliography
De Keyzer K, Van Laecke S, Peeters P, Vanholder R. Human cytomegalovirus and kidney transplantation: a clinician's update. Am J Kidney Dis. 2011;58(1):118-126. [PMID: 21684438]

Item 59   Answer: B

Educational Objective: Manage bacterial meningitis.

Continuation of current management is indicated for this patient with acute bacterial meningitis. *Streptococcus pneu-moniae* and *Listeria monocytogenes* are the most likely causative pathogens in this age group. The recommended empiric antimicrobial regimen is the combination of van-comycin, ampicillin, and a third-generation cephalosporin (either cefotaxime or ceftriaxone) pending culture results and in vitro susceptibility testing of the isolated pathogen. Because this patient may possibly have pneumococcal menin-gitis, he received adjunctive dexamethasone, which can atten-uate release of bacterial virulence components as a result of antimicrobial-induced lysis. Administration of dexam-ethasone may limit some of the pathophysiologic conse-quences of bacterial meningitis (including subarachnoid

CONT.

space inflammation, cerebral edema, and increased intracranial pressure). Although adjunctive dexamethasone has been shown to reduce the likelihood of adverse outcomes and death in adults with pneumococcal meningitis, it should be given concomitant with or just before the first dose of an antimicrobial agent to achieve these benefits.

Adding rifampin can be considered in patients with resistant pneumococcal meningitis when in vitro testing demonstrates that the organism is susceptible to this agent.

Placement of an external ventricular drain is only appropriate for treatment of hydrocephalus, which was not seen on this patient's neuroimaging studies.

Repeating the cerebrospinal fluid analysis is indicated for patients who have not improved after 36 to 48 hours of appropriate therapy, especially for patients with pneumococcal meningitis who are also being treated with adjunctive dexamethasone.

KEY POINT

- Recommended empiric therapy for bacterial meningitis is the combination of vancomycin, ampicillin, and a third-generation cephalosporin (cefotaxime or ceftriaxone), with adjunctive dexamethasone for suspected or proven pneumococcal meningitis concomitant with or just prior to the first dose of antimicrobial therapy.

Bibliography

Brouwer MC, McIntyre P, de Gans J, et al. Corticosteroids for acute bacterial meningitis. Cochrane Database Syst Rev. 2010;(9):CD004405. [PMID: 20824838]

Item 60   Answer: B

Educational Objective: Treat *Pseudomonas aeruginosa* pneumonia.

The most appropriate treatment is cefepime, tobramycin, and azithromycin. This patient has severe community-acquired pneumonia (CAP) and risk factors for *Pseudomonas aeruginosa* infection given her underlying frequent exacerbations of severe COPD and long-term corticosteroid therapy. In addition, her sputum Gram stain reveals gram-negative rods. Consequently, antibiotic therapy should include coverage for possible *P. aeruginosa* until further information is obtained from the sputum culture. Because of increasing antimicrobial resistance among gram-negative pathogens, empiric coverage for possible *P. aeruginosa* infection should include an antipseudomonal β-lactam agent with pneumococcal coverage (cefepime, imipenem, meropenem, or piperacillin-tazobactam) plus ciprofloxacin or levofloxacin; or an antipseudomonal β-lactam agent with pneumococcal coverage plus an aminoglycoside plus azithromycin; or an antipseudomonal β-lactam with pneumococcal coverage plus an aminoglycoside plus a respiratory fluoroquinolone.

Aztreonam is an alternative antipseudomonal agent that can be used for patients with severe β-lactam allergy

and would require combination with a second agent wi antipseudomonal activity, as described above.

Neither cefotaxime plus azithromycin nor the comł nation of cefotaxime, azithromycin, and levofloxacin wou provide adequate coverage against possible infection with *aeruginosa* in this critically ill patient.

KEY POINT

- Because of increasing antimicrobial resistance among gram-negative pathogens, empiric coverage for critically ill patients with possible *Pseudomonas aeruginosa* infection should include two antipseudomonal agents.

Bibliography

Mandell LA, Wunderink RG, Anzueto A, et al. Infectious Disea Society of America/American Thoracic Society consensus guidelines on the management of community-acquired pneumonia adults. Clin Infect Dis. 2007;44(suppl 2):S27-72. [PMI 17278083]

Item 61   Answer: D

Educational Objective: Manage a patient with meningoencephalitis.

Because this patient has a low probability for herpes simpl encephalitis, intravenous acyclovir should be discontinue The patient presents with meningoencephalitis, defined as altered mental status lasting at least 24 hours that is varial associated with fever, seizures, pleocytosis, and abnorm neuroimaging studies. Herpes simplex encephalitis is th most common cause of sporadic encephalitis in the Unit States and one of the few treatable causes of encephalitis. is classically associated with localized infection of the temp ral lobe; however, atypical presentations have been describe Treatment guidelines recommend initiation of empiric ac clovir in all patients with encephalitis pending diagnostic te ing for HSV. HSV polymerase chain reaction (PCR) of ce brospinal fluid (CSF) has a sensitivity of 95% and a specific of 98% for the diagnosis of herpes simplex encephalitis. Giv the excellent performance characteristics of this assay, it appropriate to discontinue acyclovir in a patient with a lo probability for herpes simplex encephalitis.

Oral formulations of acyclovir and valacyclovir do n achieve therapeutic CSF levels, which precludes treatme of encephalitis with these agents in patients with presum or confirmed herpes simplex encephalitis.

False-negative HSV PCR results may occur very ea in the course of infection. However, more than 90% patients with herpes simplex encephalitis have abnormalit on MRI of the brain. Consequently, in patients with M studies confirming temporal lobe inflammation, acyclo should be continued pending repeat testing on a secor CSF sample obtained 2 to 4 days later. However, th patient has a normal MRI and a negative HSV PCR, whi effectively excludes the diagnosis of herpes simpl encephalitis; a second HSV PCR is not needed. A positi

V PCR result is diagnostic of herpes simplex encephali-
Therefore, only patients with positive results should
ntinue to receive intravenous acyclovir for 14 to 21 days.

Staphylococcus aureus infections in adults and children. Clin Infect Dis. 2011;52(3):e18-55. Epub 2011 Jan 4. [PMID: 21208910]

EY POINT

- In patients with a low clinical suspicion for herpes simplex encephalitis, empiric acyclovir therapy may be discontinued when herpes simplex virus polymerase chain reaction results are negative.

iliography

kel AR, Glaser CA, Bloch KC, et al; Infectious Diseases Society of merica. The management of encephalitis: clinical practice guide-ines by the Infectious Diseases Society of America. Clin Infect Dis. 2008;47(3):303-327. [PMID: 18582201]

m 62   Answer: D

ucational Objective: Treat a patient with rulent cellulitis.

is patient has purulent cellulitis (cellulitis associated with rulent drainage or an exudate but without a drainable cess), and outpatient treatment with trimethoprim-sul-ethoxazole should be initiated. This infection is most ly caused by community-associated methicillin-resistant phylococcus aureus (CA-MRSA). Novel CA-MRSA ins have emerged across the United States. These strains distinct from hospital-associated or health care–associ-d MRSA strains, have different virulence factors, and en have different antimicrobial susceptibility patterns. tial cases of skin and soft tissue infections, including cel-tis with or without abscesses, occurred in children, stu-t and professional athletes, prisoners, men who have sex h men, and American Indians. CA-MRSA strains con-ue to spread throughout the community and beyond se initially defined subpopulations, and now many ients do not have identifiable risk factors. Recom-nded empiric antimicrobial agents for outpatients with CA-MRSA skin or soft tissue infection include trimetho-m-sulfamethoxazole, a tetracycline (for example, doxy-line), clindamycin, and linezolid.

Amoxicillin, cephalexin, and dicloxacillin are β-lactam nts with activity against β-hemolytic streptococci but CA-MRSA. These agents are indicated for treatment of ients with nonpurulent cellulitis.

EY POINT

- Recommended empiric antibiotic agents for outpatients with purulent cellulitis caused by community-associated methicillin-resistant *Staphylococcus aureus* include trimethoprim-sul-famethoxazole, a tetracycline (for example, doxycycline), clindamycin, and linezolid.

iliography

C, Bayer A, Cosgrove SE, et al; Infectious Diseases Society of merica. Clinical practice guidelines by the Infectious Diseases ociety of America for the treatment of methicillin-resistant

Item 63   Answer: A

Educational Objective: Manage a patient with osteomyelitis.

The most appropriate next step in management is deep bone biopsy culture before antimicrobial therapy is begun. The development of a draining sinus tract from the wound above a bone that underwent surgical instrumentation is highly suspicious for underlying contiguous osteomyelitis. The patient's current condition is presumably related to his initial open trauma or surgery 6 months ago. Microbiologic isolates from cultures obtained from a wound or draining sinus tract generally do not reliably correlate with the pathogen in the infected bone with the occasional exception of *Staphylococcus aureus*. Owing to limited utility and the possibility for providing misinformation, the use of microbiologic isolates from the culture of wounds or drain-ing sinus tracts to guide therapy, such as treatment with ampicillin-sulbactam against the organisms identified from a wound swab in this patient, is discouraged. Instead, iden-tification of the causative pathogen(s) is best attempted by bone biopsy performed surgically or percutaneously with radiographic guidance. Once the causative organism is recovered, treatment (usually consisting of at least 6 weeks of parenteral antimicrobial therapy) can be initiated. Debridement of necrotic material is often necessary, and, if feasible, removal the metallic hardware is performed to optimize the chances of microbiologic eradication and clin-ical success.

Prolonged oral ciprofloxacin has proved to be an effective therapy for bone biopsy culture–proven osteomyelitis involving susceptible gram-negative bacilli. However, oral amoxicillin would not be an adequate choice for treating the rare circumstance of enterococcal osteomyelitis.

A three-phase technetium-99m-labeled bone scan is a very sensitive imaging modality for detecting the presence of suspected osteomyelitis. However, this study lacks speci-ficity and would be expected to be abnormal owing to the patient's recent surgery and, therefore, could not reliably confirm a diagnosis of bone infection.

KEY POINT

- In patients with suspected osteomyelitis, the microbiologic isolates from cultures obtained from a wound or draining sinus tract generally do not reliably correlate with the pathogen in the infected bone with the occasional exception of *Staphylococcus aureus*.

Bibliography

Zuluaga AF, Wilson G, Saldarriaga JG, et al. Etiologic diagnosis of chronic osteomyelitis: a prospective study. Arch Intern Med. 2006;166(1):95-100. [PMID: 16401816]

H **Item 64** **Answer: C**

Educational Objective: Diagnose *Pneumocystis* pneumonia in a patient with AIDS.

The most likely diagnosis is *Pneumocystis jirovecii* pneumonia. This patient with known HIV risk factors and a reactive rapid HIV test very likely has HIV infection, although confirmation with Western blot testing still must be performed. He is most likely presenting with *Pneumocystis* pneumonia (PCP) caused by *Pneumocystis jirovecii*. His subacute presentation with dry cough and dyspnea and chest radiograph findings of diffuse interstitial disease constitute the typical presentation of PCP in patients with AIDS, which is also the most common opportunistic infection in patients not taking *Pneumocystis* prophylaxis. Bronchoscopy with lavage can be done with special stains to confirm the diagnosis. Because this patient's arterial PO_2 level is less than 70 mm Hg (9.3 kPa), treatment would include corticosteroids plus trimethoprim-sulfamethoxazole.

Although it can cause pneumonia in transplant recipients, cytomegalovirus (CMV) is an unusual cause of pneumonia in patients with AIDS. In such patients, CMV is more likely to present as retinitis or gastrointestinal disease, with CD4 cell counts less than 50/microliter.

Mycobacterium avium complex usually causes disseminated disease in patients with AIDS and CD4 cell counts less than 50/microliter who present with systemic symptoms, such as fevers, sweats, weight loss, and involvement of the liver, spleen, and lymph nodes, not as pulmonary disease.

Candida is generally a very rare cause of pulmonary infection, even in immunocompromised hosts. The presence of pseudohyphae in this patient's sputum is most likely a result of his oral candidiasis as demonstrated by his examination findings and is not evidence of pulmonary involvement.

KEY POINT

- In patients with AIDS, *Pneumocystis* pneumonia is the most common opportunistic infection in patients not taking *Pneumocystis* prophylaxis and is typically characterized by a subacute presentation with dry cough and dyspnea and chest radiograph findings of diffuse interstitial disease.

Bibliography

Carmona EM, Limper AH. Update on the diagnosis and treatment of Pneumocystis pneumonia. Ther Adv Respir Dis. 2011;5(1):41-59. [PMID: 20736243]

H **Item 65** **Answer: D**

Educational Objective: Treat mucormycosis (previously zygomycosis) in a patient with diabetic ketoacidosis.

Based on his clinical scenario and physical examination findings, this patient most likely has rhino-orbital mucormycosis (previously zygomycosis) and requires emergency surgical

debridement and intravenous amphotericin B. Because o recent change in taxonomy, the class name Zygomycetes been replaced, and, therefore, the term "zygomycosis" is longer appropriate. Classic manifestations of mucormyco are sinusitis, rhino-orbital infection, and rhinocerebral inf tion. Following inhalation of spores, infection is initially lo ized to the nasal turbinates and sinuses. Infection progress rapidly to the orbit or brain. Prompt administrati of intravenous amphotericin B and aggressive surgi debridement are essential in cases of suspected mucormy sis given the high mortality rate (25% to 62%) associated w this disorder.

Piperacillin-tazobactam is a broad-spectrum β-l tam/β-lactamase inhibitor combination that is used to tr polymicrobial bacterial infections. It does not possess ar fungal activity and, therefore, would not be appropriate the next important step in managing a life-threatening fu gal infection.

Oral posaconazole is a broad-spectrum azole antif gal agent that has in vitro activity against mucormycos This agent may have a role in step-down therapy patients who have responded to amphotericin B or as s vage therapy for patients who have not responded to fi line treatment, but it would not be appropriate first-l treatment in this patient.

The efficacy of hyperbaric oxygen treatment mucormycosis has not been definitively demonstrated clinical trials. Hyperbaric oxygen is not a first-line treatme and should not be considered in this patient.

KEY POINT

- Successful management of mucormycosis (previously zygomycosis) hinges on prompt administration of appropriate antifungal therapy coupled with aggressive surgical debridement.

Bibliography

Sun HY, Singh N. Mucormycosis: its contemporary face and mana ment strategies. Lancet Infect Dis. 2011;11(4):301-311. [PM 21453871]

Item 66 **Answer: D**

Educational Objective: Manage a patient with a epidural abscess and neurologic deficits.

This patient most likely has an epidural abscess complicat by spinal cord compression and requires emergent surg decompression. This procedure should be performed patients presenting within 24 to 36 hours of developi complete paralysis to minimize the likelihood of permane neurologic sequelae.

Empiric antimicrobial therapy should be administe intraoperatively once appropriate culture specimens obtained. Medical therapy alone can be considered patients who have only localized pain and/or radicu symptoms, but these patients require careful observati th frequent neurologic examinations and MRI studies to monstrate resolution of the abscess.

CT-guided bone biopsy might yield positive culture sults but would not treat this patient's neurologic mpromise.

Emergent radiation therapy should not be adminis- ed for a bacterial abscess or before a definitive diagnosis established. In addition, malignancy is not likely in this tient based on his initial MRI findings.

EY POINT

- **Patients with an epidural abscess and complete paralysis lasting less than 24 to 36 hours should undergo emergent surgical decompression.**

bliography

rouiche RO. Spinal epidural abscess. N Engl J Med. 2006;355(19):2012-2020. [PMID: 17093252]

em 67   Answer: B

ucational Objective: Initiate appropriate infec- on control measures in a patient with invasive dis- se secondary to *Streptococcus pyogenes* infection.

prevent dissemination of infection resulting from this tient's group A β-hemolytic streptococcal (*Streptococcus genes*) (GABHS) necrotizing fasciitis and toxic shock ndrome (TSS), contact precautions must be instituted. ce *S. pyogenes* is confirmed as the cause of infection, par- eral clindamycin and penicillin are recommended. Sec- dary transmission of GABHS-induced TSS to close con- ts of patients has been reported. Contact isolation ecautions should be initiated for patients with suspected known invasive GABHS-induced disease, including TSS d necrotizing fasciitis, until they have completed 24 urs of antibiotic therapy. Gloves and gowns should be rn by anyone entering the room. Postexposure peni- in-based prophylaxis may be considered for high-risk usehold contacts of patients with invasive GABHS infec- n, including those who are older than 65 years of age or ve conditions associated with an increased risk of devel- ing invasive infection (for example, diabetes mellitus, car- c disease, varicella infection, cancer, HIV infection, rticosteroid use, or injection drug use).

Airborne precautions are recommended for patients ected with microorganisms such as rubella virus and cobacterium tuberculosis, which are transmitted by air- rne droplet nuclei less than 5 micrometers in size. ganisms causing avian influenza, varicella, disseminated ster, severe acute respiratory syndrome, smallpox, and agents of viral hemorrhagic fever require airborne and ntact precautions. Airborne precautions include placing tients in an isolation room with high-efficiency particu- e air filtration and negative pressure. Visitors to the room uld wear appropriate respiratory protective gear when tering as should patients during transport out of the

room. Persons who are not immune to measles or varicella infection should not enter the room.

Droplet precautions are used for protection against microorganisms transmitted by respiratory droplets greater than 5 micrometers in size. These droplets can usually be trans- mitted to susceptible recipient mucosal surfaces over short dis- tances measuring less than 3 to 10 feet. Examples of other pathogens and diseases requiring institution of droplet isola- tion precautions include *Neisseria meningitidis*, pneumonic plague, diphtheria, *Haemophilus influenzae* type b, *Bordetella pertussis*, influenza, mumps, rubella, and parvovirus B19.

Standard precautions are used with all patients and include protecting breaks in the skin or mucous membranes from possible pathogenic exposures, hand washing before and after patient contact, wearing gloves when contacting blood or bodily fluids, hand washing after glove removal, and wearing a mask and eye protection when needed to decrease risk for splash- or aerosol-associated exposures. However, using only standard precautions in this patient with GABHS infection would provide inadequate protection.

KEY POINT

- **Infection control management of patients with suspected or known invasive disease caused by group A β-hemolytic streptococci, including toxic shock syndrome and necrotizing fasciitis, consists of contact precautions until completion of 24 hours of antibiotic therapy.**

Bibliography

Siegel JD, Rhinehart E, Jackson M, Chiarello L; Health Care Infec- tion Control Practices Advisory Committee. 2007 Guideline for Isolation Precautions: Preventing Transmission of Infectious Agents in Health Care Settings. Am J Infect Control. 2007;35(10 suppl 2):S65-164. [PMID: 18068815]

Item 68   Answer: D

Educational Objective: Manage HIV treatment failure.

The patient should undergo viral resistance testing while continuing his present medication regimen, with a treat- ment change based on resistance testing results. Resistance testing is appropriate in the setting of treatment failure as evidenced by suboptimally controlled HIV RNA viral loads (lack of suppressed viral loads or previously undetectable viral loads that have become detectable on repeated test- ing). This patient is adherent to his antiretroviral therapy, and his previously undetectable viral load is now repeatedly detectable, indicating treatment failure. Resistance testing should be performed to guide the selection of a new treat- ment regimen. The present regimen should be continued to sustain partial suppression of the virus pending results of resistance testing. A new regimen can be instituted once resistance testing results become available.

Continuing the same therapeutic regimen in this patient with demonstrated treatment failure would lead to development of further resistance, higher virus levels, and an eventual decline in CD4 cell count.

Resistance testing should be done while the patient continues the current regimen. Discontinuing the regimen would allow a significant increase in viral load. Resistance testing done while the patient is not receiving therapy may be unreliable without the selective pressure of the medications to maintain the presence of mutations in the predominant virus population.

This patient requires antiretroviral therapy and has been tolerating it well. The Strategies for Management of AntiRetroviral Treatment (SMART) study showed that for such patients, therapy should be maintained and a drug holiday avoided because it is associated with increased complications and mortality.

KEY POINT

- In patients with HIV infection, resistance testing is appropriate in the setting of treatment failure as evidenced by suboptimally controlled viral loads (lack of suppressed viral loads or previously undetectable viral loads that have become detectable on repeated testing).

Bibliography

Taylor S, Jayasuriya A, Smit E. Using HIV resistance tests in clinical practice. J Antimicrob Chemother. 2009;64(2):218-222. [PMID: 19535382]

Item 69   Answer: A
Educational Objective: Treat cat-scratch disease.

This patient has cat-scratch disease, and treatment with azithromycin is recommended. Cat-scratch disease most often occurs in immunocompetent children and young adults and is caused by inoculation of the fastidious gram-negative bacterium *Bartonella henselae* after the scratch or bite of a kitten or cat. A pustule or papule or erythema develops at the site of inoculation several days to 2 weeks after the injury. Significant tender regional lymphadenopathy develops 2 to 3 weeks after inoculation in areas that drain the infected site. These lymph nodes suppurate in a small number of patients. Lymphadenopathy generally resolves within months, and extranodal disease is rare. *B. henselae* infection also should be considered in the differential diagnosis of fever of unknown origin. Although cat-scratch disease is usually a self-limited illness, some experts recommend a short course of treatment with azithromycin. Other agents that can be used include doxycycline, rifampin, clarithromycin, trimethoprim-sulfamethoxazole, and ciprofloxacin.

Linezolid and dicloxacillin are used primarily to treat gram-positive bacteria such as staphylococci and streptococci and are not effective against gram-negative organisms such as *B. henselae*.

Lymphocutaneous sporotrichosis is the most common form of sporotrichosis caused by the fungus *Sporothrix*

schenckii. Following cutaneous inoculation, typically of t hand or forearm, a papule or nodule with overlying er thema develops and may ulcerate. Similar lesions devel along lymphatic channels proximal to the draining lym nodes. Itraconazole is the preferred treatment. This patie does not have findings consistent with sporotrichosis, a treatment with itraconazole is not indicated.

KEY POINT

- **Azithromycin is an effective antibiotic agent for treatment of cat-scratch disease.**

Bibliography

Stevens DL, Bisno AL, Chambers HF, et al; Infectious Diseases So ety of America. Practice guidelines for the diagnosis and manag ment of skin and soft tissue infections. Clin Infect D 2005;41(10):1373-1406. [PMID: 16231249]

Item 70   Answer: A
Educational Objective: Interpret serologic testir for *Borrelia burgdorferi* infection.

This patient requires additional evaluation for fatigue ar weakness. He has vague constitutional symptoms of seve months' duration that are nonfocal, nonspecific, and n suggestive of Lyme disease. Investigation for other possil causes is therefore indicated.

Despite this patient's low clinical suspicion for Lyr disease, serologic testing was performed. This is a co mon problem when patients are searching for answers f nonspecific, troublesome symptoms. The recommend diagnostic strategy is two-stage serologic testing for t presence of antibodies to *Borrelia burgdorferi*. The init screening test is an immunofluorescent assay or enzym linked immunosorbent assay, both of which are exqu itely sensitive but nonspecific. If the initial test is equi ocal or positive, as it was in this patient, a confirmato Western blot assay is performed. Standardized criteria a available for interpretation of Western blot IgG and Ig antibody assays based on the number of positive band Interpretation of a positive IgM antibody result with negative IgG antibody result requires clinical correlatic If symptoms are present for less than 1 month, findin may represent delayed seroconversion following acu infection, and repeat testing at a later date is reco mended to confirm the diagnosis. However, when sym toms have been present for more than 1 month, partic larly when the symptoms are nonspecific (as they are this patient), a positive IgM antibody result in t absence of IgG antibodies most likely represents a fals positive test result, and no additional testing for Lyr disease is needed.

Because the patient requires further evaluation and very unlikely to have Lyme disease, treatment of this infe tion with either ceftriaxone or doxycycline is not indicate

- Patients with nonspecific symptoms, such as fatigue, myalgia, or arthralgia, with a low pretest probability for Lyme disease, should not be tested for this disease.

Bibliography

Centers for Disease Control and Prevention (CDC). Recommendations for test performance and interpretation from the Second National Conference on Serologic Diagnosis of Lyme Disease. MMWR Morb Mortal Wkly Rep. 1995;11;44(31):590-591. [PMID: 7623762]

Item 71   Answer: B

Educational Objective: Treat pyelonephritis in a young woman in an outpatient setting.

This patient has signs and symptoms consistent with mild pyelonephritis, and because she does not require hospitalization, the optimal management is to obtain a urine culture and start a 7-day course of oral ciprofloxacin, with or without an initial loading dose of ciprofloxacin, 400 mg intravenously. Optimal treatment of acute, uncomplicated pyelonephritis depends on the severity of illness and local resistance patterns as well as host factors such as allergies. Therapy with fluoroquinolone antibiotics is indicated when the prevalence of resistance of community uropathogens to this class of medications does not exceed 10%. If the prevalence of fluoroquinolone resistance is greater than 10%, a single dose of a long-acting intravenous agent such as ceftriaxone or an aminoglycoside should be administered.

Ampicillin would not be appropriate because oral β-lactam agents are less effective than other antibiotics for treating pyelonephritis, and resistance rates are high.

Nitrofurantoin should not be used to treat pyelonephritis because it does not achieve adequate levels in renal tissue.

In a study comparing a 7-day regimen of oral ciprofloxacin with a 14-day regimen of trimethoprim-sulfamethoxazole for women with mild to moderate pyelonephritis, ciprofloxacin had significantly higher clinical and microbiologic cure rates. Trimethoprim-sulfamethoxazole would be appropriate if the pathogen was known to be susceptible.

- Standard outpatient management of mild pyelonephritis in women who are not pregnant is an oral fluoroquinolone, such as ciprofloxacin, for 7 days.

Bibliography

Gupta K, Hooton TM, Naber KG, et al; Infectious Diseases Society of America; European Society for Microbiology and Infectious Diseases. International clinical practice guidelines for the treatment of acute uncomplicated cystitis and pyelonephritis in women: a 2010 update by the Infectious Diseases Society of America and the European Society for Microbiology and Infectious Diseases. Clin Infect Dis. 2011;52(5):e103-e120. [PMID: 21292654]

Item 72   Answer: B

Educational Objective: Manage hyperlipidemia in a patient with HIV infection.

The most appropriate management of this patient is initiation of atorvastatin. Metabolic changes in patients with HIV infection can be caused by antiretroviral medications or the infection itself. HIV infection is associated with decreased total, HDL, and LDL cholesterol levels and increased triglyceride levels. Treatment with antiretroviral therapy tends to reverse some of these changes: total and LDL cholesterol increase, but HDL cholesterol remains decreased and triglycerides remain elevated. Some antiretroviral agents, including many protease inhibitors, are particularly associated with hyperlipidemia. This patient's LDL cholesterol level is still higher than goal (130 mg/dL [4.1 mmol/L]) despite diet and exercise. Treatment with a statin is therefore indicated. Atorvastatin has been shown to be effective in treating hyperlipidemia in patients with HIV infection; because of interactions with the protease inhibitor ritonavir, atorvastatin should be started at a lower dose.

This patient has a relatively healthy lifestyle except for smoking, and additional therapeutic changes would likely not have an adequately positive effect on his lipids given their current levels.

Reduction in LDL cholesterol, not triglycerides, is the primary goal of this patient's therapy, and a statin is a better choice than a fibrate for reducing LDL cholesterol levels.

Simvastatin is contraindicated in patients taking HIV protease inhibitors because of cytochrome P-450 drug metabolism interactions, which would raise simvastatin concentrations to dangerous levels.

- Atorvastatin is effective for treating hyperlipidemia in patients with HIV infection and should be started at a lower dose in patients taking protease inhibitors to avoid drug interactions.

Bibliography

Farrugia PM, Lucariello R, Coppola JT. Human immunodeficiency virus and atherosclerosis. Cardiol Rev. 2009;17(5):211-215. [PMID: 19690471]

Item 73   Answer: D

Educational Objective: Treat a patient with pneumococcal meningitis.

Vancomycin and ceftriaxone are indicated for this patient, who most likely has acute bacterial meningitis. Cerebrospinal fluid analysis was consistent with this diagnosis, and Gram stain revealed gram-positive diplococci, suggesting that *Streptococcus pneumoniae* is the bacterial pathogen. Pending in vitro susceptibility testing of the isolated organism, the patient should be presumed to have pneumococcal meningitis caused by a pathogen that is resistant to penicillin G. The combination of vancomycin and a third-generation cephalosporin (either ceftriaxone or cefotaxime) is therefore recommended because these agents have been shown to be synergistic in killing resistant pneumococci in experimental animal models of pneumococcal meningitis. Once results of in vitro susceptibility testing are available, antimicrobial therapy can be modified for optimal treatment.

Levofloxacin has not been studied in patients with bacterial meningitis, and the other antimicrobial combinations have not shown efficacy in the treatment of pneumococcal meningitis caused by highly penicillin-resistant strains.

> **KEY POINT**
> - **The recommended empiric therapy for pneumococcal meningitis is vancomycin plus a third-generation cephalosporin (either ceftriaxone or cefotaxime).**

Bibliography
Brouwer MC, Tunkel AR, van de Beek D. Epidemiology, diagnosis, and antimicrobial treatment of acute bacterial meningitis. Clin Microbiol Rev. 2010;23(3):467-492. [PMID: 20610819]

Item 74   Answer: D
Educational Objective: Diagnose *Yersinia pestis* infection.

The most likely infectious agent is *Yersinia pestis*, the causative agent of plague. *Y. pestis* is endemic to the southwestern United States where the population of reservoir rodents is dense, with transmission usually by flea bite. The bipolar staining Gram-negative bacillus giving the appearance of a closed "safety pin" is virtually pathognomonic for *Y. pestis*.

Plague typically consists of three clinical syndromes: (1) pneumonic plague, occurring with inhalation of bacteria; (2) bubonic plague, characterized by purulent lymphadenitis near the inoculation site (more common in the naturally occurring zoonotic form of infection); and (3) septicemic plague, a septic presentation that can arise from either of the other syndromes. Bubonic plague, with systemic symptoms associated with an intensely painful, swollen group of lymph nodes (bubo), is the most common form and represents 85% of all cases. Pneumonic plague is the most fulminant and lethal form of the disease, occurring primarily through direct inhalation of infectious respiratory droplets from infected animals or people or from intentional aerosol release as an act of bioterrorism. The pneumonic form of disease is virtually 100% fatal if treatment is not administered within 24 hours. Based on ease of access, the potential lethality of the aerosolized form, lack of preventive measures, and rapidity of clinical progression, the Centers for Disease Control and Prevention have designated *Y. pestis* a Category A bioterrorism agent.

Legionella infection (Legionnaires disease) generally requires the inhalation of an infectious aerosol of *Legionella pneumophila* from a contaminated water source. Although frequently associated with systemic symptoms and abnormal

laboratory findings, pneumonia is the primary clinical ma festation of infection following a few days of a nonspecific p dromal illness. *L. pneumophila* is a gram-negative bacillus a is difficult to isolate from cultures of sputum or blood; presence of gram-negative, bipolar bacilli in the blood is n consistent with Legionnaires disease.

Community-acquired   pneumonia   involvi *Pseudomonas aeruginosa* is quite uncommon in you immunocompetent hosts without underlying lung disea

Gastroenteritis is the most common presentation *Salmonella enteritidis*, with nontyphoidal strains only rar causing pleuropulmonary infections.

> **KEY POINT**
> - **Plague typically consists of three clinical syndromes: (1) pneumonic plague, occurring with inhalation of bacteria (most likely bioterrorism scenario); (2) bubonic plague, characterized by purulent lymphadenitis near the inoculation site; and (3) septicemic plague, a septic presentation arising from either of the other syndromes.**

Bibliography
Prentice MB, Rahalison L. Plague. Lancet. 2007;369(9568):11 1207. [PMID: 17416264]

Item 75   Answer: D
Educational Objective: Diagnose typhoid fever a returning traveler.

This patient most likely has typhoid fever. Most cases a diagnosed in returning international travelers. Typho fever may develop following the ingestion of *Salmone enterica* serotype Typhi, or occasionally, *S. enterica* subty paratyphi organisms. The incubation period for *S. ty* infection ranges from 1 to 4 weeks.

The clinical presentation of typhoid fever is typicall rising fever, with temperatures as high as 40.0 °C (104.0 ° accompanied by relative bradycardia and significant abdo inal pain, almost always accompanied by constipation. Di rhea may be present initially, but more often develops late the disease progresses. Approximately one third of patie develop salmon-colored, blanching, 1- to 4-cm ma lopapules on the trunk. A distended and tender abdom with splenomegaly is often present. Laboratory abnormalit include anemia, leukopenia, thrombocytopenia, and ele tions in serum bilirubin and aminotransferase levels. Hypo tremia is common. The diagnosis is mainly clinical and established by isolation of *S. typhi* or *S. paratyphi* from bloc bone marrow, stool, or skin. Two vaccines are available protection against infection with *S. typhi*, although neithe completely effective.

Brucellosis is a worldwide zoonotic infection. The cl ical manifestations are generally chronic in nature and of include fever, bone and joint symptoms, and neurolo and neuropsychiatric symptoms frequently accompanie ere weakness and malaise. Rash is not typically associated ch this infection.

Leishmaniasis is a protozoal disease transmitted to mans through the bite of a female sandfly. Patients with ceral leishmaniasis present with weight loss, fever, patosplenomegaly, pancytopenia, and hypergammaglob- nemia. The incubation period is typically several months er time of exposure in an endemic area.

Malaria is often characterized by a cyclic pattern of er without prominent gastrointestinal symptoms or rash.

EY POINT

- Typhoid fever should be considered in patients returning from endemic areas who present with a rash, rising fever, abdominal pain, and consti- pation possibly followed by diarrhea.

liography

ltzer E, Schwartz E. Enteric fever: a travel medicine oriented view. Curr Opin Infect Dis. 2010;23(5):432-437. [PMID: 20613510]

em 76   Answer: A

lucational Objective: Treat Lyme myocarditis.

ravenous ceftriaxone is the most appropriate therapy for s patient, who has complete heart block with serologic ting indicating *Borrelia burgdorferi* infection, consistent ch Lyme myocarditis. The most common cardiac mani- tation of early disseminated Lyme disease is disturbance the atrioventricular conduction system, ranging from mptomatic first-degree heart block to third-degree omplete) heart block. For patients with second- or third- gree heart block, intravenous ceftriaxone is recom- nded. In addition, symptomatic patients or those with ond- or third-degree heart block should be hospitalized cardiac monitoring during treatment.

Asymptomatic patients with first-degree heart block y be treated as outpatients with an oral regimen such as uroxime or doxycycline.

Although placement of a temporary pacemaker may be quired for symptomatic patients, the conduction abnor- lities are reversible, and use of a permanent pacemaker is t indicated.

Observation is not appropriate because antibiotic atment should be initiated immediately.

EY POINT

- Intravenous ceftriaxone is the recommended therapy for patients with Lyme myocarditis associated with second- or third-degree heart block.

liography

rmser GP, Dattwyler RJ, Shapiro ED, et al. The clinical assessment, reatment, and prevention of lyme disease, human granulocytic naplasmosis, and babesiosis: clinical practice guidelines by the nfectious Diseases Society of America. Clin Infect Dis. 006;43(9):1089-1134. [PMID: 17029130]

Item 77   Answer: A

Educational Objective: Treat nonpurulent cellulitis.

This patient has nonpurulent cellulitis that is most likely caused by β-hemolytic streptococci, and empiric outpa- tient treatment with a β-lactam agent such as cephalexin or dicloxacillin is recommended. Cellulitis is a bacterial skin infection involving the dermis and subcutaneous tis- sues. This infection is most frequently associated with dermatologic conditions involving breaks in the skin, such as eczema, tinea pedis, or chronic skin ulcers, and conditions leading to chronic lymphedema, such as mas- tectomy and lymph node dissections or saphenous vein grafts used in bypass surgery. Cellulitis should be sus- pected in patients with the acute onset of spreading ery- thema, edema, pain or tenderness, and warmth. Fever, although common, is not uniformly present. Patients with severe disease may have associated systemic toxicity. The most common pathogens are *Staphylococcus aureus* and the β-hemolytic streptococci, especially group A β- hemolytic streptococci (GABHS). GABHS is most often associated with nonpurulent cellulitis, whereas *S. aureus* may cause concomitant abscesses, furuncles, carbuncles, and bullous impetigo.

Doxycycline and trimethoprim-sulfamethoxazole have activity against community-associated methicillin-resistant *S. aureus* but are not reliably effective against β-hemolytic streptococci.

Fluconazole is an antifungal agent. Fungi do not usu- ally cause cellulitis in young, healthy persons, but fungal infection should be considered in immunocompromised patients.

Metronidazole is an antimicrobial agent used to treat some anaerobic bacterial and protozoal infections. Although metronidazole is active against some microaerophilic bacteria, it is not effective for treatment of β-hemolytic streptococci.

KEY POINT

- Outpatients with nonpurulent cellulitis should be treated empirically with a β-lactam agent such as cephalexin or dicloxacillin that is active against β-hemolytic streptococci.

Bibliography

Gunderson CG. Cellulitis: definition, etiology, and clinical features. Am J Med. 2011;124(12):1113-1122. [PMID: 22014791]

Item 78   Answer: C

Educational Objective: Manage a patient with a history of infective endocarditis before a dental procedure.

This patient with a history of infective endocarditis requires antimicrobial prophylaxis with clindamycin before her dental procedure. The American Heart Association (AHA) infective endocarditis guidelines, revised in 2007, now recommend that only patients with cardiac conditions associated with the highest risk of adverse outcome from endocarditis receive antimicrobial prophylaxis before undergoing a dental procedure involving manipulation of gingival tissue or the periapical region of teeth or perforation of the oral mucosa. These conditions include the presence of a prosthetic cardiac valve, history of infective endocarditis, unrepaired cyanotic congenital heart disease, congenital heart disease repair with prosthetic material or device for the first 6 months after intervention, presence of palliative shunts and conduits, and cardiac valvulopathy in cardiac transplant recipients. The suggested antibiotic prophylactic regimens before dental procedures for patients with these indications are agents directed against viridans group streptococci, administered as a single dose 30 to 60 minutes before the procedure. Clindamycin, azithromycin, or clarithromycin would be appropriate choices for this patient, who experienced anaphylaxis after receiving penicillin.

Amoxicillin and cephalosporins such as cephalexin should not be used in patients with a history of anaphylaxis after receiving penicillin.

Vancomycin is not required because, despite this patient's history of methicillin-resistant *Staphylococcus aureus* endocarditis, this previous infection does not influence the antibiotic choice for prophylactic endocarditis treatment.

According to the AHA guidelines, a history of infective endocarditis is one of the indications for infective endocarditis prophylaxis before a dental procedure involving gingival manipulation; consequently, providing no prophylaxis to this patient would not be appropriate.

KEY POINT

- **The indications for infective endocarditis antimicrobial prophylaxis for patients who will undergo a dental procedure involving manipulation of gingival tissue or the periapical region of teeth or perforation of the oral mucosa are (1) the presence of a prosthetic cardiac valve, (2) a history of infective endocarditis, (3) unrepaired cyanotic congenital heart disease, (4) congenital heart disease repair with prosthetic material or device for the first 6 months after intervention, (5) presence of palliative shunts and conduits, and (6) cardiac valvulopathy in cardiac transplant recipients.**

Bibliography

Wilson W, Taubert KA, Gewitz M, et al. American Heart Association Rheumatic Fever, Endocarditis, and Kawasaki Disease Committee; American Heart Association Council on Cardiovascular Disease in the Young; American Heart Association Council on Clinical Cardiology; American Heart Association Council on Cardiovascular Surgery and Anesthesia; Quality of Care and Outcomes Research Interdisciplinary Working Group. Prevention of infective endocarditis. Guidelines from the American Heart Association. A guideline from the American Heart Association Rheumatic Cardiovascular Disease in the Young, and the Council on Clinical Cardiology, Council on Cardiovascular Surgery and Anesthesia, and the Quality of Care and Outcomes Research Interdisciplinary Working Group. Circulation 2007;116(15):1736-1754. [PMID: 17446442]

Item 79   Answer: B

Educational Objective: Diagnose severe community-acquired pneumonia.

This patient requires *Legionella* and *Streptococcus pneumoniae* urine antigen assays. The role of routine diagnostic testing to determine the microbial cause of community-acquired pneumonia (CAP) is controversial. The Infectious Diseases Society of America/American Thoracic Society (IDSA/ATS) consensus guidelines suggest that diagnostic testing in outpatients, except for pulse oximetry, is optional. However, this hospitalized patient has severe CAP, defined as CAP in a patient necessitating admission to an intensive care unit or transfer to an intensive care unit within 24 hours of admission. Blood cultures, *Legionella* and *Streptococcus pneumoniae* urine antigen assays, and endotracheal aspirate for Gram stain and culture are recommended for hospitalized patients with severe CAP.

Bronchoscopy with quantitative culture can be used as a diagnostic tool in the evaluation of patients with pneumonia. When bronchoscopy was compared with evaluation using clinical features suggesting pneumonia and endotracheal aspirate for Gram stain and qualitative culture in patients with ventilator-associated pneumonia, clinical outcomes for the two approaches were equivalent. However, bronchoscopy with quantitative culture has not been prospectively studied for the management of patients with severe CAP.

Serology for atypical pathogens such as *Legionella* species is not recommended because convalescent titers would need to be obtained 6 to 8 weeks after initial testing to establish a diagnosis.

This hospitalized patient has severe CAP; consequently, providing no further evaluation would not be appropriate.

KEY POINT

- **Blood cultures, *Legionella* and *Streptococcus pneumoniae* urine antigen assays, and endotracheal aspirate for Gram stain and culture are recommended for hospitalized patients with severe community-acquired pneumonia.**

Bibliography

Niederman N. In the clinic. Community-acquired pneumonia. Ann Intern Med. 2009;151(7):ITC4-2-ITC4-14; quiz ITC4- [PMID: 19805767]

Item 80   Answer: A

Educational Objective: Diagnose a suspected brain abscess.

This patient most likely has a brain abscess, and stereotactic CT-guided aspiration of the lesion should be done next. The diagnosis of brain abscess should be considered in patients with a central nervous system mass lesion. Most of the symptoms and signs relate to the size and location of the abscess. Less than 50% of patients with a bacterial brain abscess present with the triad of headache, fever, and focal neurologic deficits. Although the most common predisposing conditions are a result of hematogenous spread or a contiguous focus of infection, 10% to 35% of brain abscesses are cryptogenic. Suspected abscesses that are greater than 2.5 cm in diameter on neuroimaging studies should be excised or aspirated under CT guidance. The specimens should then be sent for microbiologic examination (including stains and culture for bacteria, nocardia, mycobacteria, and fungi) and histopathologic examination (including special stains for identification of these organisms). Although other causes may account for this patient's mass lesion, including a neoplasm, a definitive diagnosis should be established rather than assuming that this is a malignant lesion.

Lumbar puncture is not indicated for patients with central nervous system mass lesions because of the potential complication of brain herniation.

Whole-body PET scanning or CT scanning of the chest, abdomen, and pelvis might be useful in localizing an unknown infectious or malignant focus but would not be performed before definitively diagnosing the primary central nervous system lesion, which may reveal significant information that would further guide the diagnostic evaluation and appropriate treatment.

KEY POINT

- In patients with a central nervous system mass lesion, a definitive diagnosis, such as brain abscess, should be determined rather than assuming that the lesion is malignant.

Bibliography

Lu CH, Chang WN, Liu CC. Strategies for the management of bacterial brain abscess. J Clin Neurosci. 2006;13(10):979-985. [PMID: 1705626]

Item 81   Answer: C

Educational Objective: Prevent ventilator-associated pneumonia.

The head of this patient's bed should be maintained above an angle of 30°. Ventilator-associated pneumonia (VAP) is a subset of hospital-acquired pneumonia (HAP) and refers to pneumonia that develops more than 48 to 72 hours after mechanical ventilation is begun. As in the prevention of central line–associated bloodstream infections (CLABSI), using and implementing a prevention "bundle" is a successful method for reducing the rate of VAP in a facility. A VAP prevention bundle of interventions includes: (1) maintaining the head of the patient's bed above a 30° angle, (2) daily assessments of the patient's readiness to wean from the ventilator, and (3) chlorhexidine mouth washes.

Use of chlorhexidine-based antiseptic to bathe hospitalized patients in intensive care units is a common practice. The benefit of chlorhexidine bathing has been studied relative to CLABSI prevention and spread of multidrug-resistant organisms such as *Acinetobacter baumannii*. However, controlled data pertaining to the specific role of chlorhexidine-based bathing on VAP prevention are still lacking.

Prolonged durations of perioperative surgical prophylactic antimicrobial agents have not been demonstrated to reduce the risk for VAP.

Performing early tracheotomy has not been clearly demonstrated as a method for reducing VAP.

The data regarding the role of antiseptic-coated endotracheal tubes in VAP prevention are promising, but silver-coated endotracheal tubes are not currently formally recommended for VAP prevention. In clinical studies, patients were initially intubated with silver-coated endotracheal tubes; however, the effect on VAP prevention of extubating patients and then re-intubating them with silver-coated endotracheal tubes has not been studied.

KEY POINT

- In patients receiving mechanical ventilation, maintaining the head of the bed above a 30° angle helps reduce the risk for ventilator-associated pneumonia.

Bibliography

American Thoracic Society; Infectious Diseases Society of America. Guidelines for the management of adults with hospital-acquired, ventilator-associated, and healthcare-associated pneumonia. Am J Respir Crit Care Med. 2005;171(4):388-416. [PMID: 15699079]

Item 82   Answer: E

Educational Objective: Diagnose travelers' diarrhea.

No additional diagnostic testing is indicated. This patient has travelers' diarrhea, which is an extremely common illness among visitors to developing countries, especially following ingestion of unprocessed water or raw fruits and vegetables. Travelers' diarrhea may be caused by several different pathogens. The most common pathogen is enterotoxigenic *Escherichia coli* (ETEC), which typically causes a self-limited, relatively mild diarrheal illness that can be treated symptomatically without the need for diagnostic testing.

Routine stool cultures cannot differentiate ETEC from *E. coli* organisms that are part of the normal fecal flora. However, stool cultures for bacteria should be obtained in patients with diarrhea lasting longer than 72 hours, particularly if associated with fever, tenesmus, or blood in the stool.

Stool cultures for viruses are rarely indicated for other than epidemiologic investigation because results are not useful for guiding therapy.

Symptoms lasting longer than 7 days may indicate a parasitic intestinal infection, and examination of the stool for ova and parasites is the recommended initial diagnostic test.

The presence of fecal leukocytes is suggestive of an inflammatory bacterial diarrhea; however, positive results also may be characteristic of other conditions. In this patient, who is at low risk for inflammatory diarrhea, this test would not be cost-effective because, regardless of the results, it would be unlikely to change management.

KEY POINT

- **The most common pathogen responsible for travelers' diarrhea is enterotoxigenic _Escherichia coli_, which typically causes a self-limited, relatively mild diarrheal illness that can be treated symptomatically and warrants no diagnostic testing.**

Bibliography

Hill DR, Ericsson CD, Pearson RD, et al; Infectious Diseases Society of America. The practice of travel medicine: Guidelines by the Infectious Diseases Society of America. Clin Infect Dis. 2006;43(12):1499-1539. [PMID: 17109284]

Item 83   Answer: C
Educational Objective: Treat a patient with gonococcal urethritis.

The most appropriate treatment is ceftriaxone and azithromycin. This patient presents with symptoms and signs consistent with urethritis, including laboratory findings indicating intracellular gram-negative diplococci visualized on a Gram stain of urethral discharge. If available, Gram stain results are extremely useful in the evaluation of men with symptomatic gonococcal urethritis because more than 95% of patients have this finding. Ceftriaxone is the preferred treatment option. Patients with gonococcal urethritis (or cervicitis) should also be treated for possible chlamydial infection because the risk of coinfection is high. Consequently, a single dose of azithromycin plus ceftriaxone should be given to this patient.

A high (2-g) dose of azithromycin may be sufficient for treating infection with _Neisseria gonorrhoeae_ and also _Chlamydia trachomatis_ but is limited by the high frequency of gastrointestinal side effects, increasing resistance, and expense associated with such use.

Cefoxitin has activity against penicillinase-producing _N. gonorrhoeae_ but would not be effective in a single dose without the simultaneous administration of probenecid. In addition, it would fail to cover possible coinfection with _C. trachomatis_.

The combination of ciprofloxacin and azithromycin would not be adequate therapy for this patient. Strains of

gonorrhea have become increasingly resistant to fluoro quinolones in recent years; consequently, fluoroquinolon such as ciprofloxacin are no longer recommended for trea ment of these infections.

KEY POINT

- **Patients with gonococcal urethritis (or cervicitis) should also be treated for possible coinfection with chlamydial infection with ceftriaxone plus a single dose of azithromycin.**

Bibliography

Workowski KA, Berman S; Centers for Disease Control and Preve tion (CDC). Sexually transmitted diseases treatment guideline 2010. MMWR Recomm Rep. 2010;59(RR-12):1-110. [PMI 21160459]

Item 84   Answer: A
Educational Objective: Treat possible methicillin resistant _Staphylococcus aureus_ infection in a patient with purulent cellulitis.

Empiric ceftaroline is the most appropriate β-lactam antib otic for this patient with purulent cellulitis presumab caused by methicillin-resistant _Staphylococcus aure_ (MRSA). Development of MRSA requires the acquisition a _mec_ gene, which encodes for penicillin-binding protein 2 in the bacterial membrane. Drug resistance develop because of the low affinity of penicillin-binding protein 2 for β-lactam agents. MRSA organisms are resistant t oxacillin, nafcillin, and dicloxacillin, as well as to carbapen ems (including meropenem) and monobactam antibiotic All cephalosporins, including ceftriaxone, are also inactiv against MRSA, except ceftaroline, a new fifth-generatio cephalosporin approved by the FDA for treating skin infe tions and community-acquired bacterial pneumonia. Ce taroline, unlike other β-lactam agents, has a high affinity fo penicillin-binding protein 2a. This drug also has activi against staphylococci and streptococci as well as some gran negative organisms (including _Haemophilus influenzae_) an Enterobacteriaceae (including _Klebsiella_ species an _Escherichia coli_). Ceftaroline is administered intravenous and requires dose adjustment based on kidney function.

KEY POINT

- **Ceftaroline is a new β-lactam antibiotic with significant activity against methicillin-resistant _Staphylococcus aureus_ and other aerobic and anaerobic gram-positive organisms and aerobic gram-negative bacteria, and it can be used for complicated soft tissue infections and community-acquired pneumonia.**

Bibliography

Saravolatz LD, Stein GE, Johnson LB. Ceftaroline: A no cephalosporin with activity against methicillin-resistant Staphy coccus aureus. Clin Infect Dis. 2011;52(9):1156-1163. [PMI 21467022]

Item 85   Answer: E

Educational Objective: Manage a patient with symptomatic bacteriuria.

Asymptomatic bacteriuria in the elderly does not require treatment. The prevalence of asymptomatic bacteriuria is higher among women than men and occurs more commonly in pregnant patients, patients with diabetes, and the elderly. Asymptomatic bacteriuria becomes more common among men at age 65 years or older. In asymptomatic men, symptomatic bacteriuria is defined as a single, clean-catch, voided urine specimen with one bacterial species isolated in a quantitative count of 10^5 or more colony-forming units/mL. Evidence has shown that treating asymptomatic bacteriuria in elderly patients has no effect on the incidence of symptomatic urinary tract infections, prevalence of bacteriuria, or survival. Screening or treatment of asymptomatic bacteriuria is not indicated in nonpregnant women or patients with diabetes, spinal cord injuries, or with chronic indwelling urinary catheters. Treatment of these populations puts the patients at risk for drug side effects and increases the probability of antibiotic resistance. Treating symptomatic bacteriuria is appropriate in pregnancy and before invasive urologic procedures.

Ciprofloxacin and trimethoprim-sulfamethoxazole are both appropriate choices for treating symptomatic urinary tract infection, which is not required in this patient.

Medical evaluation, such as kidney ultrasonography, is not indicated for asymptomatic bacteriuria.

Repeating a urinalysis and urine culture will likely provide similar results and will not help in managing this patient.

KEY POINT

- Except for pregnancy and prior to invasive urologic procedures, treatment of asymptomatic bacteriuria is not indicated.

Bibliography

Matthews SJ, Lancaster JW. Urinary Tract Infections in the elderly population. Am J Geriatr Pharmacother. 2011;9(5):286-309. [PMID: 21840265]

Item 86   Answer: D

Educational Objective: Diagnose selective IgA deficiency.

Selective IgA deficiency is the most likely diagnosis in this patient. Although most patients with selective IgA deficiency are asymptomatic, some have chronic or recurrent respiratory tract infections, atopic disorders (such as eczema), or a high incidence of autoimmune diseases, such as rheumatoid arthritis or systemic lupus erythematosus. Gastrointestinal and urinary tract infections may occur as well as severe anaphylactic reactions after intravenous administration of blood products or immune globulin preparations. Patients with undetectable serum levels of IgA may form antibodies directed against IgA, which rarely can be responsible for transfusion reactions.

C1-inhibitor deficiency is an autosomal dominant disorder associated with hereditary angioedema. Most patients have a family history of angioedema, and the condition often presents as recurrent episodes of subcutaneous edema, unexplained episodes of abdominal pain, or laryngeal edema. A single episode of angioedema following an erythrocyte transfusion is most compatible with selective IgA deficiency, not C1-inhibitor deficiency.

Terminal complement deficiency (C5-C9) is inherited as an autosomal co-dominant disorder and is associated with susceptibility to systemic neisserial infections, especially meningococcal disease.

Inherited defects of properdin are rare. Those with this deficiency are at risk for recurrent infection with *Neisseria meningitidis*, not anaphylaxis.

KEY POINT

- **Most patients with selective IgA deficiency are at risk for severe anaphylactic reactions after intravenous administration of blood products or immune globulin preparations.**

Bibliography

Yel L. Selective IgA deficiency. J Clin Immunol. 2010;30(1):10-16. [PMID: 20101521]

Item 87   Answer: B

Educational Objective: Manage tick-borne rickettsial infection.

Doxycycline should be started now. This patient presents with a febrile illness in the spring and a history of tick exposure, raising concern for a tick-borne infection. Results of serologic testing for any of the tick-borne rickettsial pathogens are often negative during the acute phase of the illness. Molecular testing for *Ehrlichia* and *Anaplasma* spp. by whole blood polymerase chain reaction is more sensitive during the acute phase but may be negative if the patient has received prior antibiotics. If one of these diseases is suspected based on epidemiologic and clinical data, empiric treatment should be initiated immediately without awaiting laboratory confirmation because a delay in therapy is associated with a significant increase in morbidity.

Human granulocytic anaplasmosis (HGA, caused by *Anaplasma phagocytophilum*), human monocytic ehrlichiosis (HME, caused by *Ehrlichia chaffeensis*), and Rocky Mountain spotted fever (RMSF, caused by *Rickettsia rickettsii*) present as nonfocal febrile illnesses that are variably associated with cytopenias and increased serum liver enzyme values. Clinically, these three syndromes are difficult to differentiate from each other, although a petechial skin eruption is seen in up to 85% of patients with RMSF but in many fewer adults with HME or HGA. The characteristic rash in RMSF begins as blanching erythematous

CONT.

macules around the wrists and ankles; lesions spread centripetally and become petechial. The rash is found in only 15% of patients on presentation but appears in most patients by day 4. The absence of the rash presents a diagnostic challenge because of the nonspecific nature of the presentation, but treatment should be initiated regardless of the absence of skin lesions if there is clinical concern for a tick-borne rickettsial infection.

The tick vector for HGA is the same species of tick that causes Lyme disease and is endemic to the northeastern United States and the Great Lakes region. In contrast, the tick vector for HME is distributed throughout the south central United States, and RMSF is found throughout the continental United States.

Doxycycline is the antibiotic of choice for treatment of these tick-borne illnesses; β-lactam antibiotics such as amoxicillin are not effective against these infections.

KEY POINT

- Because results of serologic testing for any of the tick-borne rickettsial pathogens are often negative during the acute phase of the illness, empiric treatment with doxycycline should be initiated immediately if one of these diseases is suspected based on epidemiologic and clinical data.

Bibliography

Chapman AS, Bakken JS, Folk SM, et al; Tickborne Rickettsial Diseases Working Group; CDC. Diagnosis and management of tick-borne rickettsial diseases: Rocky Mountain spotted fever, ehrlichiosis, and anaplasmosis—United States: a practical guide for physicians and other health-care and public health professionals. MMWR Recomm Rep. 2006;55(RR-4):1-27. [PMID: 16572105]

Item 88   Answer: D

Educational Objective: Prevent influenza virus infection in a pregnant woman.

This patient should receive trivalent inactivated influenza vaccine. Pregnant women are at higher risk for complications from seasonal influenza viruses, and severe disease has been reported during pandemics. Vaccination is the best way to prevent influenza. Ideally, vaccination with the trivalent inactivated influenza vaccine is indicated in pregnant women whose last two trimesters coincide with influenza season, but it can be administered at any time, regardless of trimester of pregnancy. The influenza vaccine should not be given to persons with anaphylactic hypersensitivity to eggs or to those with a history of Guillain-Barré syndrome, both of which are rare.

Chemoprophylaxis with antiviral medications is not a substitute for influenza vaccination when influenza vaccine is available. Oseltamivir, zanamivir, and the adamantanes (amantadine and rimantadine) are efficacious in the prevention of influenza after exposure to a household member or other close contact with confirmed influenza. Emergence

of resistance has become an issue that now limits the use the adamantanes. Antiviral therapy should be conside for those who are at higher risk for complications but w have not been vaccinated and have family or other cl contacts in whom influenza virus infection is suspected confirmed. An alternative to chemoprophylaxis is to st early therapy at the onset of signs or symptoms. Bef instituting pre-exposure chemoprophylaxis, it is import to consider that adverse effects associated with long-te use are uncertain and prolonged use of antiviral agents lead to resistance. The neuraminidase inhibitors and adamantanes are pregnancy category C agents, wh means that data from clinical studies are not adequate assess the safety of these medications for pregnant wom Pregnant women with confirmed or suspected influe should receive antiviral treatment, and pregnancy is no contraindication to oseltamivir or zanamivir use.

The live attenuated intranasal influenza vaccine is c traindicated in pregnancy as well as in patients with chro metabolic diseases, diabetes mellitus, kidney dysfuncti hemoglobinopathies, immunosuppression, and chronic eases that can compromise respiratory function or the h dling of respiratory secretions.

KEY POINT

- Vaccination with the trivalent inactivated influenza vaccine is the most effective method for preventing influenza infection and its complications in healthy persons, those with chronic medical conditions, and pregnant women.

Bibliography

Yudin MH. Optimizing knowledge of antiviral medications for p phylaxis and treatment of influenza during pregnancy. Expert Respir Med. 2011;5(4):495-501. [PMID: 21859269]

Item 89   Answer: B

Educational Objective: Diagnose familial Mediterranean fever.

This patient most likely has familial Mediterranean fe (FMF), which occurs in ethnic groups originating in t Mediterranean basin. Symptoms of this autosomal rec sive disorder typically develop in patients before the age 20 years and are characterized by acute, self-limit episodes of fever associated with abdominal, chest, or jo pain caused by serosal inflammation. Cutaneous manif tations of FMF mimic erysipelas and usually develop o a distal lower extremity (most often unilaterally but oc sionally bilaterally). A neutrophilic leukocytosis is char teristic. Elevated levels of acute phase reactants, includi the erythrocyte sedimentation rate and C-reactive prot level, are also common. The genetic association, as wel the episodic presentation of acute, self-limited episo with concomitant skin abnormalities, distinguishes cu neous manifestations caused by FMF from those caused

terial skin and soft tissue infections. The preferred
atment is colchicine.

Erythromelalgia typically manifests as paroxysmal bilat-
l erythema of the extremities with associated warmth
l burning pain. This condition is often precipitated by
rmer external temperatures and febrile episodes and is
gravated by the dependent position. The episodic pre-
tation, inciting factors, and bilateral extremity distribu-
n are helpful in distinguishing erythromelalgia from skin
l soft tissue infections. Serosal inflammation is not a fea-
re of this disease.

Staphylococcal cellulitis is less likely because of the
ateral symmetric distribution of this patient's skin find-
s and the absence of purulence and lymphadenopathy.
s history of previous episodes that resolved without
ibiotic treatment makes staphylococcal cellulitis unlikely.

Sweet syndrome, or acute febrile neutrophilic der-
titis, most commonly affects middle-aged women after
upper respiratory tract infection. Sweet syndrome may
idiopathic or may be associated with an underlying con-
ion. Patients with Sweet syndrome present with the
rupt onset of fever, arthralgia, myalgia, and cutaneous
ions. Individual lesions are tender, nonpruritic, brightly
thematous, well-demarcated papules and plaques that
pear on the neck, upper trunk, and typically, upper
remities. This patient's skin lesions are not consistent
h those of Sweet syndrome. In addition, Sweet syn-
ome is not typically associated with abdominal pain, and
loes not typically remit after several days.

EY POINT

• Familial Mediterranean fever is a hereditary
periodic fever syndrome that is characterized by
serosal inflammation in the chest, abdomen, or
joints and an erysipelas-like rash.

bliography
agas ME, Vergidis PI. Narrative reviews: Diseases that masquerade
as infectious cellulitis. Ann Intern Med. 2005;142(1):47-55.
[PMID: 15630108]

em 90   Answer: D

lucational Objective: Prevent surgical site
fection in a pregnant woman.

is patient should receive antimicrobial prophylaxis 30 to
 minutes before surgery with therapeutic levels main-
ned throughout surgery. There are several measures that
lp to prevent surgical site infections (SSIs). Antibiotic
ophylaxis should be administered 30 to 60 minutes
fore surgical incision; vancomycin and the fluoro-
inolones can be administered 60 to 120 minutes before
:ision. If the procedure is prolonged, it is important to
peat the dosage to maintain therapeutic levels throughout
e procedure depending on the agent's half-life. Preoper-
ve measures to prevent SSIs include control or elimina-
n of modifiable risk factors (for example, uncontrolled

diabetes mellitus or hyperglycemia, obesity, tobacco use,
use of immunosuppressive agents, length of preoperative
hospitalization) and antibiotic prophylaxis. Perioperative
measures to prevent SSIs are to avoid shaving of hair, provide aggressive glucose control, use chlorhexidine-based
surgical preparation, minimize traffic into and out of the
operating room, administer supplemental oxygen, and use
checklists to improve compliance with preventive processes.

Decolonization of group B *Streptococcus* vaginal/rec-
tal carriage is important for prevention of early-onset
neonatal group B streptococcal disease but has no role in
the prevention of SSIs.

Antimicrobial prophylaxis should be stopped promptly
after the procedure ends, within 24 hours following incision. Continuing antibiotics beyond this period is not recommended.

Shaving of hair prior to surgery is a risk factor for, not
a protective factor against, SSIs.

KEY POINT

• To minimize the risk for surgical site infection,
antimicrobial prophylaxis should be administered 30 to 60 minutes before surgical incision,
with therapeutic levels maintained throughout
the procedure.

Bibliography
Anderson DJ. Surgical site infections. Infect Dis Clin North Am.
2011;25(1):135-153. [PMID: 21315998]

Item 91   Answer: A

Educational Objective: Treat recurrent genital
herpes simplex virus infection in a patient with
AIDS.

The most appropriate treatment is acyclovir. This severely
immunocompromised patient with AIDS and a very low
CD4 cell count presents with recurrent genital and perianal
herpes simplex virus infection. The lesions have resolved, and
the suppressive treatment of choice is acyclovir. Chronic suppressive antiviral therapy prevents outbreaks of genital herpes
and is warranted in immunocompromised hosts or those
with frequent (>6 episodes per year) or severe recurrences.
He should be encouraged to re-initiate antiretroviral therapy
because immune reconstitution will also reduce recurrent
episodes of herpes simplex virus infection.

Cidofovir and foscarnet are intravenous preparations
reserved for treatment of acyclovir-resistant herpesvirus
infections. Cidofovir is also available as an ointment, which
can hasten healing of acyclovir-resistant lesions; however,
cidofovir can also cause mucocutaneous ulcers. The intravenous form can cause rash, neutropenia, and kidney failure. Foscarnet can also cause serious adverse effects, including kidney insufficiency, nausea, paresthesias, and seizures.

Valganciclovir is the prodrug of ganciclovir. It has
broad-spectrum activity against herpesviruses. It is currently

approved for treatment, suppression, and prevention of cytomegalovirus infections. Its principal toxicity is myelosuppression.

KEY POINT

- **Acyclovir is efficacious for treating genital herpes simplex virus infection and preventing symptomatic reactivation in immunocompromised hosts.**

Bibliography

Cernik C, Gallina K, Brodell RT. The treatment of herpes simplex infections: an evidence-based review. Arch Intern Med. 2008;168(11):1137-1144. [PMID: 18541820]

H **Item 92   Answer: D**

Educational Objective: Diagnose *Streptococcus pneumoniae* infection after transplantation.

This patient with fever, chills, cough, and pleuritic chest pain most likely has *Streptococcus pneumoniae* infection. The periods following hematopoietic stem cell transplantation (HSCT) during which opportunistic infections can occur are the pre-engraftment phase (>30 days after transplantation), the postengraftment phase (30 to 100 days after transplantation), and the late phase (>100 days after transplantation). This patient underwent HSCT 6 months ago, and this late posttransplantation time frame is associated with a high risk for infection with encapsulated bacterial organisms such as *S. pneumoniae*. Consequently, immunization with a full series of conjugated pneumococcal vaccines is indicated, beginning 3 to 6 months after transplantation.

Candida (no matter which species) is a very rare cause of pneumonia, even in immunocompromised patients.

Cytomegalovirus infection frequently occurs after the first month of transplantation but occurs less commonly 6 to 12 months after transplantation. Also, cytomegalovirus pneumonia would more likely cause diffuse interstitial infiltrates rather than lobar consolidation as demonstrated on this patient's chest radiograph.

Pneumocystis pneumonia may occur in patients following HSCT, but this patient is taking trimethoprim-sulfamethoxazole, which is very effective as prophylaxis against *Pneumocystis jirovecii*. In addition, *Pneumocystis* pneumonia would be less likely to have a lobar presentation.

KEY POINT

- **In the late posttransplantation phase (more than a few months after transplantation), hematopoietic stem cell transplant recipients are at high risk for infection with encapsulated organisms such as *Streptococcus pneumoniae*.**

Bibliography

Wingard JR, Hsu J, Hiemenz JW. Hematopoietic stem cell transplantation: an overview of infection risks and epidemiology. Infect Dis Clin North Am. 2010;24(2):257-272. [PMID: 20466269]

Item 93   Answer: B

Educational Objective: Diagnose babesiosis.

The most likely pathogen is *Babesia microti*. This patient has a febrile illness associated with clinical and laboratory evidence of hemolysis following a camping trip in New England. This presentation is highly suggestive of babesiosis, a tick-borne protozoal infection caused by *B. microti*. The vector tick is *Ixodes scapularis*, the same arthropod that transmits Lyme disease (caused by *Borrelia burgdorferi*) and human granulocytic anaplasmosis (caused by *Anaplasma phagocytophilum*). Consequently, coinfection with more than one of these tick-borne pathogens may develop. Although all three pathogens may cause a febrile illness, only *B. microti* results in significant hemolysis because of multiplication of the organisms within erythrocytes.

Because Lyme disease, human granulocytic anaplasmosis, and Rocky Mountain spotted fever (RMSF) (caused by *Rickettsia rickettsii*) are all treated with doxycycline, the onset of new symptoms in a patient taking this antibiotic would support development of another infection, such as babesiosis. This patient is unlikely to have RMSF because it is not associated with hemolysis but is often associated with a rash. The characteristic rash of RMSF begins as blanching erythematous macules around the wrists and ankles, progressing to petechiae. The rash is found in only 15% of patients on presentation but appears in 85% to 90% of patients by day 4. RMSF is more common in the southeastern and south central United States.

West Nile virus may cause a febrile illness that is variably associated with fever and central nervous system manifestations but is not associated with hemolysis. West Nile virus is usually transmitted by mosquitoes and is not a tick-borne disease.

KEY POINT

- **Because the same vector tick carries pathogens responsible for babesiosis, Lyme disease, and human granulocytic anaplasmosis, coinfection among these three entities may occur; however, only babesiosis causes hemolysis.**

Bibliography

Wormser GP, Dattwyler RJ, Shapiro ED, et al. The clinical assessment, treatment, and prevention of lyme disease, human granulocytic anaplasmosis, and babesiosis: clinical practice guidelines by the Infectious Diseases Society of America. Clin Infect Dis. 2006;43(9):1089-1134. [PMID: 17029130]

Item 94   Answer: D

Educational Objective: Manage a parapneumonic effusion.

This patient requires immediate ultrasound-guided thoracentesis. Patients such as this with community-acquired pneumonia (CAP) and a large associated pleural effusion typically defined as an effusion occupying half or more of the hemithorax on an upright chest radiograph or a fluid level of more than 1 cm on lateral decubitus films) should undergo prompt thoracentesis as part of the initial evaluation to confirm the microbial cause of the pneumonia and exclude a complicated parapneumonic effusion or empyema. Delay in the diagnosis of a complicated pleural effusion or empyema may result in a loculated effusion, often necessitating more invasive management, such as video-assisted thoracoscopic surgery or open thoracotomy.

The presence of a pleural effusion does not affect the selection of empiric antibiotic therapy; consequently, adding metronidazole or changing therapy from cefotaxime and azithromycin to cefepime and vancomycin would be unnecessary.

Pleural effusions can occur in 20% to 40% of hospitalized patients with CAP. A small pleural effusion that develops during treatment does not require thoracentesis as long as the patient is responding appropriately to antibiotic treatment.

KEY POINT

- **Patients with community-acquired pneumonia and a large associated pleural effusion should undergo prompt thoracentesis to confirm the microbial cause of the pneumonia and exclude a complicated parapneumonic effusion or empyema.**

Bibliography

Colice GL, Curtis A, Deslauriers J, et al. Medical and surgical treatment of parapneumonic effusions: an evidence-based guideline. Chest. 2000;118(4):1158-1171. [PMID: 11035692]

Item 95   Answer: A

Educational Objective: Screen for HIV infection.

The first step in the management of this patient is screening by HIV antibody enzyme immunoassay (EIA). Although this patient has no symptoms or significant risk factors for HIV infection, she has asked about receiving HIV screening. The Centers for Disease Control and Prevention (CDC) now recommend HIV screening for all persons between the ages of 13 and 64 years at least once and that those with risk factors undergo annual testing. In addition, the American College of Physicians has issued a guidance statement recommending that this age range be expanded to include patients through age 75 years because of increased rates of infection in this population. HIV antibody EIA is the appropriate first test when screening for HIV infection, and when combined with a Western blot if the EIA is positive, has 99% sensitivity and specificity for the diagnosis of HIV infection.

The Western blot assay is the confirmatory test for HIV infection and should only be used to confirm that a reactive EIA is a true positive and not a false-positive result. It should not be used as the initial step in screening.

This patient has no symptoms of acute HIV infection; consequently, there is no concern she may be in the "window period" of acute HIV infection, during which false-negative antibody testing results can occur that require HIV nucleic acid amplification testing to establish a diagnosis. In addition, HIV nucleic acid amplification testing is less sensitive and specific than standard HIV antibody EIA screening followed by Western blot confirmatory testing.

Initiating no testing for this patient, who has never had HIV screening and who has specifically requested it, would not be the most appropriate management.

KEY POINT

- **All persons between the ages of 13 and 75 years should be tested for HIV infection at least once, and those with risk factors should undergo annual testing.**

Bibliography

Branson BM, Handsfield HH, Lampe MA, et al. ; Centers for Disease Control and Prevention (CDC). Revised recommendations for HIV testing of adults, adolescents, and pregnant women in healthcare settings. MMWR Recomm Rep. 2006;55(RR-14):1-17; quiz CE1-4. [PMID: 16988643]

Item 96   Answer: C

Educational Objective: Treat a patient with bacterial meningitis following neurosurgery.

In addition to vancomycin, meropenem is the most appropriate antimicrobial agent for this patient, who has most likely developed bacterial meningitis following a neurosurgical procedure. The most common pathogens that cause meningitis in this setting are gram-positive organisms (such as *Staphylococcus aureus* and coagulase-negative staphylococci) and gram-negative bacilli. Based on the possibility of staphylococcal meningitis, including that caused by methicillin-resistant strains, vancomycin should be included in the empiric therapeutic regimen. Multiple gram-negative bacilli must also be considered, including *Pseudomonas aeruginosa* and *Acinetobacter* species. Of the possible choices listed, meropenem is the best agent to treat the most likely gram-negative bacilli in a patient with nosocomial meningitis.

Ceftriaxone and trimethoprim-sulfamethoxazole are not active against *P. aeruginosa*.

Although gentamicin has activity against many gram-negative bacilli, it does not achieve adequate cerebrospinal fluid concentrations after parenteral administration to treat gram-negative meningitis.

Metronidazole is only active against anaerobic bacteria.

Bibliography

van de Beek D, Drake JM, Tunkel AR. Nosocomial bacterial meningitis. N Engl J Med. 2010;362(2):146-154. [PMID: 20071704]

Item 97   Answer: E

Educational Objective: Prevent travelers' diarrhea in a patient with inflammatory bowel disease.

This patient should be given prophylactic rifaximin to reduce her risk for travelers' diarrhea. Travelers' diarrhea is the most common illness in persons visiting developing countries, with an overall incidence of about 20% to 60%. The risk of acquiring this condition correlates directly with the geographic region visited. The highest risk is associated with travel to Mexico, South and Central America, Asia, and countries in Africa other than South Africa. Travelers' diarrhea is defined as the occurrence of three or more unformed stools per day with abdominal pain or cramps, nausea or vomiting, bloody stools, or fever. Diarrhea is usually self-limited, generally lasting 1 to 4 days, although in some patients, symptoms persist longer. Bacteria such as enterotoxigenic *Escherichia coli* cause most episodes of travelers' diarrhea. Other causative bacterial organisms include *Salmonella, Shigella, Campylobacter, Aeromonas*, and *Vibrio* species. Protozoan pathogens are isolated in less than 10% of patients. Travelers' diarrhea caused by viral diseases is uncommon, but in certain circumstances such as on cruise ships, it may be caused by norovirus infection. No definitive microbiologic agent is identified in about 30% of patients.

Reducing the risk for travelers' diarrhea involves multiple modalities. The use of prophylactic antibiotics has proved effective but is not recommended for the average traveler owing to potential side effects. Antibiotics may be warranted in some instances, such as this patient whose inflammatory bowel disease could be greatly exacerbated by an episode of travelers' diarrhea, and others with immunocompromising illnesses and chronic diseases that could be exacerbated in the setting of dehydration or electrolyte imbalance. Historically, the fluoroquinolone class of antibiotics has been used to treat travelers' diarrhea, although the development of fluoroquinolone resistance has led to increased interest in alternative agents. Rifaximin, a nonabsorbed antibiotic, is effective and safe when prescribed at doses of 200 mg, once or twice daily for 2 weeks, particularly when *E. coli* will be the most likely acquired pathogen during travel.

Although it may seem logical that avoiding tap water that is potentially contaminated with diarrhea-producing microorganisms would decrease the risk for travelers' diarrhea, this practice has only been shown to confer a small benefit. Nonetheless, instituting water purification techniques, such as boiling tap water for 3 minutes and then cooling it to room temperature, are highly recommended.

Taking bismuth subsalicylate at the high dose required to diminish the incidence of travelers' diarrhea is not convenient and could lead to salicylate toxicity.

The effectiveness of probiotics in reducing the risk for travelers' diarrhea remains uncertain, with results varying depending on the preparation studied.

The use of antimotility medications, such as loperamide or diphenoxylate, to prevent travelers' diarrhea has not been shown to be effective as a prophylactic intervention.

Bibliography

DuPont HL, Ericsson CD, Farthing MJ, et al. Expert review of the evidence for prevention of travelers' diarrhea. J Travel Med. 2009;16(3):149-160. [PMID: 19538575]

Item 98   Answer: A

Educational Objective: Diagnose giardiasis.

The study most likely to establish a diagnosis is a stool assay for *Giardia* antigen. This patient's clinical presentation of a prolonged gastrointestinal illness characterized by watery diarrhea and weight loss and his history of camping in the preceding month are strongly suggestive of infection with *Giardia lamblia*. This parasitic infection is typically transmitted by ingestion of *Giardia* cysts found in natural bodies of water. Giardiasis can be prevented by boiling or filtering water or by iodine treatment. Most infections are asymptomatic. Symptomatic infection often involves the small bowel and is characterized by large-volume liquid stools and bloating or belching. Although fever is rare, weight loss due to anorexia and malabsorption is an almost universal finding. A monoclonal antibody assay that detects *Giardia* antigen directly on a stool sample is recommended for diagnosis.

Stool cultures for bacteria have a low yield in diagnosing a diarrheal illness lasting more than 7 to 10 days and, in addition, would not be useful in this patient who has protozoal infection.

Although giardiasis may be diagnosed by microscopic examination for ova and parasites identifying *Giardi*

phozoites or cysts, the intermittent shedding of these
ganisms makes this a less sensitive test than the *Giardia*
tigen assay. In situations in which antigen testing is not
dily available, examination of three stool specimens for
a and parasites may be diagnostic.

Modified acid-fast staining of a stool sample is needed
visualize *Cryptosporidium*, *Isospora*, and *Cyclospora*
ganisms but is not indicated for the diagnosis of *Giardia*.

EY POINT

- The most sensitive test for diagnosing giardiasis
  is a stool assay for *Giardia* antigen.

bliography

vlowski SW, Warren CA, Guerrant R. Diagnosis and treatment of
acute or persistent diarrhea. Gastroenterology. 2009;136(6):1874-
1886. [PMID: 19457416]

em 99   **Answer: B**

lucational Objective: Diagnose the acute retro-
al syndrome.

ie most appropriate next diagnostic test is an HIV
cleic acid amplification test. This patient's medical his-
ry and timing of symptoms are typical of acute HIV
fection. Although his symptoms could also represent
ectious mononucleosis or syphilis, preliminary results
those conditions are negative. Most persons in whom
IV infection develops experience an acute symptomatic
hess within 2 to 4 weeks of infection. Symptoms typi-
ly last for a few weeks and range from a simple febrile
hess to a full-blown mononucleosis-like syndrome.
cause patients lack an immune response during this
riod, virus levels tend to be very high, resulting in high
els of infectivity. Symptoms of acute HIV infection
solve with or without treatment, and most acute infecns are undiagnosed. Patients presenting with sympto-
ttic acute HIV infection (the acute retroviral syndrome)
usually in the "window period," which may extend for
to 6 weeks, during which time seroconversion of the
ease has not yet occurred and results of HIV antibody
ting are negative. However, viral-specific tests, such as
ose for nucleic acid, are usually positive at quite high
els during this time frame and can be used to establish
e diagnosis.

Measurement of CD4 cell counts is neither sensitive
r specific for HIV infection and should be performed
ly after the diagnosis of HIV is already established. The
D4 cell count can be normal in HIV infection, and con-
rsely, can be depressed from many other conditions that
n present similarly to acute HIV infection.

During the window period of acute HIV infection,
tibody testing is unreliable. Therefore, antibody-based
ting, whether by repeat enzyme immunoassay or West-
1 blot, would not be useful.

KEY POINT

- Most persons in whom HIV infection develops
  experience an acute symptomatic illness within
  2 to 4 weeks of infection, with symptoms ranging from a simple febrile illness to a mononucleosis-like syndrome.

Bibliography

Cohen MS, Gay CL, Busch MP, Hecht FM. The detection of acute
HIV infection. J Infect Dis. 2010;202(suppl 2):S270-S277.
[PMID: 20846033]

Item 100   Answer: D

Educational Objective: Prevent malaria in a pregnant patient.

This patient should receive chemoprophylaxis with
mefloquine. Because malaria in a pregnant woman can be
very deleterious to both the mother and the fetus, it is
advisable that travel to malaria-endemic areas be delayed
until after delivery of the fetus. However, when pregnant
travelers cannot or will not defer travel, chemoprophylaxis with mefloquine during the second and third
trimesters of pregnancy has been found to be safe and is
the recommended drug for travel to areas of the world
where chloroquine-resistant malaria is found. Safety data
on the use of this medication during the first trimester
are less available.

Owing to the predominance of chloroquine-resistant
Plasmodium falciparum species in Africa, chemoprophylaxis with chloroquine would be inadequate, even though
this drug has been deemed safe during pregnancy.

Doxycycline, although active against all malaria species,
including chloroquine resistant-strains, should not be used
during pregnancy. Potential adverse effects of doxycycline
to the fetus include inhibition of bone growth, dysplasia,
and dental discoloration.

Atovaquone-proguanil, a preferred agent for preventing malaria in chloroquine-resistant zones, is not recommended for prophylaxis in pregnant women owing to insufficient data.

KEY POINT

- Chemoprophylaxis with mefloquine during
  the second and third trimesters of pregnancy
  is safe and recommended for pregnant travelers who cannot defer travel to areas of the
  world where chloroquine-resistant malaria is
  found.

Bibliography

Schlagenhauf P, Petersen E. Malaria chemoprophylaxis: strategies for
risk groups. Clin Microbiol Rev. 2008;21(3):466-472. [PMID:
18625682]

Item 101   Answer: B

Educational Objective: Treat a patient with ventilator-associated, methicillin-resistant *Staphylococcus aureus* pneumonia.

This patient requires discontinuation of vancomycin and initiation of intravenous linezolid. Linezolid is an oxazolidinone drug with bacteriostatic activity against gram-positive aerobic bacteria, including methicillin-resistant *Staphylococcus aureus* (MRSA) and vancomycin-resistant enterococci, and it has performed well in randomized controlled trials compared with vancomycin. The pharmacokinetics of linezolid in the lung are favorable, and it is an excellent alternative to vancomycin for treatment of MRSA. An important side effect of linezolid is myelosuppression, notably thrombocytopenia. Weekly complete blood counts should be obtained in patients treated with linezolid.

Daptomycin is effective in treating staphylococcal bacteremia and right-sided infective endocarditis in addition to skin and skin structure infections. It is equally effective for methicillin-susceptible *Staphylococcus aureus* (MSSA) and MRSA infections. Although daptomycin is no more effective than β-lactams for treating MSSA infections, it may be a useful alternative to vancomycin for treating MRSA infections in patients with fluctuating kidney function or in patients who require a relatively high (≥2 micrograms/mL) vancomycin minimal inhibitory concentration (MIC). Daptomycin is bound by surfactant, and it is not effective in the treatment of pneumonia.

Rifampin often has good in vitro activity against *S. aureus* but should not be used as a single agent because resistance to this agent can emerge rapidly.

Tigecycline is indicated for the treatment of community-acquired pneumonia but not for hospital-acquired (or ventilator-associated) pneumonia. An FDA warning reported increased mortality rates among patients treated with tigecycline in randomized controlled trials of patients with hospital-acquired pneumonia. Consequently, tigecycline should not be used for treatment of ventilator-associated pneumonia unless there are no alternative therapies.

KEY POINT

- **Linezolid is an FDA-approved option for treating methicillin-resistant *Staphylococcus aureus* pneumonia, including ventilator-associated pneumonia, as well as vancomycin-resistant enterococci.**

Bibliography
Liu C, Bayer A, Cosgrove SE, et al. Clinical practice guidelines by the Infectious Diseases Society of America for the treatment of methicillin-resistant Staphylococcus aureus infections in adults and children: executive summary. Clin Infect Dis. 2011;52(3):285-292. [PMID: 21217178]

Item 102   Answer: A

Educational Objective: Treat a patient with nonpurulent cellulitis with systemic symptoms.

This patient has nonpurulent cellulitis with associated fever and leukocytosis and should be treated with clindamycin to provide coverage for both β-hemolytic streptococci and community-associated methicillin-resistant *Staphylococcus aureus* (CA-MRSA). Although β-hemolytic streptococci are most likely causing his infection, coverage for CA-MRSA is also recommended by some experts because of the patient's associated systemic symptoms. Known risk factors for lower-extremity cellulitis include tinea pedis, onychomycosis, chronic leg ulcerations, varicose veins of the leg, phlebitis, obesity, type 2 diabetes mellitus, and heart failure. Treatment of this patient's tinea pedis is an appropriate intervention to prevent recurrent cellulitis.

Doxycycline and trimethoprim-sulfamethoxazole are active against CA-MRSA but do not provide reliable coverage for β-hemolytic streptococci. If either of these agents is used, a β-lactam agent such as amoxicillin should be added to provide coverage for β-hemolytic streptococci.

Although rifampin is active against staphylococci and streptococci, it should never be used as monotherapy because of the development of resistance. Only limited data are available to recommend the use of rifampin as an adjunctive agent for treatment of skin and soft tissue infections.

KEY POINT

- **In an outpatient with nonpurulent cellulitis and associated systemic symptoms, treatment with clindamycin is recommended to provide activity against both β-hemolytic streptococci and community-associated methicillin-resistant *Staphylococcus aureus*.**

Bibliography
Liu C, Bayer A, Cosgrove SE, Daum RS, et al; Infectious Diseases Society of America. Clinical practice guidelines by the Infectious Diseases Society of America for the treatment of methicillin-resistant Staphylococcus aureus infections in adults and children. Clin Infect Dis. 2011;52(3):e18-55. Epub 2011 Jan 4. [PMID: 21208910]

Item 103   Answer: C

Educational Objective: Choose the appropriate site of care for a patient with community-acquired pneumonia.

The patient needs to be started on empiric antibiotic treatment for community-acquired pneumonia (CAP) and admitted to the medical ward. Rules that predict mortality risk can be used to guide site-of-care decisions in patients with CAP. The CURB-65 score estimates mortality based on the following indicators: confusion, blood urea nitrogen level greater than 19.6 mg/dL (7.0 mmol/

piration rate 30/min or more, systolic blood pressure
s than 90 mm Hg or diastolic blood pressure 60 mm Hg
less, and age 65 years or older. One point is scored for
ch positive indicator. Patients with a score of 0 or 1 have
ow mortality risk and can be considered for outpatient
atment. Those with a score of 2 or more should be hos-
alized. Patients with a score of 3 or more should be con-
ered for admission to the intensive care unit (ICU). This
tient's CURB-65 score is 3, and his predicted mortality
k is 17%; hospitalization is generally recommended for
rsons with scores of 2 or higher.

Discharging this patient on oral antibiotic therapy after
piric treatment with intravenous antibiotic therapy
uld not be appropriate because, in addition to empiric
tibiotic therapy, this patient requires hospitalization.

Admission to the ICU should be considered in
ients with CURB-65 scores of 3 or higher. To help fur-
er define the population of patients who would benefit
m admission to the ICU, the Infectious Diseases Society
America/American Thoracic Society (IDSA/ATS) con-
nsus guidelines for the management of community-
quired pneumonia have proposed major and minor crite-
for ICU admission. Major criteria include the need for
sopressor support or mechanical ventilation. Minor crite-
include confusion, hypothermia, respiration rate of
/min or more (or the need for noninvasive positive-pres-
re ventilation), hypotension requiring aggressive fluid
uscitation, multilobar infiltrates, arterial PO_2/FIO_2 ratio
250 or less, leukopenia, thrombocytopenia, and blood
ea nitrogen level of greater than 20 mg/dL (7.1
mol/L). This patient has two minor criteria; ICU admis-
n should be considered in patients with three or more
nor criteria.

Because the patient's CURB-65 score predicts a sig-
icant mortality risk, outpatient therapy would not be
propriate.

EY POINT

- In patients with community-acquired pneumonia, the CURB-65 score assigns one point for
  each positive indicator (confusion, blood urea
  nitrogen level >19.6 mg/dL [7.0 mmol/L],
  respiration rate ≥30/min, systolic blood pressure <90 mm Hg or diastolic blood pressure
  ≤60 mm Hg, and age ≥65 years), with a score
  of 0 or 1 indicating consideration for outpatient management, and a score of 2 or more
  indicating the need for hospitalization.

bliography

ndell LA, Wunderink RG, Anzueto A, et al. Infectious Diseases
Society of America; American Thoracic Society. Infectious Diseases
Society of America/American Thoracic Society consensus guide-
ines on the management of community-acquired pneumonia in
dults. Clin Infect Dis. 2007;44(suppl 2):S27-72. [PMID:
7278083]

Item 104   Answer: B

Educational Objective: Treat a patient with
tuberculous meningitis.

This patient has tuberculous meningitis and requires treatment for 9 to 12 months. He has several characteristic features of this infection, including headache, fever, and
lethargy. Results of lumbar puncture show an increased
opening pressure and a cerebrospinal fluid (CSF) lymphocytic pleocytosis, an elevated CSF protein level, and a
decreased CSF glucose level. A CT scan shows basilar
meningeal involvement (hydrocephalus may be seen also).

In general, the recommendations for treatment of
extrapulmonary tuberculosis are the same as those for
treatment of pulmonary disease. For most patients with
extrapulmonary tuberculosis caused by strains that are
fully susceptible to all drugs, the recommended treatment
duration is 6 to 9 months. This includes a 2-month initial
phase of isoniazid, rifampin, pyrazinamide, and ethambutol followed by a continuation phase of isoniazid and
rifampin for 4 or 7 months. The 7-month continuation
phase is recommended when pyrazinamide cannot be
administered during the initial phase. However, treatment
of tuberculous meningitis is an exception to these recommendations. The American Thoracic Society, Centers for
Disease Control and Prevention, and the Infectious Diseases Society of America consensus guidelines recommend
that patients with tuberculous meningitis be treated for 9
to 12 months rather than the standard 6 to 9 months.
Adjunctive corticosteroids are also recommended. Serial
lumbar punctures should be considered to assess the
response of the CSF cell count and protein and glucose
levels to therapy.

Four months of therapy is inappropriate because at
least 6 months of treatment is recommended for patients
with any form of extrapulmonary tuberculosis.

Therapeutic durations longer than 9 to 12 months are
recommended for patients with various patterns of multidrug-resistant tuberculosis.

KEY POINT

- **The recommended duration of antituberculous
  treatment in patients with tuberculous meningitis is 9 to 12 months.**

Bibliography

American Thoracic Society; CDC; Infectious Diseases Society of
America. Treatment of tuberculosis. MMWR Recomm Rep.
2003;52(RR-11):1-77. [PMID: 12836625]

Item 105   Answer: A

Educational Objective: Diagnose invasive
aspergillosis after transplantation.

This patient has aspergillosis. *Aspergillus* species is the most
common cause of invasive fungal infection after transplantation, especially following lung transplantation and during

CONT.

the neutropenic phase after hematopoietic stem cell transplantation (HSCT). Invasive aspergillosis involves the lungs more often than the sinuses, and patients typically have fever, and possibly, dry cough or hemoptysis, and chest pain. Dissemination to the brain may be characterized by headache, focal deficits, or mental status changes. This patient's risk factors for invasive fungal disease include profound neutropenia of prolonged duration, persistent fever while receiving broad-spectrum antibacterial coverage, and pulmonary nodules. The treatment of choice is voriconazole. This patient has been taking fluconazole prophylaxis, which provides coverage for most *Candida* species but not for *Aspergillus* species.

Cytomegalovirus (CMV) pneumonia is less likely to occur in the first few weeks after HSCT (pre-engraftment phase) than in the period after the first few weeks through the first few months following transplantation (postengraftment phase). CMV infection would also be unlikely to cause pulmonary nodules on imaging.

Mucormycosis (zygomycosis) is a rapidly progressive fungal infection that most commonly occurs in patients with hematologic malignancies or other disorders associated with prolonged neutropenia or immunosuppression, severe burns or trauma, or diabetic ketoacidosis. Corticosteroids, cytotoxic agents, or deferoxamine also confers an increased risk. Rhinocerebral or pulmonary involvement occurs most commonly. Invasive aspergillosis is much more commonly associated with early fungal infections following stem cell transplantation than is mucormycosis.

Pneumocystis jirovecii infection is less likely to occur in the acute setting immediately following transplantation. The chest radiograph typically shows bilateral interstitial infiltrates, but rarely, findings can vary from a normal radiograph to consolidation, cysts, nodules, pleural effusions, or a pneumothorax.

KEY POINT

- Invasive aspergillosis is a common fungal infection following transplantation (especially of the lung and during the neutropenic phase after hematopoietic stem cell transplantation) and may be characterized by fever, dry cough, or hemoptysis.

Bibliography

Asano-Mori Y. Fungal infections after hematopoietic stem cell transplantation. Int J Hematol. 2010;91(4):576-587. [PMID: 20432074]

Item 106   Answer: C

Educational Objective: Manage postcoital urinary tract infection.

The most appropriate next step in preventing recurrent urinary tract infections (UTIs) in this patient is postcoital ciprofloxacin. Recurrent UTIs in young, sexually active women are more commonly a reinfection rather than

relapse and are often associated with sexual intercour[se]. Consequently, a detailed sexual history should be obtain[ed] from female patients with a presentation such as that in t[his] patient. Symptoms of UTI are often related to the use [of] spermicidal agents because spermicides decrease the nu[m]ber of healthy vaginal lactobacilli and predispose women [to] UTIs. However, this patient does not use spermici[dal] agents. The recommended prophylaxis against recurr[ent] UTI is liberal fluid intake and postcoital voiding. Althou[gh] these recommendations are not evidenced-based, they [are] unlikely to be harmful. If UTIs continue to occur desp[ite] these measures as they have in this patient, prophylaxis w[ith] a postcoital antibiotic such as ciprofloxacin is appropria[te].

Chronic suppressive antibiotic therapy can be an eff[ec]tive method for preventing postcoital UTI, but patients m[ay] have difficulty adhering to this regimen, and it is associa[ted] with increased costs, resistance, and candidal superinfectio[n].

Randomized clinical trials have not demonstrated t[hat] drinking cranberry juice reduces the incidence of recurr[ent] UTI, including postcoital UTI.

Removal of this patient's intrauterine device (IUD) [is] not warranted because IUDs are not associated with UTI[s].

Adding a spermicide is likely to increase, not decrea[se] this patient's incidence of UTI.

KEY POINT

- **Antibiotic prophylaxis following intercourse is appropriate for preventing recurrent postcoital urinary tract infections in women.**

Bibliography

Dielubanza EJ, Schaeffer AJ. Urinary tract infections in women. M[ed] Clin North Am. 2011;95(1):27-41. [PMID: 21095409]

Item 107   Answer: D

Educational Objective: Treat early-latent syphilis.

The Centers for Disease Control and Prevention (CD[C]) recommends a single dose of intramuscular benzath[ine] penicillin G for the treatment of primary, secondary, a[nd] early-latent syphilis. This regimen is appropriate for in[di]viduals with coexisting HIV infection as well.

This asymptomatic patient who has serologic evide[nce] of syphilis now but had negative serologic results [for] syphilis 6 months ago has early-latent syphilis. Recent e[pi]demiologic data have shown that the rates of syphilis a[nd] other sexually transmitted infections (STIs) are increas[ing] among men who have sex with men, especially amo[ng] younger men, those in urban areas (particularly members [of] racial and ethnic minorities), and men who use drugs d[ur]ing sex. Periodic screening for STIs in persons at risk is [an] important part of HIV primary care. This patient sho[uld] receive counseling regarding STI risk reduction and sho[uld] be encouraged to refer his sexual partners for evaluati[on]. Persons exposed to sexual partners diagnosed with prima[ry]

ondary, or early-latent syphilis within the preceding 90
⟩s should be treated, regardless of serologic results. Indi-
uals exposed to sexual partners with syphilis more than
⟩ days before a diagnosis was established should receive
atment if there is any concern regarding whether they
ll undergo follow-up serologic testing.

The recommended treatment for late-latent syphilis,
ich is defined as syphilis of more than 1 year in duration
⟩ syphilis of unknown duration, consists of three doses of
ramuscular benzathine penicillin G.

Aqueous crystalline intravenous penicillin G is the
atment of choice for patients with neurosyphilis, but this
ient does not have evidence of central nervous system
olvement. The need for cerebrospinal fluid (CSF) exam-
tion in all patients with HIV infection and syphilis is con-
versial. CSF abnormalities suggestive of neurosyphilis are
⟩re likely in individuals with rapid plasma reagin titers of
⟩2 or higher and those with CD4 cell counts of 350
ls/microliter or less; however, the CDC guidelines do
t recommend routine CSF examination in patients with
V infection who do not have neurologic symptoms.

Doxycycline is an alternative treatment in patients who
 allergic to penicillin. This patient does not have a peni-
in allergy.

EY POINT

- **The Centers for Disease Control and Prevention recommends a single dose of intramuscular
  benzathine penicillin G for the treatment of
  primary, secondary, and early-latent syphilis.**

oliography

rkowski KA, Berman S; Centers for Disease Control and Preven-
ion (CDC). Sexually transmitted diseases treatment guidelines,
2010. MMWR Recomm Rep. 2010;59(RR-12):1-110. [PMID:
21160459]

em 108   Answer: D

ucational Objective: Treat invasive pulmonary
⟩ergillosis in a patient with leukemia.

is patient should be treated with voriconazole. She has
⟩bable invasive pulmonary aspergillosis, for which acute

leukemia with profound and prolonged neutropenia is a
risk factor. She has classic symptoms and signs of an
angioinvasive fungal infection, including fever, cough,
chest pain, hemoptysis, and pulmonary nodules on chest
radiograph. In addition, her CT scan demonstrates evidence of the "halo sign," which is an area of low attenu-
ation surrounding a nodule, reflecting hemorrhage into
the tissue surrounding the fungus. The halo sign is not
diagnostic of aspergillosis and may occur in infection
caused by other angioinvasive fungi. Evidence from a
large randomized controlled trial supports voriconazole as
the treatment of choice in patients with invasive
aspergillosis. Standard procedures for establishing a definitive diagnosis of pulmonary aspergillosis are bronchoalveolar lavage with or without biopsy, transthoracic
percutaneous needle aspiration, or video-assisted thoracoscopic biopsy. The galactomannan antigen immunoassay is an important non–culture-based method of diagnosing invasive aspergillosis. It has good sensitivity in
detecting invasive aspergillosis in patients with hematologic malignancy. When combined with early use of CT,
the serum galactomannan antigen immunoassay permits
early treatment with antifungal therapy.

Liposomal amphotericin B may be considered an alternative primary therapy for some patients. Amphotericin B
formulations, itraconazole, posaconazole, and echinocandin agents such as caspofungin and micafungin are appropriate as salvage therapy in patients who are refractory to,
or intolerant of, voriconazole.

KEY POINT

- **Voriconazole is the drug of choice for immunocompromised patients with invasive pulmonary
  aspergillosis.**

Bibliography

Walsh TJ, Anaissie EJ, Denning DW, et al; Infectious Diseases Society
of America. Treatment of aspergillosis: clinical guidelines of the
Infectious Diseases Society of America. Clin Infect Dis.
2008;46(3):327-360. [PMID: 18177225]

Index

Note: Page numbers followed by f and t denote figures and tables, respectively. Test questions are indicated by Q.

A | **NAME AND ADDRESS (Please complete.)**

Last Name _____ First Name _____ Middle Initial _____

Address _____

Address cont. _____

City _____ State _____ ZIP Code _____

Country _____

Email address _____

ACP | AMERICAN COLLEGE OF PHYSICIANS
INTERNAL MEDICINE | *Doctors for Adults*

**Medical Knowledge
Self-Assessment
Program® 16**

TO EARN *AMA PRA CATEGORY 1 CREDITS*™ YOU MUST:

1. Answer all questions.
2. Score a minimum of 50% correct.

===

TO EARN *FREE* SAME-DAY *AMA PRA CATEGORY 1 CREDITS*™ ONLINE:

1. Answer all of your questions.
2. Go to **mksap.acponline.org** and access the appropriate answer sheet.
3. Transcribe your answers and submit for CME credits.
4. You can also enter your answers directly at **mksap.acponline.org** without first using this answer sheet.

To Submit Your Answer Sheet by Mail or FAX for a $10 Administrative Fee per Answer Sheet:

1. Answer all of your questions and calculate your score.
2. Complete boxes A–F.
3. Complete payment information.
4. Send the answer sheet and payment information to ACP, using the FAX number/address listed below.

B | **Order Number**

(Use the Order Number on your MKSAP materials packing slip.)

[| | | | | | | | | | | | | | | |]

C | **ACP ID Number**

(Refer to packing slip in your MKSAP materials for your ACP ID Number.)

[| | | | | | | | | | | | | | | |]

COMPLETE FORM BELOW ONLY IF YOU SUBMIT BY MAIL OR FAX

Last Name | First Name | MI

[| | | | | | | | | | | | | | | | | | | | | | | | | | | | | | | |]

Payment Information. Must remit in US funds, drawn on a US bank.

The processing fee for each paper answer sheet is $10.

☐ Check, made payable to ACP, enclosed

Charge to ☐ **VISA** ☐ **MasterCard** ☐ **AMERICAN EXPRESS** ☐ **DISCOVER**

Card Number _____

Expiration Date _____ / _____ Security code (3 or 4 digit #s) _____
　　　　　　　　　MM　　　YY

Signature _____

Fax to: 215-351-2799

Questions?
Go to **mskap.acponline.org** or email **custserv@acponline.org**

Mail to:
Member and Customer Service
American College of Physicians
190 N. Independence Mall West
Philadelphia, PA 19106-1572

1 Ⓐ Ⓑ Ⓒ Ⓓ Ⓔ   46 Ⓐ Ⓑ Ⓒ Ⓓ Ⓔ   91 Ⓐ Ⓑ Ⓒ Ⓓ Ⓔ   136 Ⓐ Ⓑ Ⓒ Ⓓ Ⓔ
2 Ⓐ Ⓑ Ⓒ Ⓓ Ⓔ   47 Ⓐ Ⓑ Ⓒ Ⓓ Ⓔ   92 Ⓐ Ⓑ Ⓒ Ⓓ Ⓔ   137 Ⓐ Ⓑ Ⓒ Ⓓ Ⓔ
3 Ⓐ Ⓑ Ⓒ Ⓓ Ⓔ   48 Ⓐ Ⓑ Ⓒ Ⓓ Ⓔ   93 Ⓐ Ⓑ Ⓒ Ⓓ Ⓔ   138 Ⓐ Ⓑ Ⓒ Ⓓ Ⓔ
4 Ⓐ Ⓑ Ⓒ Ⓓ Ⓔ   49 Ⓐ Ⓑ Ⓒ Ⓓ Ⓔ   94 Ⓐ Ⓑ Ⓒ Ⓓ Ⓔ   139 Ⓐ Ⓑ Ⓒ Ⓓ Ⓔ
5 Ⓐ Ⓑ Ⓒ Ⓓ Ⓔ   50 Ⓐ Ⓑ Ⓒ Ⓓ Ⓔ   95 Ⓐ Ⓑ Ⓒ Ⓓ Ⓔ   140 Ⓐ Ⓑ Ⓒ Ⓓ Ⓔ

6 Ⓐ Ⓑ Ⓒ Ⓓ Ⓔ   51 Ⓐ Ⓑ Ⓒ Ⓓ Ⓔ   96 Ⓐ Ⓑ Ⓒ Ⓓ Ⓔ   141 Ⓐ Ⓑ Ⓒ Ⓓ Ⓔ
7 Ⓐ Ⓑ Ⓒ Ⓓ Ⓔ   52 Ⓐ Ⓑ Ⓒ Ⓓ Ⓔ   97 Ⓐ Ⓑ Ⓒ Ⓓ Ⓔ   142 Ⓐ Ⓑ Ⓒ Ⓓ Ⓔ
8 Ⓐ Ⓑ Ⓒ Ⓓ Ⓔ   53 Ⓐ Ⓑ Ⓒ Ⓓ Ⓔ   98 Ⓐ Ⓑ Ⓒ Ⓓ Ⓔ   143 Ⓐ Ⓑ Ⓒ Ⓓ Ⓔ
9 Ⓐ Ⓑ Ⓒ Ⓓ Ⓔ   54 Ⓐ Ⓑ Ⓒ Ⓓ Ⓔ   99 Ⓐ Ⓑ Ⓒ Ⓓ Ⓔ   144 Ⓐ Ⓑ Ⓒ Ⓓ Ⓔ
10 Ⓐ Ⓑ Ⓒ Ⓓ Ⓔ   55 Ⓐ Ⓑ Ⓒ Ⓓ Ⓔ   100 Ⓐ Ⓑ Ⓒ Ⓓ Ⓔ   145 Ⓐ Ⓑ Ⓒ Ⓓ Ⓔ

11 Ⓐ Ⓑ Ⓒ Ⓓ Ⓔ   56 Ⓐ Ⓑ Ⓒ Ⓓ Ⓔ   101 Ⓐ Ⓑ Ⓒ Ⓓ Ⓔ   146 Ⓐ Ⓑ Ⓒ Ⓓ Ⓔ
12 Ⓐ Ⓑ Ⓒ Ⓓ Ⓔ   57 Ⓐ Ⓑ Ⓒ Ⓓ Ⓔ   102 Ⓐ Ⓑ Ⓒ Ⓓ Ⓔ   147 Ⓐ Ⓑ Ⓒ Ⓓ Ⓔ
13 Ⓐ Ⓑ Ⓒ Ⓓ Ⓔ   58 Ⓐ Ⓑ Ⓒ Ⓓ Ⓔ   103 Ⓐ Ⓑ Ⓒ Ⓓ Ⓔ   148 Ⓐ Ⓑ Ⓒ Ⓓ Ⓔ
14 Ⓐ Ⓑ Ⓒ Ⓓ Ⓔ   59 Ⓐ Ⓑ Ⓒ Ⓓ Ⓔ   104 Ⓐ Ⓑ Ⓒ Ⓓ Ⓔ   149 Ⓐ Ⓑ Ⓒ Ⓓ Ⓔ
15 Ⓐ Ⓑ Ⓒ Ⓓ Ⓔ   60 Ⓐ Ⓑ Ⓒ Ⓓ Ⓔ   105 Ⓐ Ⓑ Ⓒ Ⓓ Ⓔ   150 Ⓐ Ⓑ Ⓒ Ⓓ Ⓔ

16 Ⓐ Ⓑ Ⓒ Ⓓ Ⓔ   61 Ⓐ Ⓑ Ⓒ Ⓓ Ⓔ   106 Ⓐ Ⓑ Ⓒ Ⓓ Ⓔ   151 Ⓐ Ⓑ Ⓒ Ⓓ Ⓔ
17 Ⓐ Ⓑ Ⓒ Ⓓ Ⓔ   62 Ⓐ Ⓑ Ⓒ Ⓓ Ⓔ   107 Ⓐ Ⓑ Ⓒ Ⓓ Ⓔ   152 Ⓐ Ⓑ Ⓒ Ⓓ Ⓔ
18 Ⓐ Ⓑ Ⓒ Ⓓ Ⓔ   63 Ⓐ Ⓑ Ⓒ Ⓓ Ⓔ   108 Ⓐ Ⓑ Ⓒ Ⓓ Ⓔ   153 Ⓐ Ⓑ Ⓒ Ⓓ Ⓔ
19 Ⓐ Ⓑ Ⓒ Ⓓ Ⓔ   64 Ⓐ Ⓑ Ⓒ Ⓓ Ⓔ   109 Ⓐ Ⓑ Ⓒ Ⓓ Ⓔ   154 Ⓐ Ⓑ Ⓒ Ⓓ Ⓔ
20 Ⓐ Ⓑ Ⓒ Ⓓ Ⓔ   65 Ⓐ Ⓑ Ⓒ Ⓓ Ⓔ   110 Ⓐ Ⓑ Ⓒ Ⓓ Ⓔ   155 Ⓐ Ⓑ Ⓒ Ⓓ Ⓔ

21 Ⓐ Ⓑ Ⓒ Ⓓ Ⓔ   66 Ⓐ Ⓑ Ⓒ Ⓓ Ⓔ   111 Ⓐ Ⓑ Ⓒ Ⓓ Ⓔ   156 Ⓐ Ⓑ Ⓒ Ⓓ Ⓔ
22 Ⓐ Ⓑ Ⓒ Ⓓ Ⓔ   67 Ⓐ Ⓑ Ⓒ Ⓓ Ⓔ   112 Ⓐ Ⓑ Ⓒ Ⓓ Ⓔ   157 Ⓐ Ⓑ Ⓒ Ⓓ Ⓔ
23 Ⓐ Ⓑ Ⓒ Ⓓ Ⓔ   68 Ⓐ Ⓑ Ⓒ Ⓓ Ⓔ   113 Ⓐ Ⓑ Ⓒ Ⓓ Ⓔ   158 Ⓐ Ⓑ Ⓒ Ⓓ Ⓔ
24 Ⓐ Ⓑ Ⓒ Ⓓ Ⓔ   69 Ⓐ Ⓑ Ⓒ Ⓓ Ⓔ   114 Ⓐ Ⓑ Ⓒ Ⓓ Ⓔ   159 Ⓐ Ⓑ Ⓒ Ⓓ Ⓔ
25 Ⓐ Ⓑ Ⓒ Ⓓ Ⓔ   70 Ⓐ Ⓑ Ⓒ Ⓓ Ⓔ   115 Ⓐ Ⓑ Ⓒ Ⓓ Ⓔ   160 Ⓐ Ⓑ Ⓒ Ⓓ Ⓔ

26 Ⓐ Ⓑ Ⓒ Ⓓ Ⓔ   71 Ⓐ Ⓑ Ⓒ Ⓓ Ⓔ   116 Ⓐ Ⓑ Ⓒ Ⓓ Ⓔ   161 Ⓐ Ⓑ Ⓒ Ⓓ Ⓔ
27 Ⓐ Ⓑ Ⓒ Ⓓ Ⓔ   72 Ⓐ Ⓑ Ⓒ Ⓓ Ⓔ   117 Ⓐ Ⓑ Ⓒ Ⓓ Ⓔ   162 Ⓐ Ⓑ Ⓒ Ⓓ Ⓔ
28 Ⓐ Ⓑ Ⓒ Ⓓ Ⓔ   73 Ⓐ Ⓑ Ⓒ Ⓓ Ⓔ   118 Ⓐ Ⓑ Ⓒ Ⓓ Ⓔ   163 Ⓐ Ⓑ Ⓒ Ⓓ Ⓔ
29 Ⓐ Ⓑ Ⓒ Ⓓ Ⓔ   74 Ⓐ Ⓑ Ⓒ Ⓓ Ⓔ   119 Ⓐ Ⓑ Ⓒ Ⓓ Ⓔ   164 Ⓐ Ⓑ Ⓒ Ⓓ Ⓔ
30 Ⓐ Ⓑ Ⓒ Ⓓ Ⓔ   75 Ⓐ Ⓑ Ⓒ Ⓓ Ⓔ   120 Ⓐ Ⓑ Ⓒ Ⓓ Ⓔ   165 Ⓐ Ⓑ Ⓒ Ⓓ Ⓔ

31 Ⓐ Ⓑ Ⓒ Ⓓ Ⓔ   76 Ⓐ Ⓑ Ⓒ Ⓓ Ⓔ   121 Ⓐ Ⓑ Ⓒ Ⓓ Ⓔ   166 Ⓐ Ⓑ Ⓒ Ⓓ Ⓔ
32 Ⓐ Ⓑ Ⓒ Ⓓ Ⓔ   77 Ⓐ Ⓑ Ⓒ Ⓓ Ⓔ   122 Ⓐ Ⓑ Ⓒ Ⓓ Ⓔ   167 Ⓐ Ⓑ Ⓒ Ⓓ Ⓔ
33 Ⓐ Ⓑ Ⓒ Ⓓ Ⓔ   78 Ⓐ Ⓑ Ⓒ Ⓓ Ⓔ   123 Ⓐ Ⓑ Ⓒ Ⓓ Ⓔ   168 Ⓐ Ⓑ Ⓒ Ⓓ Ⓔ
34 Ⓐ Ⓑ Ⓒ Ⓓ Ⓔ   79 Ⓐ Ⓑ Ⓒ Ⓓ Ⓔ   124 Ⓐ Ⓑ Ⓒ Ⓓ Ⓔ   169 Ⓐ Ⓑ Ⓒ Ⓓ Ⓔ
35 Ⓐ Ⓑ Ⓒ Ⓓ Ⓔ   80 Ⓐ Ⓑ Ⓒ Ⓓ Ⓔ   125 Ⓐ Ⓑ Ⓒ Ⓓ Ⓔ   170 Ⓐ Ⓑ Ⓒ Ⓓ Ⓔ

36 Ⓐ Ⓑ Ⓒ Ⓓ Ⓔ   81 Ⓐ Ⓑ Ⓒ Ⓓ Ⓔ   126 Ⓐ Ⓑ Ⓒ Ⓓ Ⓔ   171 Ⓐ Ⓑ Ⓒ Ⓓ Ⓔ
37 Ⓐ Ⓑ Ⓒ Ⓓ Ⓔ   82 Ⓐ Ⓑ Ⓒ Ⓓ Ⓔ   127 Ⓐ Ⓑ Ⓒ Ⓓ Ⓔ   172 Ⓐ Ⓑ Ⓒ Ⓓ Ⓔ
38 Ⓐ Ⓑ Ⓒ Ⓓ Ⓔ   83 Ⓐ Ⓑ Ⓒ Ⓓ Ⓔ   128 Ⓐ Ⓑ Ⓒ Ⓓ Ⓔ   173 Ⓐ Ⓑ Ⓒ Ⓓ Ⓔ
39 Ⓐ Ⓑ Ⓒ Ⓓ Ⓔ   84 Ⓐ Ⓑ Ⓒ Ⓓ Ⓔ   129 Ⓐ Ⓑ Ⓒ Ⓓ Ⓔ   174 Ⓐ Ⓑ Ⓒ Ⓓ Ⓔ
40 Ⓐ Ⓑ Ⓒ Ⓓ Ⓔ   85 Ⓐ Ⓑ Ⓒ Ⓓ Ⓔ   130 Ⓐ Ⓑ Ⓒ Ⓓ Ⓔ   175 Ⓐ Ⓑ Ⓒ Ⓓ Ⓔ

41 Ⓐ Ⓑ Ⓒ Ⓓ Ⓔ   86 Ⓐ Ⓑ Ⓒ Ⓓ Ⓔ   131 Ⓐ Ⓑ Ⓒ Ⓓ Ⓔ   176 Ⓐ Ⓑ Ⓒ Ⓓ Ⓔ
42 Ⓐ Ⓑ Ⓒ Ⓓ Ⓔ   87 Ⓐ Ⓑ Ⓒ Ⓓ Ⓔ   132 Ⓐ Ⓑ Ⓒ Ⓓ Ⓔ   177 Ⓐ Ⓑ Ⓒ Ⓓ Ⓔ
43 Ⓐ Ⓑ Ⓒ Ⓓ Ⓔ   88 Ⓐ Ⓑ Ⓒ Ⓓ Ⓔ   133 Ⓐ Ⓑ Ⓒ Ⓓ Ⓔ   178 Ⓐ Ⓑ Ⓒ Ⓓ Ⓔ
44 Ⓐ Ⓑ Ⓒ Ⓓ Ⓔ   89 Ⓐ Ⓑ Ⓒ Ⓓ Ⓔ   134 Ⓐ Ⓑ Ⓒ Ⓓ Ⓔ   179 Ⓐ Ⓑ Ⓒ Ⓓ Ⓔ
45 Ⓐ Ⓑ Ⓒ Ⓓ Ⓔ   90 Ⓐ Ⓑ Ⓒ Ⓓ Ⓔ   135 Ⓐ Ⓑ Ⓒ Ⓓ Ⓔ   180 Ⓐ Ⓑ Ⓒ Ⓓ Ⓔ